AF556810

ADVANCES IN GYNAECOLOGICAL SURGERY

To my wife, Carmel, and my children James, Olivia, Charles and Niamh
P. J. O'D.

To my wife, Louise, and my children George and Lily
E. G. R. D.

ADVANCES IN GYNAECOLOGICAL SURGERY

Edited by

Peter J. O'Donovan
Consultant Gynaecologist, MERIT Centre, Bradford Royal Infirmary, UK

Ellis G. R. Downes
Consultant Gynaecologist, Chase Farm Hospital, Enfield, Middlesex, London, UK

Associate Editor

Paul McGurgan
Karl Stortz Research Fellow
The MERIT Centre
Bradford Royal Infirmiry
Bradford

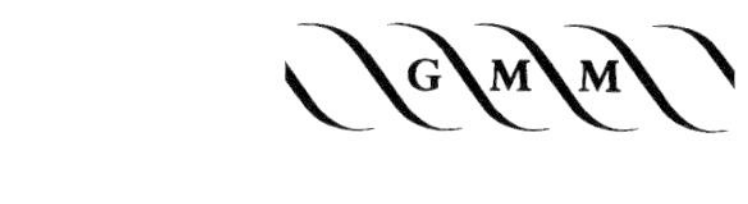

LONDON • SAN FRANCISCO

Greenwich Medical Media Ltd
4th Floor
137 Euston Road
London
NW1 2AA

870 Market Street, Ste 720
San Francisco
CA 94109, USA

ISBN: 1 900 151 499

First Published 2002

www.greenwich-medical.co.uk

A catalogue record for this book is available from the British Library.

Designed and Typeset by
Saldatore Limited and Phoenix Photosetting Ltd, Chatham

Printed by The Bath Press

CONTENTS

LIST OF CONTRIBUTORS

N N Amso
Senior Lecturer/Honorary Consultant
University of Wales College of Medicine
Department of Obstetrics and Gynaecology
Cardiff, UK

J Bidmead
Urogynaecology Research Fellow
King's College Hospital
London, UK

L Cardozo
Professor of Urogynaecology
Kings College Hospital
London, UK

C Chapron
Service de Gynecologie Obstetrique II
A Orientation Gynecologique
Groupe Hospitalier Cochin
Paris, France

R A F Crawford
Consultant Gynaecologist
Addenbrooke's Hospital
Cambridge, UK

Ellis Downes
The Kings Oak Hospital
Chase Farm
Enfield

J B Dubuisson
Service de Gynecologie Obstetrique II
A Orientation Gynecologique
Groupe Hospitalier Cochin
Paris, France

A Fauconnier
Service de Gynecologie Obstetrique II
A Orientation Gynecologique
Groupe Hospitalier Cochin
Paris, France

M Farrugia MRCOG
Research Fellow
Whipps Cross Hospital
London

G M Filshie MD FRCOG
Formerly Reader/Consultant
Queens Medical Centre
Nottingham

AJ Gallagher
Consultant
Department of Psychology
David Keir Building
Queens University
Belfast, UK

M J Gannon
Consultant Obstetrician and Gynaecologist
Gynaecology Out-Patients Department
Pinderfields Hospital
Wakefield, UK

JK Gupta MD MRCOG
Senior Lecturer
Birmingham Women's Hospital
Edgebaston
Birmingham

R Hawthorn MD FRCOG
Consultant
Southern General Hospital
Glasgow

P Hogston
Consultant Gynaecologist
Saint Mary's Hospital
Portsmouth, UK

S M F Ismail MRCOG
Research Fellow
MERIT Centre
Consultant Gynaecologist
MERIT Centre
Bradford Royal Infirmary
UK

D A Johns
Clinical Associate Professor
Texas Health Care
Fort Worth
Texas, USA

T C Li
Consultant Obstetrician and Gynaecologist
Jessop Wing
Royal Hallamshire Hospital
Sheffield, UK

N McClure
Senior Lecturer
Academic Dept of Obstetrics and Gynaecology
Queen's University of Belfast
Belfast, UK

J A McGuigan
Consultant Thoracic Surgeon
Royal Victoria Hospital
Belfast, UK

P McGurgan MB BA MRCOG MRCPI
Karl Stortz Research Fellow
The MERIT Centre
Bradford Royal Infirmary
Bradford, UK

L McMillan FRCOG
Consultant
Whipps Cross Hospital
London

P J O'Donovan
Consultant Gynaecologist
MERIT Centre
Bradford Royal Infirmary
Bradford, UK

D E Parkin
Consultant in Obstetrics and Gynaeocology
Aberdeen Maternity Hospital
Aberdeen, UK

S Pringle
Specialist Registrar in Obstetrics and Gynaecology
Southern General Hospital
Glasgow, UK

N Sharp
Consultant Obstetrician and Gynaecologist
Royal United Hospital
Combe Park
Bath, UK

S S Sheth
Consultant Gynaecologist
Breach Candy Hospital
Sir Hurkisondas Hospital
India

A R B Smith
Consultant Obstetrician and Gynaecologist
St Mary's Hospital
Whitworth Park
Manchester, UK

J G Thornton
Research School of Medicine
Centre for Reproduction, Growth and Development
University of Leeds
Leeds, UK

E Tsakos
Consultant Obstetrician and Gynaecologist
St Luke's Hospital
Thessaloniki
Greece

FOREWORD

The final quarter of the last century witnessed a revolution in gynaecological surgery when the traditional approach by laparotomy was replaced by minimal access surgery. After dramatic improvements in safety in the final quarter of the preceding century, most pelvic operations changed very little in the ensuing 100 years and most advances were due to extrinsic factors, such as the introduction of fluid replacement and blood transfusion and the introduction of prophylaxis with antibiotics and anticoagulants. The actual approach to the surgery remained static until the introduction of laparoscopy and hysteroscopy, which enabled the inside of the abdominal cavity and the inside of the uterus to be visualised with remarkable detail and visualisation.

That final quarter of the 20th Century was an exciting time to be involved in this particular branch of surgery and scarcely a year went past without the introduction of some new technique or energy source. Within a remarkably short space of time, it became possible to perform all procedures in the gynaecological repertoire, with the exception of operations for advanced malignancy which were essentially palliative and of questionable benefit in the long term.

I recall a conversation I had with an expert in feto-maternal medicine in 1985, when we were trying to get minimal access surgery accepted by the Royal College as a sub-specialty in its own right. I was told in no uncertain terms that the literature on laparoscopic and hysteroscopic surgery was scant, at best, and the quality was extremely poor with very little published in the form of randomised, controlled trials. Little did he know that in the ensuing years there would be an avalanche of publications, not merely addressing the technical minutiae, but also addressing safety issues and increasingly using well-designed studies to justify the superiority of minimal access therapy, according to the principles of evidence-based medicine.

This time has now come to look at ourselves in a mirror and ascertain our present strengths and weaknesses and this is exactly what this book sets out to do. The Editors are both enthusiastic young surgeons who learned minimal access techniques during their training and are therefore able to look at these developments from a healthy distance. It has enabled them to produce an excellent volume of essays which are largely written by the "Young Turks" in the battalion rather than the “Old Guard”, although I am happy to see that the latter are well represented by Shirish Sheth from India, who looks at his lifetime experience with vaginal surgery and Alan Johns from Fort Worth in Texas who was one of the pioneers of laparoscopic hysterectomy and the laparoscopic repair of uterovaginal prolapse.

The volume looks at new methods of access with special emphasis on miniaturisation and also endeavours to show the reader that many of the operations no longer need to be performed in the hospital operating department and that the development of office-based procedures will certainly decrease the cost of minimal access surgery. Hysterectomy for menorrhagia will increasingly be replaced by ablative procedures and the best of these are certain to be those that can be performed in the out-patient setting with local anaesthesia and oral analgesia. The different methods available for thermal ablation are well reviewed as well as newer techniques that might be available in the future, such as photodynamic therapy and virtual reality surgery.

I was also fascinated by the chapter on Decision Analysis in Surgery and since our decision of when and when not to perform a certain procedure has a profound effect on the lives of our patients, it is interesting to analyse the various steps that we go through in an almost intuitive way and there will be few readers who will not be fascinated by the analysis of this process.

All in all, this is an excellent volume of essays by a wide variety of practising endoscopic surgeons as well as urogynaecologists and oncologists and provides an excellent bouncing board for our first leap into the new millennium.

Professor Christopher Sutton
Professor of Gynaecological Surgery
Royal Surrey County Hospital

PREFACE

Despite the massive changes in our specialty, gynaecology remains fundamentally a surgical discipline. As working gynaecologists, we have been concerned about the predomination of endoscopic meetings demonstrating the technical brilliance of a few highly-gifted surgeons which may actually inhibit rather than encourage "surgical gynaecologists" working at the clinical cutting edge.

Because of this, we decided to initiate a series of annual meetings known as "IMRAGS" - The International Meeting of Recent Advances in Gynaecological Surgery, at which the best and latest aspects of surgery – both endoscopic and non-endoscopic – were highlighted.

This volume of invited chapters is the result of our series to date. They are topical, clinical chapters which we hope gynaecologists will find stimulating and challenging to the point that they may just change their clinical practice.

P. J. O'D.
E. G. R. D.
July 2001

About the Editors

Mr Peter J. O'Donovan is a Consultant Obstetrician and Gynaecologist at the Bradford Hospitals NHS Trust. He is also the Executive Co-director of the Micro-Endoscopy Research, Innovation and Training Centre (MERIT) at the hospital. He has a wide interest in new operative techniques, and is currently Vice President (President Elect) of the British Society for Gynaecological Endoscopy. He is also on the Safety Committee of the Medical Devices Agency (MDA), Department of Health and is also a member of the Minimal Access Surgery Committee of the Royal College of Obstetricians and Gynaecologists. He travels widely and has spoken at meetings both nationally and internationally.

Mr Ellis G. R. Downes is a Consultant Obstetrician and Gynaecologist at Barnet & Chase Farm Hospitals NHS Trust, based at Chase Farm Hospital, Enfield. He has a special interest in endoscopic surgery and uro-gynaecology. He is a board member and trustee of the British Society of Gynaecological Endoscopy and referees widely for a number of gynaecological academic journals. He has travelled widely and presented at many national and international meetings. He is also a non-executive director of Microsulis Medical Ltd, the manufacturer and distributor of Microwave Endometrial Ablation.

ACKNOWLEDGEMENTS

We would like to thank our colleagues for their patience with our enthusiastic attempts at academic prowess; we would also like to thank our publishers, Greenwich Medical Media Ltd for their patience and professionalism at guiding two novices through the book production stage.

INTRODUCTION

Gynaecological Surgery - Where Are We Going ?

"From inability to leave well alone;
From too much zeal for what is new and contempt for what is old;
From putting knowledge before wisdom, ·
Science before art, cleverness before commonsense;
From treating patients as cases; and
From making the cure of a disease more grevious than its endurance,
Good Lord Deliver us"

Hutchinson, 1871–1960
Cited in Bailey & Love's "A Short Practice of Surgery"

Introduction

As our speciality of gynaecology develops and grows, so does the range of surgical procedures we have to offer our patients. Surgery of course, is not merely about performing an operation, it is about careful history taking, meticulous examination and careful use of investigations to reach a diagnosis. Only then can the management strategies be discussed with the patient. If surgical options are considered, the age and medical condition of the patient will influence exactly what is performed.

But how do we learn surgery, and how does this influence what we do. Traditionally of course, we have learnt from our teachers during our training, the operation is done like this "because it has always been done this way". Increasingly this approach must be complemented with the foundation of evidence-based practice, structured formal training and carefully supervised surgical technique.

As we move forward into this new millennium, it is therefore timely to review where we have come from to reach the surgical standards we achieve today. In addition we must reflect on the challenges ahead, how they may be faced and how we can continue to improve our techniques to offer the highest level of care to our patients.

General considerations

Place of surgery
Traditionally surgical procedures have always taken place in an operating theatre. Increasingly, we are seeing procedures that may be performed in the out-patient or office setting. As technology improves and the morbidity and pain of surgical procedures can be reduced, it may be that more operations need no longer be performed in the operating theatre setting.

There has been a growth in "day surgery units", "office-based procedure units" and the like, as the benefits of less medically-intensive treatment areas are appreciated. Hysteroscopy is increasingly performed under local anaesthetic in the out-patient setting. Diagnostic and therapeutic colposcopy is also nearly always performed in the out-patient setting. Other surgical procedures such as some bladder neck suspensions can be performed away from the traditional operating theatre environment. Global ablative technology in the treatment of menorrhagia is also another area where the treatments are increasingly leaving the operating theatre and moving into the office environment.

Such fundamental changes in operating practice have many advantages. Firstly for the patient, not going into an operating theatre may be less stressful and anxiety provoking. For the surgeon, there is often a greater turnaround in the out-patient setting where the patients are waiting outside rather than the operating theatre where patients may have to travel from hospital wards, meaning a greater work-rate is possible.

Financially, such an approach away from the operating theatre has many advantages. Operating theatres are expensive to run, and performing procedures in the out-patient setting is much cheaper. This is highly attractive both to purchasers and insurers.

The operating theatre of the future is not, and of course never will be, redundant. Despite the development of alternative procedures major surgery will always be performed in gynaecology, needing extensive conventional operating theatre facilities.

Analgesia
The majority of gynaecological surgical procedures are performed under general anaesthesia. As these procedures develop, and as our understanding of analgesia grows, so it is becoming increasingly possible to undertake many procedures under local or regional anaesthetic.

Endometrial ablation, anterior colporraphy, bladder neck procedures can now all be performed under local anaesthetic[1]. Not only does this reduce the need for conventional anaesthetic support; by avoiding general anaesthetic, the sickness and post-operative nausea can be abolished.

In anterior colporraphy for example, traditionally an operation needing a 2–3 day in-patient stay, performing the procedure under local anaesthetic allows patients to go home the same day. Why should this be? The operation is the same, surely it is the abolition in general anaesthetic morbidity coupled with the expectations by surgeon, nurse and patient that the patient will go home that day. Fifteen years ago patients undergoing hysterectomy would routinely spend up to 12 days in hospital, now it is only 3 or 4, and some colleagues perform the operation of on a "day case" basis[2].

Our expectations of what patients are able to do, and when they can be safely discharged is therefore changing. We must make sure, however, that we are discharging patients home earlier after surgery than we would traditionally for the right reasons and not merely because it saves money.

Instrumentation
One only has to wander through a medical exhibition at a conference to be aware of the massive developments in medical instrumentation in the last 10 years. Are we as surgeons being "hoodwinked" by the equipment companies that all of these new instruments, many of them disposable, are essential to the development of good surgical skills? Or have there been genuine developments which we must examine carefully in order to improve our surgical skills. The answer of course is somewhere between these two views.

The developments in the quality of surgical endoscopes in gynaecology, the laparoscope and hysteroscope, has been nothing short of awesome. Not only is the visual quality improving to give brilliantly clear detail, the size of the scopes is reducing dramatically thus making hysteroscopy and less so laparoscopy entirely feasible under local anaesthesia. These factors coupled with the developing growth of the camera and monitor technology, with the new single chip cameras being almost as good as a triple chip camera, are leading to a level of visual clarity that allows advanced laparoscopic surgical dissection in anatomically challenging areas to be entirely feasible and possible.

Equipment companies are trying to persuade us to buy disposable equipment since it boosts their profits if we have to keep coming back and purchasing from them rather than a one-off purchase. Some of the disposable equipment is useful, for example, the Veress needle whose sharp point makes trocar insertion easier and safer than if performed with a blunt instrument. However, a considerable number of disposable gadgets add little to our conventional equipment inventory and are, in my opinion, a waste of money. Interestingly some equipment companies have recognised this and now market their equipment with a "reposable" description - the bulk of it is reusable, just a small part is disposable.

Training

We are slowly seeing the change of training structures in medicine. Traditionally we have had the apprenticeship structure. We have worked with consultants and their skills have been informally transferred to us (see one, do one, teach one as the cynic would say!). Training has been poorly monitored and supervised and the skills of trainees at the end of their training have varied. The beauty of our speciality is that those people who do not enjoy surgery or are not adept at it can be pointed into another area. The challenge is to maintain and develop surgical skills in those trainees who want to practice gynaecological surgical technique.

In the United Kingdom the length of training is being shortened. This factor, coupled with the reduction in doctors hours leads to an obvious paradox. How is clinical training maintained if clinical exposure is shortened? Nowhere is this more difficult than in teaching surgical skills.

Formal training schemes in which trainees are taught and assessed are slowly being developed. Instead of a trainee guessing (or exaggerating) how many hysterectomies they have done, these are now all recorded in the trainees log book.

One of the biggest challenges with new training schemes is teaching surgical skills. A surgeon needs to know the capabilities of the trainee; having trainees flitting in and out of theatre due to on-call commitments and days off does not help build close relationship essential to fostering teacher-student skill. The person who must never be forgotten is the patient who must have her operation carefully and skilfully carried out. In the future, we may see greater use of simulation technology to teach trainees the basics of surgery away from patients both conventional and laparoscopic surgery.

Clinical considerations

Menorrhagia

Menstrual problems remain the cornerstone of gynaecological practice, being one of the commonest gynaecological reasons for women to consult doctors. While menorrhagia can be treated either medically or surgically, many women ultimately will need a surgical solution which has traditionally been hysterectomy. The hysterectomy rate varies considerably world-wide and is dependent on many factors including economics, the type of health-care system, cultural factors and physician preference and training.

Since it was first described in 1843, hysterectomy has become the "gold-standard" treatment for menorrhagia. While it is an excellent treatment, it does have a greater morbidity and mortality than endometrial ablative techniques. Since the vast majority of women with menorrhagia do not have either an enlarged uterus or a structural abnormality[3], increasingly, the need to perform hysterectomy in menorrhagia must be challenged. Since the uterus is about 90% myometrium and 10% endometrium, the logic of performing a major operation to remove an organ, 90% of which is not contributing to the pathology must be questioned.

Over the last 10 years a variety of different ablative techniques have been described ranging from endometrial resection, roller-ball ablation to newer techniques such as balloon therapies or microwave endometrial ablation. While these techniques will never have the success rates of hysterectomy where 100% amenorrhoea is virtually guaranteed, they offer high patient acceptance rates and have obvious advantages in terms of cost, complication rate and in-patient stay compared to hysterectomy[4].

In the future we will see more ablative procedures being performed with fewer hysterectomies. Globally the world-wide hysterectomy rate is already starting to fall. The challenging question remains: which ablative technique will become pre-eminent? The answer is impossible to speculate and will surely be those techniques which have had careful scientific evaluation and have been shown to be efficacious and safe, have a relatively rapid learning curve and increasingly importantly, are highly cost-effective.

Prolapse surgery

We have made relatively little progress in our speciality until comparatively recently, in techniques for prolapse surgery. Since it was first described, our pelvic reconstructive surgical techniques have remained largely unchanged. Increasingly we are realising that although our surgery may improve the consequence of the defect, i.e. abolish the bulge, it may not treat the cause of the defect. It is understanding the types of anatomical defects, and the symptoms they cause that will in future underpin our surgical repair principles[5].

If one considers the operative procedure of posterior repair. For many years the concept has been to repair the bulge and oppose the levator ani muscles in order to support the perineum. Few surgeons follow-up their prolapse surgery results long-term. Recently the long-term success of this conventional surgery has been examined and worryingly unacceptable rates of bowel symptoms, recurrent prolapse and dyspareunia have been found[6].

The laparoscope allows us to more closely identify anatomical sites of prolapse by demonstrating defects in fascial planes which can be repaired. While these results, and the anatomical landmarks shown laparoscopically are truly eye-opening, there will undoubtedly be a long-period of flux until many more surgeons develop the necessary skills to undertake this sort of surgery.

Until that time "conventional repair" techniques will continue to be used, although one must consider what sort of modifications are important. What exactly is the role of mesh, be it collagen or synthetic in strengthening and reducing the risk of recurrence? Some workers are also undertaking repair techniques under local anaesthesia, allowing patients to return home much sooner than conventionally.

Oncology

As our speciality moves slowly towards sub-specialisation, the advances in oncological surgery will surely improve survival rates from gynaecological malignancies. It is likely in the future that our existing dogmas will be challenged and surgery will develop to the extent that it will be less morbid, and still remove the affected malignancy and lymph nodes.

In endometrial cancer for example, many of our patients are old and frail. Conventional teaching is that these patients should have an abdominal hysterectomy and removal of ovaries. The question of which women should undergo lymph node removal remains controversial. There are an increasing group of surgeons who are performing laparoscopic lymphadenectomies and then removing the uterus and adnexae vaginally reducing the morbidity for the operation and speeding recovery compared to the conventional abdominal approach[7].

Likewise in cervical carcinoma, Schauta's radical vaginal hysterectomy is finding renewed popularity as surgeons appreciate its beauty and elegance coupled with good patient recovery. The laparoscope is used by some to assist the dissection of the upper aspects of the procedure.

The management of adnexal masses laparoscopically remains controversial. But as greater experience is gained, what was thought to be a contra-indication to an endoscopic approach is now much less so. Many would argue that as ovarian cancer *per se* is often a peritoneal disease there are few roles apart from perhaps the initial staging procedure in early disease, for the laparoscopic approach.

Ovarian cysts which are strongly suspected to be benign are increasingly managed laparoscopically. Careful pre-operative assessment is vital including ultra-sonography and tumour marker assays, but many of those lesions which conventionally would have needed a laparotomy are being treated laparoscopically. As our-experience grows, even quite large lesions may be treated laparoscopically. Dermoid cysts were once thought to be not suitable for a laparoscopic approach due to the possibility of mucous spillage causing a sterile peritonitis. These concerns have not been borne out in practice provided meticulous lavage is performed.

REFERENCES

1. Ulmsten U, Johnson P, Rezapour M. A three-year follow up of tension free vaginal tape for surgical treatment of female stress urinary incontinence. *Br J Obstet Gynaecol* 1999 Apr; 106(**4**): 345–350.
2. Moore J. Vaginal hysterectomy. Its success as an outpatient procedure. *AORN J* 1988 Dec; 48; **6**: 1114, 1116–1120.
3. Shaw R W & Duckitt K. Management of menorrhagia in women of childbearing age. In: *Menorrhagia*, eds Seth & Sutton, 1999; Isis Medical, pp79–98.
4. O'Connor H, Magos AL. Endometrial resection for menorrhagia: Evaluation of the results at 5 years. 1996, *N Eng J Med,* **335**: 151–156.

5. DeLancey JO. Structural anatomy of the posterior pelvic compartment as it relates to rectocele. *Am J Obstet Gynecol* 1999 Apr; 180; **4**: 815–823.
6. Kahn MA, Stanton SL. Posterior colporrhaphy: its effects on bowel and sexual function. *Br J Obstet Gynaecol* 1997 Jan; 104; **1**: 82–86.
7. Querleu D. Laparoscopically assisted radical vaginal hysterectomy. *Gynecol Oncol* 1993 Nov; 51(**2**): 248–254.

1

Microendoscopy in Gynaecology

P. J. O'Donovan
J. K. Gupta

Introduction

During the past decade technological advances have led to the development of small fibre-optic endoscopes with diameters as low as 0.3 mm **(Figure 1.1)**. These have been used in fields such as cardiology and vascular surgery.

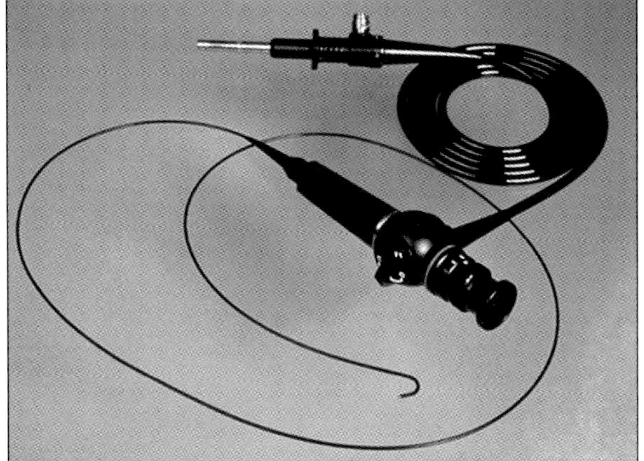

Figure 1.1 1.4 mm angioscope (KeyMed, UK) used in vascular surgery.

They offer clinicians a unique opportunity to inspect inaccessible parts of the body that would normally have required an open surgical procedure. Examples of this include angioscopy, endoscopy of the eustachian tube for evaluation of the middle ear,[1] spinal endoscopy,[2] falloposcopy,[3,4] using different extremely small flexible fibre-optic endoscopes ranging from 0.4 to 1 mm diameter depending on the applications. **(Figure 1.2)**.

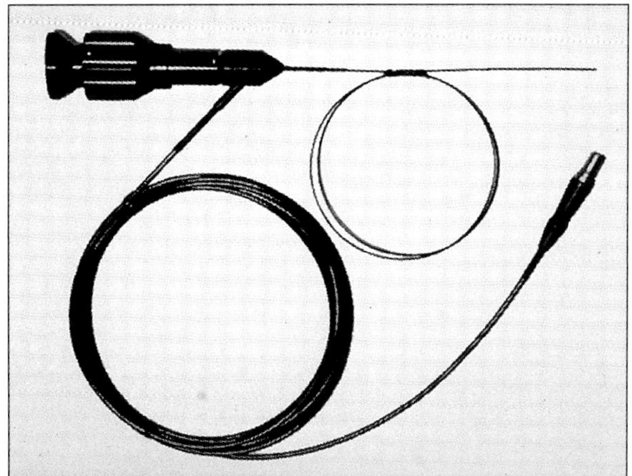

Figure 1.2 0.9 mm fibre-optic catheter (Myelotec, US) used for spinal endoscopy (visualisation of the epidural space). A micro-fibre-optic spinal endoscope.

In gynaecology, laparoscopy and hysteroscopy have been performed for decades. Currently, the vast majority of laparoscopic procedures are performed in operating theatres under general anaesthetic using conventional optical laparoscopes (5–10 mm). Nowadays, even smaller diameter instruments as low as 0.3 mm are under evaluation. It has been suggested that even smaller endoscopes may be able to perform diagnostic procedures without the need for general anaesthesia. These smaller endoscopes requiring smaller ports are now available, but do not yet have the optical resolution found in conventional diameter endoscopes.

However, significant improvements in optical systems, illumination, video equipment and operating instruments have resulted in expanding indications for these new procedures. An example of this is falloposcopy which allows the total length of the fallopian tube to be visualized using small endoscopes inserted via the transvaginal approach.[4,5]

In this chapter, we will discuss an overview of microendoscopy in gynaecology. Our title will conflict with our proposed new terminology but we feel that it should be maintained as it is easily recognised to identify the topic as a whole. We shall also discuss the organisation required in setting up microendoscopic services, indications and contraindications and role of anaesthesia. Finally, we shall speculate if this is the way forward, and the need for future research.

Definitions and terminology

The introduction of small diameter endoscopes has seen an explosion of publications with different, often confusing, definitions in this new subspeciality. A number of proposals have previously been made, but there is no universal agreement between gynaecologists and surgeons in the use of standard terminology. Dorsey & Tabb[5] defined the use of fine endoscopes as minilaparoscopy. They, however, said that the prefix 'mini' referred to the fact that the incisions placed in the abdomen were 3 mm in length.[5] Subsequently, microlaparoscopy became the popular usage with many authors.[6–9] Other suggested terminologies include small diameter laparoscopy[10] and miniscopes.[11] Similarly, general surgeons have also used the term minilaparoscopy[12] and also microlaparoscopy.[13] The terminology used in hysteroscopy is also just as confusing.

Manufacturing companies who produce small diameter endoscopes have suggested different terms i.e. miniature laparoscope (Storz), minilaparoscope (Wolf), microlaparoscope (Circon), minihysteroscope (Storz) or microhysteroscope (Circon). In all instances the diameter that is considered for small endoscopes is not defined and the variation depends on each surgical speciality.

Suggested new terminology

Since the term microendoscopy has been used for many years in several specialities, and since this term has not given rise to confusion, we feel that it should overall be retained to define endoscopy using small diameter endoscopes. However, a clearer definition is required and we propose that new terminology should be universally standardised across all fields of surgery where endoscopes are used. (**Table 1.1**). Microendoscopy is not just about the instrument size, it is also about the philosophy which is being applied to the overall patient management. Sub-division of the terminology should depend on the size of the outer sheath diameter of the endoscope.

Table 1.1

Outer sheath diameter (mm)	Endoscope classification
> 5 mm	Conventional
2–5 mm	Mini
< 2 mm	Micro

In the case of hysteroscopy, however, a separate classification is proposed. Hysteroscopes 2–5 mm in diameter should be referred to as "mini" hysteroscopes. Microhysteroscopy should be confined to hysteroscopy using endoscopes with an outer sheath of less than or equal to 2 mm.

By the nature of the manufacturing process, microendoscopes are likely to have fibre-optic flexible bundles for image collection, whereas standard rigid endoscopes would probably use rod lens systems. As an example, a 0.5 mm flexible endoscope used for investigation of lachrymal ducts should be classified as a micro-fibre-optic endoscope and a 4 mm rigid endoscope for hysteroscopy should be termed minihysteroscope. However, a rigid 1.2 mm semi-rigid hysteroscope is called a microhysteroscope. Microcolpohysteroscopy is a separate entity described by Hamou. Microcolpohysteroscopy refers to a technique described by Hamou[14] using a contactmicrocolpohysteroscope which has an endoscope diameter of 4 mm and a magnifying capacity of up to 150 fold.

Microendoscopy in obstetrics and gynaecology

There are several indications for the use of microendoscopic instruments in obstetrics and gynaecology. These include:

1. Endoscopic uterine surgery in obstetrics such as transabdominal diagnostic and operative fetoscopy.

2. Diagnostic and operative office microhysteroscopy and microcolpohysteroscopy.

3. Diagnostic and operative outpatient microlaparoscopy. The latter includes endoscopic adhesiolysis, endoscopic distal tubular disease

surgery such as salpingostomy, endoscopic reversal of sterilisation and pain mapping (pelvic). In the management of infertility it includes microculdoscopy and falloposcopy.

4. New microelectrodes including bipolar devices have been developed to allow uterine surgery to be performed using saline medium.

OUTPATIENT MICROHYSTEROSCOPY

Set-Up, personnel and equipment

It is necessary to identify a room where these procedures can be done which has access to oxygen and a resuscitation trolley. A room for counselling and also a recovery room are important. Personnel should be fully trained in standard endoscopic procedures prior to embarking on microendoscopic procedures. Outpatient hysteroscopic equipment includes either a flexible hysteroscope or 1.2 mm microendoscope with a 2.5 mm diagnostic sheath. A 150 W cold light source is sufficient for vision but a 175 W Xenon light source enables a good depth of field. A carbon dioxide hysteroflator is optional and saline can be used as an alternative for uterine distension. A Xenon light source of 175–300 W and a video camera monitor is an advantage as the image generated on a monitor allows participation and education of nursing staff and the patient herself. The purchase of an additional electrically powered table/chair is an option to allow easier patient manoeuvrability.

When performing outpatient microhysteroscopy, as the image obtained is quite small, it is preferable to have a camera with a zoom system to select the appropriate picture size. Using too high a magnification can result in the magnification of the pixels. The single chip endoscope camera is sufficient for diagnostic hysteroscopic procedures and also permits minor operative hysteroscopic procedures to be performed. A three chip camera will not bring more improvement, unless it incorporates additional features such as filters to eliminate the pixelisation and digitalisation of the image. In terms of durability, although the new generation of semi-rigid fibre optic microendoscopes are more durable and more user friendly with superior light transmission compared with similar diameter rod lens telescopes, extra care is needed by nursing staff when handling these fine instruments. The majority are not currently autoclavable and have to be soaked in sterilising solution. When autoclavable the lifetime of the microendoscope is reduced. Furthermore, with microendoscopy it is recommended that one uses fluid distension, rather than gaseous medium, as very mild contamination of the lens by blood or mucus obscures the picture quality. This problem may be overcome by having the scope outside the sheath by 1 mm. However, a significant advantage of microhysteroscopy over standard hysteroscopy is that its narrower outer sheath diameter makes it easier to insert in nulliparous or post-menopausal women without prior cervical dilatation.

The role of anaesthesia for microhysteroscopy

Even before the advent of microhysteroscopy, surgeons reported that no anaesthesia/analgesia was required in the vast majority of patients undergoing standard outpatient hysteroscopy.[15] Non-steroidal anti-inflammatory drugs are sometimes given for the mild cramps which occasionally accompany the procedure.[16] In one study, 65% of patients reported that the local anaesthetic intracervical injection was more painful than the hysteroscopic examination itself.[17] In another study, the use of para-cervical block for routine outpatient hysteroscopy in pre-menopausal women had no advantage,[18] It has been our experience that the performance of microhysteroscopy examination causes less patient discomfort than endometrial biopsy.[18]

Outpatient microhysteroscopy

Hysteroscopy is now being used to replace dilatation and curettage as the current technique to evaluate and treat abnormal uterine bleeding. Due to technological advances and the introduction of microhysteroscopes, over 80% of all diagnostic hysteroscopies can be performed in an outpatient setting.

In a series of 2500 diagnostic hysteroscopies using 4 mm hysteroscopes, more than 50% of women presenting with a history of abnormal bleeding had abnormal findings. The procedure was successfully completed in 96% of patients and a complete view of the uterine cavity was obtained in 89% of patients.[19] Similarly, 1000 outpatient microhysteroscopic procedures have been described using a 1.2 mm semi-rigid microhysteroscope **(Figure 1.3)** with normal saline as the distending medium. The procedure was successful in 97% of patients **(Figure 1.4)** and a satisfaction survey revealed a 98% approval rating from patients.[20]

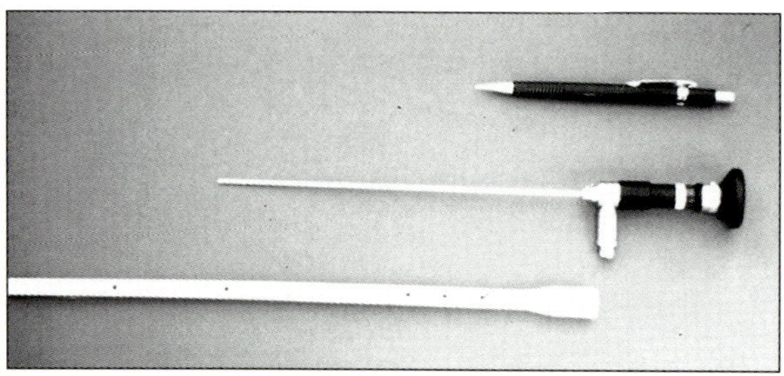

Figure 1.3 1.2 mm fibre-optic hysteroscope 0° lens with protective sheath (Karl Storz, Germany). A micro-fibre-optic hysteroscope.

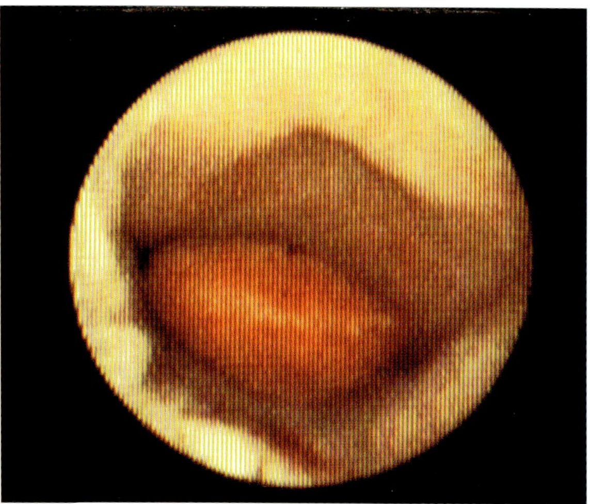

Figure 1.4 View of the uterine cavity obtained with a micro-fibre-optic hysteroscope showing a large polyp-1.2 mm fibre-optic hysteroscope 0° lens (Karl Storz, Germany).

Similar success rates have been achieved with the flexible 2.9 mm or 3.6 mm hysteroscope.[21]

Operative outpatient microhysteroscopy procedures

It is possible to perform simple hysteroscopic procedures such as polypectomy in the outpatient setting using microhysteroscopy. This is a problem encountered in approximately 20% of women presenting to the outpatient clinic.[20,21] However, one of the shortcomings is that due to the small image any bleeding encountered during surgery obscures the visual field. The use of a continuous flow channel can resolve this problem. Bipolar microelectrodes that work in a saline medium could

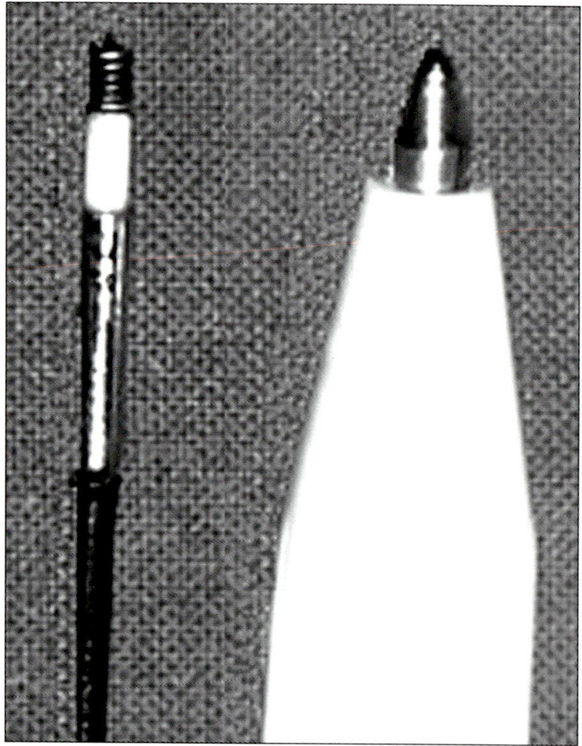

Figure 1.5 A Versapoint Bipolar electrode 5 Fr diameter (Ethicon, UK) used for operative outpatient microhysteroscopy alongside a biro.

be a useful tool to reduce the need for subsequent inpatient operative hysteroscopy[22,23] (Figure 1.5).

Learning curve and accreditation

In the United Kingdom, there are recognised training courses in hysteroscopic surgery which have Royal College approval. A survey of training in minimal access surgery in the West Midlands region supports the strong link between supervision of appropriate training and complications in minimal access surgery and stresses the crucial role of the supervisor and the need for formal training.[24] This study revealed that only 25% of trainees attended a formal training course.

Of the trainees, 26% encountered hysteroscopic complications in their total experience. In general, microhysteroscopes that are rigid or semi-rigid are easier to insert and have a shorter learning curve; 2.5–3 mm flexible hysteroscopes can also be used. The advantage of such instruments is flexibility, the disadvantage is that insertion of flexible hysteroscopes into the cervical canal require a longer learning curve.

Conclusions: are patients better off?

Both standard and microhysteroscopy can be done in the outpatient setting with little or no anaesthetic. However, microhysteroscopy with its finer instruments may be better suited to a subgroup of patients where no prior cervical dilatation is required; post-menopausal and nulliparous women. Significant cervical stenosis makes the insertion of a conventional hysteroscope more difficult as opposed to those with a diameter of 2 mm or less. The drawbacks, however, are that as microhysteroscopes usually contain fibre-optic systems, the image quality is not as clear. Although it is possible to do operative procedures with both, microhysteroscopy is more likely to be limited to minor procedures. Furthermore, microhysteroscopes are fragile and they need careful handling from all personnel.

Summary

After considering the advantages and disadvantages it can be concluded that the place for microhysteroscopy requires further evaluation but initial results do suggest that it has a role in selected patients where the use of standard hysteroscopy with large diameter might be more difficult. Further work needs to be performed on the potential non-invasive advantage of vaginal scanning versus outpatient hysteroscopy particularly in the post-menopausal patient.[25]

OUTPATIENT MICROLAPAROSCOPY

Evolution of operative endoscopy has led to the development of microlaparoscopy with endoscopes of less than 2 mm diameter.[26] The evolution towards microendoscopic techniques has been supported by:

1. The desire to perform minimal access surgery.
2. The desire to avoid large trocar incisions as these may lead to herniation or incarceration of bowel.
3. The desire to perform endoscopic techniques with the patient under conscious sedation.
4. The desire to perform outpatient endoscopic procedures.

We would recommend the following progression for gynaecologists who wish to offer their patients outpatient microendoscopy:

1. Become proficient at performing a variety of laparoscopic procedures with standard size instruments in hospital or in the operating theatre.

2. Attend a formal comprehensive course in performing microendoscopy in the outpatient setting. The programme should consist of both lectures and hands-on training.

3. Practice these newly learned skills by performing microendoscopy in the hospital operating room or procedure room. If possible, have a mentor, instructor attend your first few cases.

4. Once you become adept at microendoscopic techniques transfer these procedures into the outpatients setting.

Indications for microlaparoscopy

Indications for outpatient microlaparoscopy under local anaesthetic can be expanded to cover many circumstances:

1. Safety in trocar placement in patients with intra-abdominal adhesions, and primary trocar placement as an alternative to open laparoscopy.[26–28]

2. Diagnostic laparoscopy. Used in the diagnosis of the acute abdomen[29] and also for conscious pain mapping.[30] Patients need to be awake to map out painful areas. This is a new and evolving area that has not been well defined so far.

3. Operative laparoscopy may be used. The micro-laparoscope may be used for bilateral tubal occlusion,[31] endometriosis therapy and assisted reproductive technology.[32] Operative laparoscopy may also be used for tubal surgery for simple diagnostic procedures, operative salpingostomy[33] and second look laparoscopy for the diagnosis of patients with suspected malignancy.[34]

Contra-indications to microlaparoscopy

Contra-indications for the use of microlaparoscopy are the same as those for routine laparoscopy with only a few exceptions:

1. Contra-indications whether medical or surgical as applied to routine laparoscopy.

2. Enlarged uterus over 12–14 weeks size with the placement of a microlaparoscope in the mid point between the symphysis and umbilicus. A large uterus could feasibly get in the way of examination of the adnexa and cul-de-sac.

3. Obesity. Due to the length of the microlaparoscope, it is obvious that the thickness of the abdominal wall would limit its use.

4. Multiple abdominal incisions. In those patients with multiple abdominal incisions where open laparoscopy would ordinarily be chosen, a microlaparoscope inserted in a closed fashion could feasibly be unsafe. However, insertion of the microlaparoscope at Palmer's Point in the left upper quadrant is an alternative that allows the insertion of secondary trocars under direct vision.[27,28]

5. Already planned operative laparoscopy. Any patient on whom one already plans to perform an operative laparoscopy under general anaesthetic would not require microlaparoscopy unless it is to visualise insertion of secondary trocars in a patient with a previously scarred abdomen.

Instrumentation for microlaparoscopy

At present, the new generation of fibre-optic microlaparoscopes are more durable and more user friendly with superior light transmission compared to glass rod endoscopes of comparable diameter. Microlaparoscopes which can be fitted to existing operating room equipment such as

camera light sources are advantageous. It is our experience that a single chip endoscopic camera produces an image quality that is sufficient for adequate diagnosis and surgery.[35] Trocars and cannulas of varying design have been produced to match these new generation microendoscopes. We use 2 mm cannulas but insufflating ports have been designed using a standard 15 cm long Veress needle.

After inserting the Veress needle into the abdominal cavity, the cannula is removed and a 2 mm laparoscope **(Figure 1.6)** introduced into the abdominal cavity.

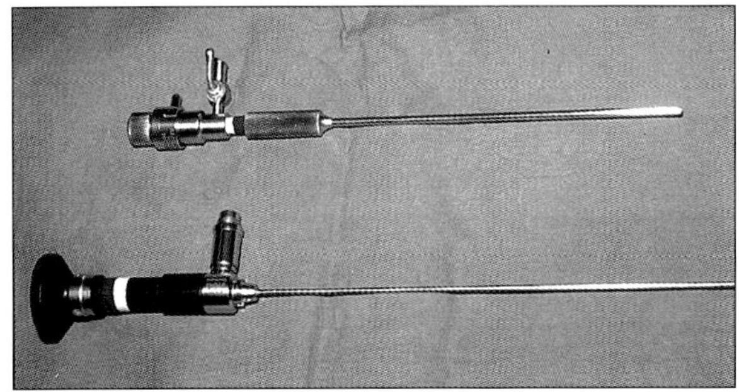

Figure 1.6 2 mm fibre-optic laparoscopewith a 3.2 mm optic Veress needle (Karl Storz, Germany). A fibre-optic mini-laparoscope.

This introducer is fitted with a rectangular flange which can be activated to prevent it from being pulled out inadvertently from the abdominal cavity. Constant CO_2 insufflation can then be instituted through the insufflation port to keep the abdomen distended at a constant pressure.

Small instruments, as small as 1 mm, have been designed for surgical procedures. These include, micro-scissors, graspers, dissectors and probes. These instruments are either conventional in design or modified hysteroscopic instruments. Mechanical failure can occur especially during long surgical procedures owing to their small size and semi-rigid construction.

Image quality and accuracy

The diagnostic accuracy of microlaparoscopes (1.2–2 mm) has been compared with 5–10 mm rodless systems.[7,10,35,36] It has been shown that although microendoscopes are adequate for diagnostic and minor operative procedures and the images obtained were comparable with those obtained with conventional laparoscopy, this is not achievable in all cases.[7,36] Under these circumstances, conventional laparoscopy has to be used, and for these purposes it has been shown that the use of a 5 mm endoscope with modern optics and video will provide maximum utility and at the lowest cost.[36] Furthermore, operative gynaecological endoscopic surgery is only possible to levels I and II with microlaparoscopes.[33] This raises the question of what major advantage micro-laparoscopy might have over conventional laparoscopy.[37]

The role of anaesthesia for microlaparoscopy

Laparoscopy has been performed under local anaesthetic for many years.[38] The surgeons' skills are keenly tested when performing microlaparoscopy under local anaesthetic. This is mainly because of using the low insufflation pressures (6–8 mmHg) required to minimise pain. As a result of the limited operating time, the surgeon must also be able to work quickly and accurately in a highly 'protocalised' framework.[39] Perhaps the most important ingredient in performing microlaparoscopy under local anaesthesia is a sense of trust and rapport between the patient and physician. It is important to realise, however, that no amount of medication would make the procedure acceptable for a patient who is inappropriate for the procedure. Patients for outpatient microlaparoscopy should be selected because they are motivated to have the procedure done under these conditions or are at least very receptive to the possibility that outpatient microlaparoscopy under local anaesthetic will provide information that cannot easily be obtained in any other way.

Outpatient operative microlaparoscopy

The limitations include the fact that image quality is not as good as the rod lens system, which is the gold standard, but is still adequate to perform to level II procedures.[33] In addition the size of the image is smaller. Potential problems include the fact that there is shown to be a decreased performance of skill of the laparoscopic surgeon using a microlaparoscope versus a standard laparoscope.[39] These results demonstrate that there is an increased difficulty in performing laparoscopy with 2 mm instruments, which underscores the importance of formal training and objective skill assessment. Currently, as there are no guidelines for outpatient procedures, surgeons can perform almost anything they desire in the outpatient setting. This highlights the importance of attending a formal training course. It is generally agreed, however, that most first procedures should be performed in the hospital environment, particularly in operating theatre where there are facilities for resuscitation available, in case complications do arise. However, despite the many precautions and training procedures for performing outpatient microlaparoscopy, complications are occasionally unavoidable, particularly if resuscitation is required. For this reason, surgeons performing outpatient laparoscopy would be best advised to be in a hospital setting. A very careful selection of patients with informed consent is essential and the most advanced procedure one would consider performing is tubal sterilisation or minor adhesiolysis. Patient preferences as regards local versus general anaesthesia needs to be assessed.

Conclusions – are patients better off?

Conventional laparoscopy has reached its current state of sophistication and utility because it offers clear and indisputable advantages over laparotomy. For the vast number of gynaecological surgical indications, laparoscopy can accomplish, without therapeutic compromise, the same task that previously would have demanded a large abdominal incision, and offer a milder convalescence and superior cosmesis in return. Similarly, the benefits of advanced operative laparoscopy are now being exploited with low associated risks. Microlaparoscopy currently provides potentially similar benefits but using much smaller instruments. It has, however, to be questioned if there are any major benefits if this procedure gives a poorer video image (the instrument needs to be held very close to the organ to obtain adequate resolution), especially if the lens is contaminated by blood or peritoneal fluid, misses small pelvic lesions and underscores endometriosis. Furthermore, most microlaparoscopists suggest that conventional laparoscopy is required if adequate imaging is not obtained with microlaparoscopy. Clearly, more research is required to evaluate microlaparoscopy and determine if it does have advantages over conventional laparoscopy especially in the outpatient setting where only very minor procedures are achievable.

SUMMARY

Microendoscopy in gynaecology

The growth of endoscopy is occurring as part of a larger shift from open surgery to closed procedures. The role of microendoscopy is being evaluated in order to take the daycase, inpatient role of endoscopy to a (local anaesthetic) outpatient environment.

Outpatient hysteroscopy can now be achieved with little or no discomfort and without the need for local anaesthesia in most cases. The use of microhysteroscopy has allowed this to occur safely. We believe that very few of these procedures need to be performed under general anaesthesia in a hospital setting. The advent of new bi-polar diathermy instruments that can work in saline medium may mean that simple procedures such as polypectomy or division of intrauterine adhesions will be able to be performed in the outpatient setting. The broader question, in the context of women presenting with abnormal uterine bleeding, of whether hysteroscopy is required or is superior to lesser invasive procedures such as transvaginal scanning has yet to be evaluated. We await further clinical trials to answer this question.

The promise of microlaparoscopy in comparison to conventional laparoscopy is still debatable. Conventional daycase laparoscopy utilising 5–10 mm scars have been a major advantage over large open abdominal wall incisions. Massive scale outpatient local anaesthetic laparoscopic sterilisations using conventional endoscopes have been done successfully.[40] Does the use of even smaller scars for microlaparoscopy result in less pain and faster discharge from hospital? Outpatient local anaesthesia microlaparoscopic procedures may have this advantage but not all patients will tolerate such procedures particularly in developed countries. These patients have to be carefully selected and motivated to undergo such procedures. The indications for microlaparoscopy are currently to assess safety in trocar placement in patients with intra-abdominal adhesions[41] and also for conscious pain mapping.[30] The value of reduced operative morbidity, earlier return to work and improved quality of life have yet to be evaluated by larger studies. More importantly, the cost-effectiveness of such procedures has to be addressed.[42]

Microlaparoscopy will need to be scrutinised in this manner before it is widely accepted as the norm over conventional laparoscopy for clinical practice in the next millennium. In order to more clearly define the area covered we propose a new terminology which should be universally standardised across all fields of surgery where endoscopes are used.

REFERENCES

1. Edelstein DR, Magnan J, Parisier SC, *et al.* Microfiberoptic evaluation of the middle ear cavity. *Am J Otol* 1994; **15**: 50-55.
2. Saberski LR, Kitahata LM. Direct visualization of the lumbosacral epidural space through the sacral hiatus. *Anesth Analg* 1995; **80**: 839–840.
3. Kerin J, Daykhovsky L, Segalowitz J, *et al.* Falloposcopy: a microendoscopic technique for visual exploration of the human fallopian tube from the uterotubal ostium to the fimbria using a transvaginal approach. *Fertil Steril* 1990; **54**: 390-400.
4. Scudamore IW, Dunphy BC, Cooke ID. Outpatient falloposcopy: intra-luminal imaging of the fallopian tube by trans-uterine fibre-optic endoscopy as an outpatient procedure. *Br J Obstet Gynaecol* 1992; **99**: 829–835.
5. Dorsey JH, Tabb CR. Mini-laparoscopy and fibre-optic lasers. *Obstet Gynecol Clin North Am* 1991; **18**: 613–617.
6. Barisic D, van der Ven H, Prietl G, Strelec M. The diagnostic accuracy of a 1.2 mm mini-laparoscope. *Gynaecol Endosc* 1996; **5**: 283–286.
7. Risquez F, Pennehouat G, Fernandez R, Confino E, Rodriquez O. Microlaparoscopy: a preliminary report. *Hum Reprod* 1993; **8**: 1701–1702.
8. Phipps JH, Hassanien M, Miller R. Microlaparoscopy: diagnostic and sterilization without general anaesthesia: a safe, practical and cost-effective technique. *Gynaecol Endosc* 1996; **5**: 223–224.
9. Haeusler G, Lehner R, Hanzal E, Kainz C. Diagnostic accuracy of 2mm microlaparoscopy. *Acta Obstet Gynecol Scand* 1996; **75**: 672–675.
10. Bauer O, Devroey P, Wisanto A, Gerling W, Kaisi M, Dredrich K. Small diameter laparoscopy using a microlaparoscope. *Hum Reprod* 1995; **10**: 1461–1464.
11. van Herendael BJ, Slangen T, Mencaglia L, Palfijn J. Use of rigid miniscopes in endoscopy. *J Am Assoc Gynecol Laparosc* 1995; **2** (Suppl): 556.
12. Cuschieri A, Hennessy TP, Stephens RB, Berci G. Diagnosis of significant abdominal trauma after road accidents: preliminary results of a multicentre trial comparing minilaparoscopy with peritoneal lavage. *Ann R Coll Surg Eng* 1988; **70**: 153–155.
13. Schwaitzberg SD. Use of microlaparoscopy in diagnostic procedures. *Surg Laparosc Endosc* 1995; **5**: 407–409.
14. Hamou J, Frydman R, Fernandez H, Capella S, Taylor S. Can microcolpohysteroscopy be used to

screen cervical lesions? *Contracept. Fertil Sex*. 1997; **25**: 358–62

15. Wamsteker K. Office Hysteroscopy: Complications and management. In: Isaacson KB. *Office Hysteroscopy* 1996; Mosby: St Louis.

16. Downes E. Goodbye D&C welcome hysteroscopy. *Br J Hosp Med* 1992; **48**: 75–77.

17. Vercellini P, Colombo A, Mauro F, Oldeni S, Bramate T, Crosignani PG. Paracervical anesthesia for outpatient hysteroscopy. *Fertil Steril* 1994; **62**: 1083–1085.

18. McElligott AJ, Jones SE, O'Donovan P, Ludkin H, Quinn P. Pain scores in outpatient microhysteroscopy. *Gynaecol Endosc* 1997; (Suppl): 222 (Abstract).

19. Nagele F, O'Connor H, Davies A, Badawy A, Mohamed H, Magos AL. 2500 outpatient diagnostic hysteroscopies. *Obstet Gynecol* 1996; **88**: 87–92.

20. O'Donovan PJ, Jones SE, Quinn P, Ludkin H. What is the place of out-patient microhysteroscopy in the management of abnormal vaginal bleeding? Experience with 1000 patients using a 1.2 mm semi-rigid hysteroscope. *Gynecol Endosc* 1997; **6** (Suppl): 226 (Abstract).

21. Coats PM, Haines P, Kent ASH. Flexible hysteroscopy: an outpatient evaluation in abnormal uterine bleeding. *Gynaecol Endosc* 1997; **6**: 229–235.

22. O'Donovan PJ, Jones SE. Versapoint: Operative microhysteroscopy using bipolar electrosurgery in a saline medium. *Gynecol Endosc* 1997; **6** (Suppl): 73 (Abstract).

23. Vleugels MPH. First clinical results with the new bipolar electrosurgical device versapoint in hysteroscopic surgery. *Gynecol Endosc* 1997; **6** (Suppl): 74 (Abstract).

24. Chin K, Newton J. Survey of training in minimal access surgery in the West Midlands Region of the UK. *Gynaecol Endosc* 1996; **5**: 329–333.

25. Gupta JK, Wilson S, Desai P, Hau C. How should we investigate women with postmenopausal bleeding? *Acta Obstet Gynecol Scand* 1996; **75**: 475–479.

26. O'Donovan PJ. Microlaparoscopy in gynaecology. *Gynecol Endosc* 1997; **6** (Suppl): 46 (Abstract).

27. Okeahialam MG, Gupta JK. O'Donovan PJ, Palmer's point: A safe microlaparoscopic technique for patients with suspected intra-abdominal adhesions. *Gynaecol Endosc* 1999; **8**: 115–116.

28. Lang PFJ, Tamussino K, Honigl W. Palmer's point: an alternative site for inserting the operative laparoscope in patients with intra-abdominal adhesions. *Gynaecol Endosc* 1993; **2**: 35–37.

29. Palter SF, Olive DL, Rosser JC. Diagnosis of acute appendicitis by microlaparoscopy under local anesthesia. *J Am Assoc Gynecol Laparosc* 1995; **2**: S40 (Abstract).

30. Palter SF, Olive DL. Office microlaparoscopy under local anesthesia for chronic pelvic pain. *J Am Assoc Gynecol Laparosc* 1996; **3**: 359–364.

31. Love BR, McCorvey R, McCorvey M. Low cost office laparoscopic sterilization. *J Am Assoc Gynecol Laparosc* 1994; **1**: 379–382.

32. Downing BG, Wood C. Initial experience with a new microlaparoscope 2 mm in external diameter. *Aust N Z J Obstet Gynaecol* 1995; **35**: 202–204.

33. van der Wat J. Microendoscopy in the operating room. *Gynecol Endosc* 1997; **6**: 265–268.

34. Childers JE, Hatch KD, Surwit EA. Office laparoscopy and biopsy for evaluation of patients with intraperitoneal carcinomatosis using a new optical catheter. *Gynecol Onc* 1992; **47**: 337–342.

35. Faber BM, Coddington CC. Microlaparoscopy: a comparative study of diagnostic accuracy. *Fertil Steril* 1997; **67**: 952–954.

36. Fuller PN. Microendoscopic surgery: A comparison of four microendoscopes and a review of the literature. *Am J Obstet Gynecol* 1996; **174**: 1757–1762.

37. Pelosi MA, Pelosi MA. Minilaparoscopy: Post hoc, ergo propter hoc. *Gynaecol Endosc* 1997; **6**: 251.

38. Gordon AG. Laparoscopy under local anaesthesia. *J Roy Soc Med* 1984; **77**: 540-541.

39. Rosser JC, Olive DL, Zreik T, Duleba A, Arici A, Rutherford T, Palter SF. Decreased performance of skilled laparoscopic surgeons at microlaparoscopy versus traditional laparoscopy. *J Am Assoc Gynecol Laparosc* 1996; **3**: S44 (Abstract).

40. Metha PV. A total of 250,136 laparoscopic sterilizations by a single operator. *Br J Obstet Gynaecol* 1989; **96**: 1024–1034.

41. Steege JF. Repeated clinic laparoscopy for the treatment of pelvic adhesions: a pilot study. *Obstet Gynecol* 1994; **83**: 276–279.

42. Hasson HM. Endoscopic surgery, cost-effectiveness, and the quality of life. *J Am Assoc Gynecol Laparosc* 1995; **2**: 115–121.

2

Laparoscopy in Urogynaecology

A. R. B. Smith

The role of laparoscopy in urogynaecology

The results reported by Marshall *et al* [1] in 1949 and Burch[2] in 1961 demonstrated that the abdominal approach to bladder neck surgery produced a greater chance of success and a lower risk of recurrence. This has led the majority of gynaecologists and urologists to adopt the suprapubic approach to bladder neck surgery, though a reluctance to move from the vaginal route was derived at least in part from concern about the increased morbidity produced by an abdominal incision. Similarly, the surgical treatment of vaginal vault prolapse can be achieved by an abdominal or vaginal approach. One randomised trial comparing abdominal sacrocolpopexy with vaginal sacrospinous fixation has been published and demonstrated a reduced risk of recurrence with the sacrocolpopexy, but sacrospinous fixation has the advantage that a laparotomy is not required.[3] Thus, in both types of pelvic reconstructive surgery the abdominal approach appears to confer some benefits, but has the disadvantage that the abdominal wall needs to be opened. This will inevitably increase the post-operative discomfort for the patient and in the obese woman can make surgery technically more demanding. The development of the laparoscopic approach to reproduce the techniques performed through an abdominal wall incision has the potential to provide maximum benefit with least disturbance to the patient. This chapter will cover the literature of laparoscopic reconstructive pelvic surgery, a description of the techniques including some of the author's own experience and the lessons and needs for the future.

Laparoscopic colposuspension

The first report on laparoscopic colposuspension by Vancaillie and Schuessler[4] demonstrated that the procedure was possible but not without technical difficulty, illustrated by two bladder injuries in this report of nine cases. Bladder injury is the most frequently reported intra-operative problem indicating that the technique has some inherent difficulties. My own experience suggests that there are ways to minimise the risk of bladder injury. The reports published following the Vancaillie paper have no uniformity of surgical technique and many different surgical materials are used (e.g. sutures, bone anchors and meshes). Apart from bladder injury, intra-operative difficulties are little mentioned in the reports. Few details of immediate post-operative morbidity in terms of pyrexia, the need for transfusion or infective morbidity are reported. Liu[5] reported results from a series of 58 women and found no cases of post-operative fever; all the women were able to return to work one week after surgery. Post-operative pain is not critically analysed in the published reports. In a retrospective record review in Manchester of 50 open and 116 laparoscopic colposuspensions, opiate analgesia was administered twice as frequently following open surgery indicating that immediate post-operative pain is greater with a laparotomy incision than laparoscopic port wounds. Length of stay in hospital after surgery is difficult to compare between Europe and North America where financial imperatives dictate early hospital discharge. Post-operative voiding difficulties are often responsible for longer hospitalisation after bladder neck surgery. Different catheter regimes, including routine use of intermittent self-catheterisation will influence time of discharge. In Manchester, our results show that short term voiding difficulty is less frequent following laparoscopic surgery but in the longer term voiding problems are equally distributed between laparoscopic and open surgery. **Table 1.1** illustrates a meta-analysis of published complications of laparoscopic colposuspension.

Apart from Burton[7] all the published studies are retrospective reviews. Burton performed a randomised, prospective study comparing laparoscopic with open colposuspension and demonstrated that operating time was longer, recovery time from surgery shorter and successful cure of stress incontinence was only 74% at 12 months compared to 93% with the open approach. There was one bladder injury in each group. At 3-year follow-up, the difference in success is more marked with 60% for

Table 1.1 Meta-analysis of complications of laparoscopic colposuspension

Haemorrhage	0.5%
Transfusion	< 1%
Bladder injury	3.7%
Ureteral injury/kinking	< 0.1%
Voiding dysfunction	5%
Detrusor instability	5%
Prolapse	3%
Incisional hernia	< 0.1%

the laparoscopic approach compared to 94% for the open approach. The main criticism of this study apart from the number of patients recruited is that Burton had not gained sufficient experience in laparoscopic surgery before starting the study. It does, however, give information about what success rates a novice laparoscopic surgeon might expect to achieve if attempting laparoscopic colposuspension.

Retrospective reports on laparoscopic colposuspension have included 2-year follow up with different results. Lobel and Sand[8] reported a cure rate of 89% at 3 months, 86% at 1 year and 69% at 2 years. The series included a number of different techniques and an average operating time of 190 minutes was recorded. Ross[9] conducted a retrospective review of 40 cases over 2 years and reported success rates of 98% at 6 weeks and 90% at 2 years. Thus, one series suggests a marked decline in efficacy and the other a sustained effect on longer-term follow up. It is interesting to note that Lobel and Sand frequently used a Stamey needle to assist in their technique and appear to be producing results similar to the Stamey type colposuspension with a higher risk of recurrence.

The main advantage of laparoscopic surgery is said to be the rapid post-operative recovery. This is supported in the report by Liu[5] that all patients had returned to normal activity within 1 week of surgery. There is no comparative data available for open surgery in these series. It is not known whether it is good for the longevity of the bladder neck support for patients to return to normal activity sooner. Post-operative return to normal activity appears to vary between countries, with North American studies indicating that when there is sufficient financial pressure, early return home and to normal activity is commonplace. MacKenzie[10] illustrated, in patients recovering from hysterectomy, that pre-operative information given to patients has a major influence on time for recovery. The apparent rapid recovery following laparoscopic surgery may, at least in part, be produced by the patient's and physician's expectations. The Sheffield cholecystectomy study[11] illustrated that when patients were blinded to the method of gall bladder removal their recovery rates were the same for open and laparoscopic techniques. A similar study is required to assess whether there is any difference in immediate post-operative recovery from colposuspension when the patients and attendant nursing staff do not know by which technique the operation was performed.

In the author's experience of over 200 cases, the main differences from open surgery are the new operative skills required and the immediate post-operative recovery.

Laparoscopy is a surgical technique that all gynaecologists learn in training. Similarly, minor surgical procedures such as sterilisation and minor adhesiolysis are learnt in training. The most difficult new skill of laparoscopic colposuspension is laparoscopic suturing. For this reason mesh, stapling techniques, and the Stamey needle have been used to try to overcome the suturing difficulties. Suturing skills can be learnt with training and practice.

In a review of the first 50 cases the author performed, the operating time halved, largely due to improved suturing skills, but also due to improved familiarity with the procedure by all members of the theatre team . The laparoscopic approach now takes, on average, 15 min longer than the open approach.

Surgical technique for laparoscopic colposuspension

Position on the operating table

The most convenient position, that allows the surgeon to insert fingers in the vagina to aid mobilisation of the paraurethral fascia, is the reverse Trendelenberg with an assistant sitting in between the patient's legs.

Access to retropubic space

All laparoscopic surgeons need to be aware of the vessels of the anterior abdominal wall. The inferior epigastric artery is most at risk when using the transperitoneal approach.

Advantages of the transperitoneal approach

- Intraperitoneal procedures may be performed including treatment of enterocele.
- Larger operating field.
- There is easier access to the upper lateral vaginal wall which is important for paravaginal repair.

Disadvantages of transperitoneal approach

- Risk of injury to inferior epigastric artery.
- Risk of bowel or other vascular injury with port insertion.
- Risk of bladder injury when opening the peritoneum.
- Risk of hernia from port wounds.
- Intraperitoneal adhesions from previous surgery may limit access to an anterior abdominal wall.

Extraperitoneal approach

Under normal conditions the loose areolar connective tissue of the retropubic space can be divided easily with blunt dissection. Balloon devices are available and may prove helpful.

Difficulties

The main difficulty is avoiding bladder injury. Adhesions from previous pelvic surgery can lead to the bladder being adherent to the anterior abdominal wall. This can best be overcome by dissection first into the retropubic space lateral to the midline since most adhesions from previous surgery occur centrally and are easier to identify when the space has been opened laterally.

Mobilisation of peri-urethral fascia

The surgeon's index finger is placed in the vagina lateral to the bladder neck whilst the bladder is mobilised medially with the aid of a pledget. It is advisable to tie a long suture to the pledget to avoid losing it. Disposable pledgets fixed to a holder are available.

Fixation of peri-urethral fascia to Cooper's ligament

Using a straight needle attached to a suture of choice two bites of the peri-urethral fascia are taken and a single bite of Cooper's ligament taken and the needle withdrawn. When the tissues are poor a full thickness bite of the fascia is advisable to reduce the risk of tearing. A Roeder knot is tied and pushed down with an assistant's finger elevating the fascia. It is not always possible to attain direct approximation of fascia to ligament, particularly when an anterior vaginal repair has been performed previously. The author places two sutures on each side to ensure a strong fixation and two bites of the fascia are taken with the first suture. The main difference from open colposuspension is that a narrower area of fascia is elevated with the laparoscopic route although the difference is not obvious on vaginal examination after the procedure.

If a paravaginal repair is performed less bladder mobilisation is required, but a curved needle is necessary to enable access for fixation of the endopelvic fascia to the fascia on the pelvic side wall.

Suprapubic catheterisation

The author uses suprapubic catheterisation on account of the ease of management of patients with post-operative voiding difficulties. The bladder is filled via the urethral catheter which is present throughout surgery on free drainage. The suprapubic catheter is inserted under direct vision into the bladder. A Bonnano catheter is suitable, but other types equally serve the purpose.

Peritoneal closure

The anterior abdominal peritoneum may be closed, but this is not necessary if the peritoneal incision is large. A narrow gap in the peritoneum could lead to bowel entrapment. In three out of the four cases in which the author has re-entered the peritoneal cavity some months after laparoscopic colposuspension the peritoneum had healed normally. In one case the retropubic space remained open, but had become peritonealised.

Wound closure

There is a significant risk of hernia formation in port wounds of more than 5 mm diameter. A full thickness closure is therefore required in lateral wounds of more than 5 mm. Disposable and re-usable devices are available for this.

Post-operative care

The author clamps the suprapubic catheter 36 h after surgery and removes the suprapubic catheter when the residual urine is less than 150 ml. In the author's experience, most catheters can be removed by the fourth day, but voiding problems after this are not uncommon. Rarely, long-term intermittent self catheterisation is required.

In Manchester we have found that the incidence of post-operative pyrexia is reduced from 31–11%, wound infection from 8–1% and the doses of narcotic analgesia required halved after laparoscopic colposuspension when compared, retrospectively, to 50 women who underwent open colposuspension in the unit during a similar time period.[9]

The average time for post-operative catheterisation was also reduced, but voiding problems were not uncommon in both groups, and so length of hospital stay, (since women in the UK are reluctant to return home with a catheter in place), was only reduced by 3 days on average. At 6-months review with urodynamics the objective cure rate was similar but women said that return to normal took 9 weeks after laparoscopic colposuspension compared to 19 weeks after open colposuspension. There was no statistical difference in the incidence of new detrusor instability on urodynamics at 6 months between the two groups. A 2-year questionnaire review has been performed, this has revealed that 58% of the laparoscopic group never leak urine, and 50% of the open group never leak. Ninety-four percent of the laparoscopic group said they were satisfied with the result of their surgery compared with 80% of the open group. This retrospective review is flawed in many ways with the potential for bias (in both directions) in a number of areas but it indicates that, at 2-year follow up of two demographically and clinically similar groups of women, there is no major difference in cure rate between the open and laparoscopic techniques. This highlights the need for a randomised prospective study involving a large number of patients

Laparoscopic sacrocolpopexy

A number of abdominal procedures have been described for the treatment of vaginal vault prolapse, including anchorage of the vaginal vault to the anterior abdominal wall with fascial strips or non-absorbable sutures[12] or elevation of the vault towards the sacrum. Several techniques for anchoring the vaginal vault to the sacrum have been described and one of the earliest was that by Lane[13] in which a synthetic graft is sutured from the vaginal vault to the sacral promontory. Different materials have been used to anchor the vaginal vault; Teflon mesh,[14] Marlex mesh,[15] Mersilene[1,6–18] or fascia lata,[19] These procedures have resulted in success rates ranging from 91–100%.

Laparoscopic sacrocolpopexy was first reported by Nezhat *et al.*[20] Fifteen cases were included in which a 2.5 cm by 10 cm piece of Mersilene or Gore-Tex® mesh (WL Gore & Associates, Inc, Phoenix, AZ) was sutured to the vaginal apex and sutured or stapled to the sacrum. Follow up from 3–40 months is reported with "complete relief" of their symptoms in all cases. One woman required a laparotomy for bleeding from the pre-sacral area. In 1995 a series of 29 cases was reviewed retrospectively by Mahendran *et al* from Manchester.[21] In this series one recurrence of vault prolapse was reported in follow up ranging from 6 months to 2 years. Of interest was the finding of low rectocoeles in ten of the women when examined 6 months post-operatively, although the women were not always aware of the prolapse. In an attempt to reduce the incidence of recurrence of posterior vaginal wall prolapse the author performed a number of procedures in which prolene mesh was introduced vaginally during a conventional posterior repair thereby reinforcing the full length of the posterior vaginal wall. A series of 29 cases illustrated that this is generally followed by an uncomplicated recovery, but trimming of the mesh in the out-patient clinic was required in one in four cases. In one case a mesh was removed after a perineal abscess developed, but this was thought to be related to an anal sphincter repair rather than the mesh. Subsequently a more extensive dissection between the vagina and rectum has been employed laparoscopically, enabling the mesh to be placed down to the level of the perineum without opening the vagina. This dissection can be difficult particularly since most women have undergone previous surgery in the region. In one case, a hole was made in the rectum but after laparoscopic repair the sacrocolpopexy was uncomplicated, as was the recovery. Since patients who have vaginal vault prolapse are often frail, elderly and obese, the benefits of laparoscopic surgery are often more obvious than for colposuspension.

Ross[22] published a 12-month review of 19 women following laparoscopic surgery for post-hysterectomy "vault eversion." All 19 women underwent sacrocolpopexy, modified culdoplasty and Burch urethropexy. Six paravaginal and 13 posterior vaginal repairs were performed. Prolene mesh was sutured to the circumference of the vaginal apex and passed through a peritoneal tunnel to be sutured to the anterior sacral ligaments. Bladder injury occurred in three cases but all women were discharged within 24 h of surgery and no patient had a catheter in place for more than 4 days. At 1 year after surgery one woman had "mild" stress incontinence (compared to 17 pre-operatively), two women had cystocoeles and three rectocoeles. This represents quite a high recurrence rate of lower vaginal prolapse at short-term follow up despite extensive repair surgery.

Technique

Once anaesthetised, the patient is placed in the reverse Trendelenberg position with the legs in Lloyd-Davies stirrups. The bladder is then catheterised with a size 18 Foley catheter. A pneumoperitoneum is created by inserting a Veress needle suprapubically. A subumbilical 10 mm port is used for the laparoscope and two further ports introduced; a left lateral 5 mm port and a right lateral 12 mm port. Particular care is taken not to damage the inferior epigastric artery. These two lateral ports are used to introduce the instruments used to perform the procedure. The peritoneum over the vaginal vault is opened using the diathermy scissors and the bladder dissected anteriorly and the rectum posteriorly to expose the vaginal vault and posterior vaginal wall. This dissection is made easier by the introduction of a vaginal dilator into the vagina by an assistant to elevate the vault. On occasions a rectal probe can be of assistance. A prolene mesh graft is inserted into the pelvis through one of the ports. The graft is sutured to the vaginal vault using a No."0" PDS Endoknot (Ethicon, Scotland). Initially four sutures were used to secure the graft over an area 3 cm × 3 cm. With increasing experience, this area has been extended to include the whole of the posterior vaginal wall including beyond the rectal reflection. Anchorage of the graft along the full length of the vagina to the perineum will reduce the risk of posterior vaginal wall prolapse post-operatively. In cases where there is an obvious deficit in the upper anterior vaginal wall this area is also covered with mesh.

The sacral promontory is identified and the peritoneum over the promontory is incised over an 8 cm vertical area using diathermy scissors. The retroperitoneal tissue is dissected away from the periosteum of the promontory. This length of incision is required to mobilise sufficient peritoneum to cover the mesh after fixation to the vagina and sacrum. Careful identification of the rectum to the left of the incision, and the right internal iliac artery and right ureter is carried out during this dissection. Care is also taken with vessels running over the sacral promontory.

The graft is then secured to the sacrum using a hernia stapling device (either Autosuture UK Ltd, England or Ethicon UK). The open weave type of graft has been found to be easier to suture and staple through than materials of a closer weave (e.g. Gore-Tex®). The graft can be sutured to the sacral promontory, but this can be difficult. The stapler is a much quicker and easier method and would appear to provide a secure attachment. The authors have found that it is easier to achieve the appropriate tension in the graft by fixation to the vagina first. The vagina is then supported by a dilator, whilst the mesh is aligned over the sacrum and the staples inserted. Any excess mesh can then be trimmed away. Having anchored the graft, the peritoneum over the graft is closed using the staples in order to close off any potential gap that could lead to an internal hernia. The patients are given an intra-operative bolus dose of co-amoxiclav 1.2 g intravenously.

Results

A series of 29 patients who underwent laparoscopic sacrocolpopexy has been published.[21] This paper demonstrates that the technique is safe and effective. Few intra-operative problems were encountered, although bladder injury occurred on two occasions. One of these occurred during colposuspension when there were adhesions from previous surgery. The mean theatre time was 123 min (including anaesthesia time) which is longer than open surgery although this time includes the "learning curve" times. Post-operative recovery was markedly different from the author's experience of open surgery where ileus is not uncommon. 17 of the 29 cases returned home within 72 h of surgery with a range of 1–8 days (mean 3 days). At follow up, the main problem has been recurrence of lower posterior vaginal wall prolapse (10 cases) and this has led to modification of the technique as described above. All the women have been questioned about dyspareunia and this has not been a problem at 6 months or beyond in those women who were sexually active. Stress incontinence has been reported post-operatively and the author now performs a colposuspension when there has not been any previous retropubic surgery.

Laparoscopic repair of enterocoele and rectocoele

The first published report of the laparoscopic repair of an enterocoele in 1993[23] included 18 women in whom the enterocoele repair was performed in combination with a posterior repair, a laparoscopic Burch colposuspension and in some cases a hysterectomy. In one case the enterocoele repair was not possible due to intra-peritoneal adhesions from previous surgery. Medial displacement of the ureter was noted in six of the 17 cases but no detriment to function occurred. In one case a suture was placed through the ureter but recognised and removed immediately.

Most patients were discharged within 48 h but voiding difficulties kept a few women hospitalised for up to 5 days. Follow up was 12 months in one case but less in the remainder. No evidence of enterocoele was seen on examination but two of the women were troubled by dyspareunia.

A descriptive report of a new laparoscopic approach to enterocoele repair[24] detailed a technique based upon the principles of the Zacharin abdomino-perineal repair. Forty women underwent surgery which included major concomitant surgery in 37 cases. Bladder perforation occurred in one case but the intra-operative blood loss was only 40 ml on average. Twenty-five out of the 40 women experienced low back pain post-operatively and 20 out of the 40 women complained of constipation. The average length of hospitalisation was 2.2 days (range 1–7 days) and all women were reported as being able to return to normal activity within 1–2 weeks. For reasons that are not made clear there were no details of further follow up.

The only published series of laparoscopic rectocoele repair is a series of 20 women in whom a polyglactin mesh was sutured into the plane between vagina and rectum.[25] All 20 women underwent laparoscopic colposuspension and McCall colpopexy, 16 underwent paravaginal repair, 12 supracervical hysterectomy, 4 sacrocolpopexy, 3 rectopexy and 3 perineorrhaphy. No intra-operative problems were reported, with the average estimated blood loss being 5 ml. There were no cases of fever, anaemia or re-hospitalisation and all women were discharged within 24 h. At a 12-month review, no woman reported dyspareunia and a 95% rate of "symptom relief " was given without any details of findings on examination.

Conclusions

Laparoscopic pelvic reconstructive surgery is still in its infancy, particularly with regard to evaluation. It is clear that reproduction of the open techniques are possible but this does not equate to reproduction of results. Prospective randomised comparative studies are required for a meaningful evaluation.

REFERENCES

1. Marshall VF, Marchetti AA, Krantz KE. The correction of stress incontinence by simple vesicoureteral suspension. *Surg Gynaecol Obstet* 1949; 88–509.
2. Burch JC. Urethrovaginal Fixation to Cooper's Ligament for Correction of Stress Incontinence, Cystocoele and Prolapse. *Am J Obstet Gynaecol* 1961; 81–281.
3. Benson JT, Lucente V, McClellan E. Vaginal versus abdominal reconstructive surgery for the treatment of pelvic support defects: A prospective randomized study with long-term outcome evaulation. *Am J Obstet Gynecol* 1996; **175**: 1418–22.
4. Vancaillie TG, Schuessler W. Laparoscopic bladder neck suspension. *J Laparoendosc Surg* **3**: 169–73.
5. Liu CY. Laparoscopic retropubic colposuspension (Burch procedure). *J Reprod Med* 1993; **38**: 526–530.
6. Lavin JM, Lewis CJ, Foote AJ, Hasker GL, Smith ARB. Laparascopic Burch Colposuspension Paper. *Gynae Endoscopy* 1998; **7**: 251–258.
7. Burton G. A three year prospective randomised urodynamic study comparing open and laparoscopic colposuspension. *Continence Foundation Australia*. Ann Scientific Meeting Melbourne. 1996 (August).
8. Lobel RW, Sand PK. Long term results of laparoscopic Burch colposuspension. *Neurourology & Urodynamics* 1996; **15**: 398–399
9. Ross JW. Two year objective follow up of laparoscopic Burch colposuspension. *Proceedings of the 1996 International Continence Society* (Athens) 364–365.
10. McKenzie IZ. Reducing hospital stay after abdominal hysterectomy. *Br J* Obstet Gynaecol 1996; **103**: 175–178.
11. Majeed AW, Troy G, Nicholl JP, Smythe A, Reed MW, Stoddard CJ, Peacock J, Johnson AG. Randomised, prospective, single-blind comparison of laparoscopic versus small-incision cholecystectomy. *The Lancet* 1996; **347**: 989–994.
12. Conran W, Morgan HR. Abdominal sacral colopexy *Am J Obstets Gynaecol* 1980; **138**: 348–350.
13. Lane FE. Repair of post-hysterectomy vaginal vault prolapse. *Obstets & Gynaecol* 1962; **20**: 72–77.
14. Birnbaum SJ. Rational therapy for the prolapsed vagina. *Am J Obstets & Gynaeco* 1973; **115**: 411–419.

15. Grundsell H, Larsson G. Operative management of vaginal vault prolapse following hysterectomy.*BJ Obstets & Gynaecol* 1984; **91**: 808–811.

16. Yates MJ. An abdominal approach to the repair of post-hysterectomy vaginal invasion. *B J Obstets & Gynaecol* 1975; **82**: 817–819.

17. Addison WA, *et al* . Abdominal sacral colpopexy with mersilene mesh in the retroperitoneal position in the management of post-hysterectomy vaginal vault prolapse and enterocoele. *Am J Obstets & Gynecology* 1985; **153**: 140–146.

18. Creighton SM, Stanton SL. The surgical management of vaginal vault prolapse. *B J Obstets & Gynaecol* 1991; **98**: 1150–1154.

19. Ridley JH, Botte JM, Howlett RJ. A composite vaginal vault suspensions using fascia lata. *Am J Obstet Gynecol* 1976; **126**: 590–595.

20. Nezhat CH, Nezhat F, Nezhat CR. Laparoscopic sacral colpopexy for vaginal vault prolapse *Obstet Gynaecol* 1994; **84**(5): 885–888.

21. Mahendran D, Prashar S, Smith ARB, Murphy D. Laparoscopic sacrocolpopexy in the management of vaginal vault prolapse. *Gynaecological Endoscopy* 1996; **5**: 217–222.

22. Ross JW. Techniques of laparoscopic repair of total vault eversion after hysterectomy. *J Am Assoc Gynaecologic Laparoscopists* Feb 1997; **4**(2): 173–183.

23. Vancaillie TG, Butler DJ. Laparoscopic enterocoele repair – description of a new technique. *Gynaecological Endoscopy* 1993; **2**: 211–216.

24. Lam A, Rosen D. A new laparoscopic approach for enterocoele repair. *Gynaecological Endoscopy* 1997; **6**: 211–217.

25. Lyons TL, Winer WK. Laparoscopic rectocoele repair using polyglactin mesh. *J Am Assoc Gynae Laparoscopists* May 1997; **4**(3): 381–384.

3

Decision Analysis in Surgery

J. G. Thornton

Introduction

Imagine a man with localised prostate cancer. Radical surgery reduces mortality but inevitably impairs sexual function to some degree, and often causes complete impotence. Some tumours never spread beyond the prostate, and those that do can be treated with hormones that also cause impotence. A policy of observation and delayed hormone treatment if spread occurs carries a mortality rate intermediate between radical surgery and no treatment. All the risks vary with the tumour grade and stage, and individual men vary in the importance they give to sexual function. It is impossible to make a sensible decision without having some logical way to both estimate risks correctly and take into account individual preferences.

Decision analysis

Decision analysis provides a solution.[1–3] It involves breaking the decision down into its component parts, analysing these in detail separately and then combining them to identify the course of action that in prospect will be of the most value.

The steps of decision analysis

1. Define the decision problem.
2. Model it over time in a flow diagram, identifying the possible choices, the uncertainties resulting from these choices, and the outcomes which may differ in value (utility).
3. Measure the probabilities and utilities of each outcome.
4. Combine the two to identify the choice with the maximum expected utility.
5. Measure the effects of plausible changes in the various uncertainties by sensitivity analysis.

Advantages
The whole process is analytical, structured, and transparent. It permits correct weighting to be given to all probabilities, and avoids the biases that affect subjective estimates of probability.[4] It is particularly suited to those decisions where personal values matter, since it allows the values of the individual most affected by the decision to be given correct weighting, and provides a check against the doctors' values being given undue prominence. It is prescriptive. Its underlying basis, expected utility theory, provides a rational way to choose how to act under uncertainty. Decision-makers should choose the course of action with the maximum expected utility, defined as the product of the utility of the outcome (correctly measured) and its probability.[5,6]

Disadvantages
Decision analysis has limitations. It takes time and intellectual effort, which may be better spent elsewhere. It is best suited to relatively complex but well structured decisions. If the decision is too simple the effort is unnecessary. If the decision is unstructured it may be impossible to reach a clear decision. Its very openness may offend some people. Sometimes people prefer decisions to be opaque.

Nevertheless, surgeons tend to like explicit and open analysis, so it is not surprising that decision analysis is being increasingly used in this field. In this chapter the author will illustrate decision analysis with one detailed example, cancer surgery that will destroy fertility, and describe briefly some other areas where decision analysis has been used.

Cancer surgery that will destroy fertility

The scenario
A 29–year-old nurse had an abnormal cervical smear and a cone biopsy had revealed a moderately differentiated squamous cancer, invading 2 mm below the basement membrane and with lymphatic involvement. The primary tumour was completely

excised and the pathologist reported a wide margin of normal tissue around the tumour. The nurse has no children. What treatment should she choose?

The treatment options lie between no further therapy, and extended hysterectomy with lymphadenectomy. Simple hysterectomy would not remove tumour metastases, is unlikely to improve survival, and would automatically render her infertile. The possible outcomes are survival with fertility retained, immediate death from surgical complications, delayed death from cancer, and infertile survival.

Decision tree

We first structure the problem using a decision tree. This is a flow diagram in which decisions and outcomes are represented in order, with early events to the left and later events to the right.

Decision points are represented by square nodes and points where outcomes occur by chance, by round nodes. The decision node represents the choice between no further surgery and radical hysterectomy. The upper chance node represents the chance that the patient may die of cancer or survive in full health having retained her fertility if the "no surgery" option is chosen. The other nodes are self-explanatory. The order of events in this decision tree needs to be chosen with care. The chance outcome of "spread" or "no spread" occurs before operation but will only become known to the clinician when the excised specimen has been examined. It is therefore placed after the operation.

Probabilities and utilities

Probabilities

The next step is to fill in the probabilities and utilities of each outcome. There are no randomised trials to provide these, so we base our estimates on observational studies, just as we would do if we were not using decision analysis. After literature review we estimated surgical mortality as 5 per 1000, the likelihood of disease spread beyond the cone biopsy as 2% and the chance of cure by surgery if it had done so as 50%.[7]

Surgery thus has the lowest expected mortality of 1.5% (0.5% operative mortality plus half of 2% mortality from disease spread not cured by radical surgery). No surgery carries a 2% mortality.

Utilities

However, this does not mean that radical hysterectomy is the best treatment. We need also to consider the patient's preference for delayed death from cancer versus immediate death from surgery, and the desire to conserve fertility. We need to know the patients' relative value or utility of being rendered infertile and of suffering a delayed death from cancer. She ranked them as follows: the best was fertile life, the worst delayed death, with infertile life and immediate death rated intermediate (**Figure 3.1**).

We need to know where exactly the intermediate states fall on this scale. There are a number of possible ways to do this although only one is correct. Let us consider the utility of being rendered infertile.

Measuring utility

We could ask the patient to mark on the line the point that she believes corresponds to this health state. This is quick and easy to do but may be misleading. Even if people really believe that a health state is valued at the extreme end of the scale they

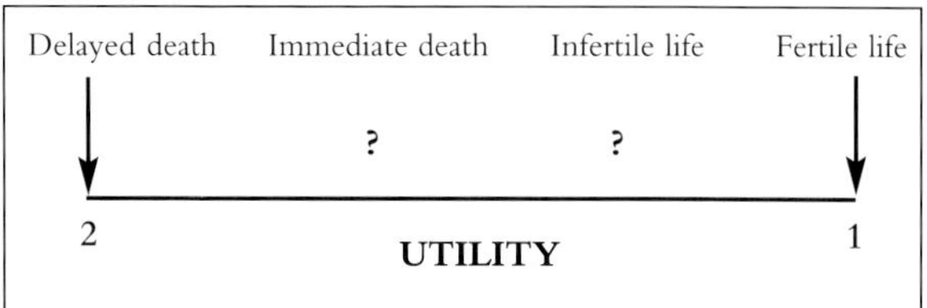

Figure 3.1 A scale of values for the cervical cancer decision.

typically mark it towards the middle section. We could ask her to express the utility of infertility in terms of some other natural scale such as money or years of her own life. For example we could ask her how much money she would pay or how many years of her own life she would sacrifice to retain fertility. For health interventions that people are used to paying, these methods may be effective, but usually people find them too hypothetical. Another problem with measuring utility on such scales is that they are usually non-linear. Typically, people are risk-averse for both money and years of life, and value the first monetary increment proportionally more than later ones, and years immediately ahead proportionally more than years far in the future. Instead, we ask patients directly how much risk of dying they would be prepared to take to avoid infertility. The process is called the basic reference lottery. It goes as follows.

We ask her to imagine two doors, one of which she must go through. Behind the left hand door there was no risk of death but she would be rendered infertile. Behind the right hand door she would encounter a 50% chance of fertile survival but also a 50% risk of death. She chose the left-hand door. The risks of death through the right hand door were decreased until a point was reached where she could not decide which door to choose. This occurred when the risk of death through the right-hand door was 5% and of fertile survival 95%. She valued survival with infertility as 0.95 on a scale where full health was valued 1 and immediate death valued 0. A second similar lottery between delayed death from cancer and various chances of full health or immediate death gave a utility for delayed death of 0.05.

Combining probabilities and utilities

Having measured the utilities we need to combine them with the probabilities to select a preferred course of action, i.e. that with the greatest expected utility. We start by estimating the utility of each chance node.

This is calculated as the weighted average of the utilities of its possible outcomes, where the weights are the probabilities of each outcome. The utility of the upper chance node wis thus:

$$(0.02 \times 0.05) + (0.98 \times 1.0) = 0.981$$

Where there is a sequence of chance nodes in the tree we use the weighted utility of the distal chance node in calculating the expected utility of the proximal node. The utility of a decision node is the maximum of the utilities of its component branches since a rational decision-maker should choose this strategy. We call the process of pruning all but the most advantageous branches at decision nodes "folding back" and the process of calculating utilities at a chance node "averaging". By a combination of both processes it is possible to select the course of action with the highest expected utility.

Expected utilities are shown in lozenges with arrows pointing to the node or branch to which they apply. Branch utilities are shown in grey lozenges and are the product of the outcome utility and its probability. Chance node utilities are shown in white lozenges and are the sum of the relevant branch utilities. It is clear that the expected utility of no further surgery (0.981) is greater than radical hysterectomy (0.936) and this is the option our patient should choose.

The difference in expected utility between the different courses of action may not appear very great, but on this scale the difference 0.045 represents 4.5% of the value of her entire remaining life in full health! Moreover, if the axioms of expected utility theory are accepted by our patient (most people do agree that this is how they wish to make decisions), and if the probability and value estimates are the best possible, it would be perverse to choose the course of lower utility however small the difference.

Sensitivity analysis

We have now shown how the problem is structured, probabilities are selected, values measured and the course of maximum expected utility identified.

The final part of a full decision analysis should include a sensitivity analysis, because conclusions are dependent on the probabilities and utilities used and in real life we are rarely, if ever, certain what these are. In a sensitivity analysis, each of the key probabilities and values are varied in turn within the range of reasonable uncertainty to test the robustness of the conclusion. **Figure 3.2** shows a one-way sensitivity analysis to show the effect of varying the utility of infertility. Each straight line on the graph represents the expected utility of the relevant strategy at each level of infertility utility. The strategy lines intersect at an infertility utility of 0.995; therefore above this value radical surgery is the preferred option while below it no further surgery is preferred. The point at which the strategy lines intersect is called a decision threshold. This threshold will vary itself if other variables such as operative mortality and recurrence risk are changed. The effect of changing more than one variable can be shown in a threshold analysis (**Figure 3.3**). Here the decision threshold is plotted against recurrence risk and utility of infertility for three different operative mortality rates. For each patient the utility of infertility and probability of disease spread is plotted. If this point falls below and to the left of the relevant threshold line the patient should not undergo surgery and if above and to the right she should. The effect of varying utilities and probabilities can be seen at a glance. Since our conclusions are very sensitive to the value placed on retaining fertility it is important to explore this issue carefully with the patient.

Other examples

Oophorectomy

Whether to remove the ovaries at hysterectomy has been long debated. If hormone replacement therapy is available, and since ovarian removal adds little to operative mortality and prevents ovarian cancer, the conclusion has usually been that bilateral oophorectomy is best. However, even taking a tablet a day to replace oestrogen is an inconvenience, and for those who will not comply it may be safer to leave the ovaries to prevent heart disease and osteoporosis. Decision analysis confirms this; for women of average drug taking compliance ovarian conservation is the preferable course.[8] The question of prophylactic oophorectomy as well as mastectomy also arises for women with a high risk of breast cancer due to the BRCA1 or BRCA2 gene mutations. Here, survival has to be traded against quality of life.

It turns out that prophylactic surgery improves survival, with prophylactic mastectomy giving much greater gains than oophorectomy.[9] However, when quality of life is taken into account the overall benefit is restricted to the highest risk patients.[10]

Sometimes decision analysis provides a surprising slant on an old question. Generally, gynaecologists remove the uterus if they are already removing both ovaries, the argument being that leaving it behind serves no useful purpose and carries a risk of endometrial cancer. However, when decision analysis takes into account the additional short-term morbidity of hysterectomy, the benefits are marginal and the optimal choice sensitive to the patient's attitude to risk.[11]

Cervical cancer prevention

Is it better to repeat borderline smears or proceed directly to colposcopy? If colposcopy reveals an abnormality, is it better to treat this immediately or to await histological confirmation? In both cases there is a difference in survival and convenience from the competing policies, and decision analyses show clearly both that immediate colposcopy is preferable to repeating the smear,[12] and that for apparently high-grade colposcopic lesions "see and treat immediately" is preferred to awaiting histology.[13]

Route of hysterectomy

The choice between the abdominal and vaginal route for hysterectomy may appear an obvious topic for decision analysis. However, the lack of

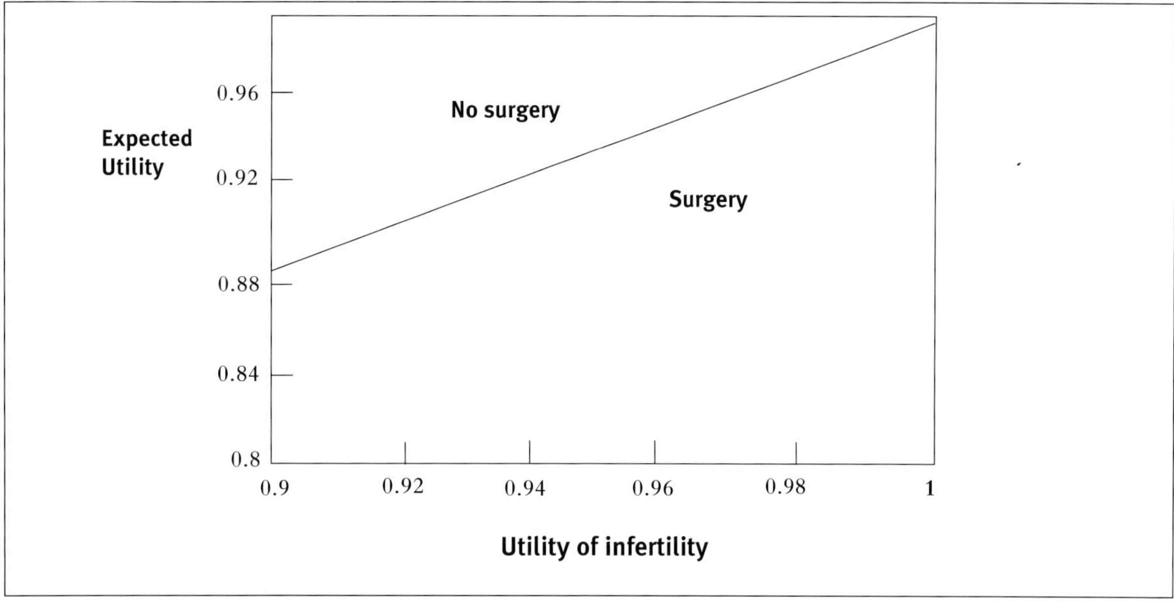

Figure 3.2 A one-way sensitivity analysis for the cervical cancer decision.

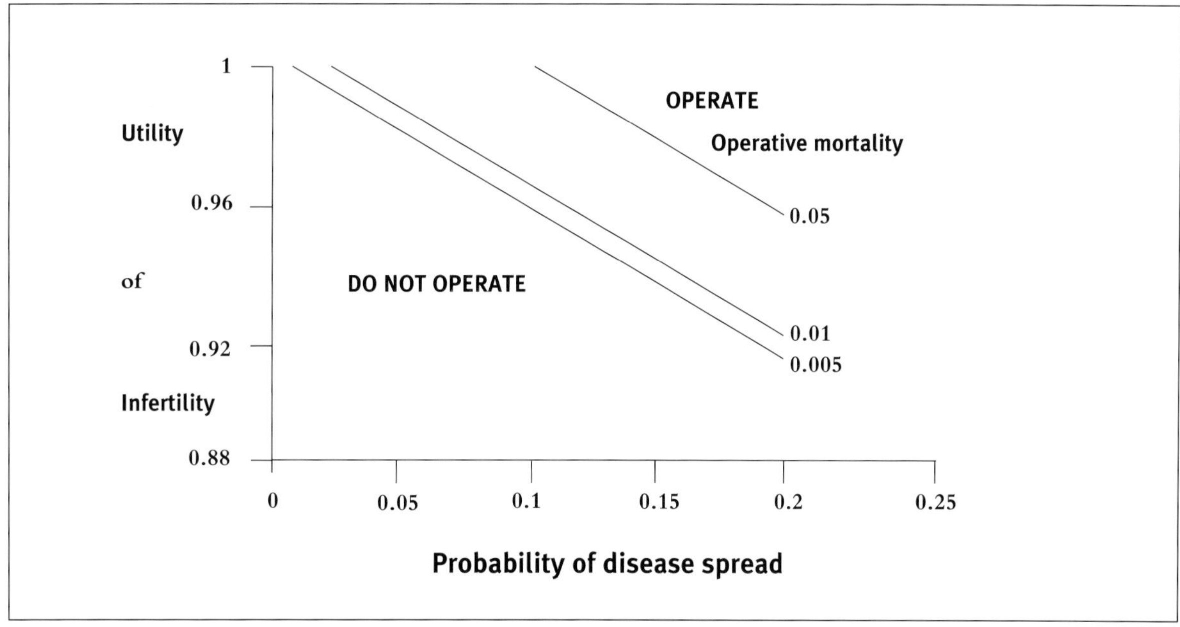

Figure 3.3 A threshold analysis for the cervical cancer decision.

unbiased data on the relative short-term morbidity from the two procedures limits the conclusions that may be drawn. Although most analyses suggest that the vaginal route should be encouraged plausible changes in the uncertainties would change the conclusions.[14] Decision analysis works best on well structured, albeit complicated problems.

Non-gynaecological surgery

Prostate cancer

The example in the introduction of early prostate cancer, has been the subject of a number of analyses. It turns out that although surgery increases life expectancy slightly, when individual values are taken into account, quality-adjusted life expectancy is often reduced so that watchful waiting is sometimes the best policy. Nevertheless the overall effect on the quality-adjusted life expectancy is sensitive to individual utilities, and men who place relatively little value on sexual function may benefit from radical surgery.[15] The clarity introduced by decision analysis has considerably enhanced the quality of debate over this complex management decision.[16]

Neuro- and vascular surgery

A famous example of decision analysis concerns whether to operate on patients with incidental intra-cranial saccular aneurysms. The aneurysm may rupture at any time and cause death or stroke, but surgery also carries a risk of immediate death and brain damage. The optimum choice depends on the age and general health of the patient, the chance of rupture, surgical mortality and morbidity, and the patient's relative preference for immediate or long-term risks. For an otherwise healthy woman of 45, surgery has the greatest expected utility.[17] Later analyses have not seriously questioned this conclusion,[18] although if anti-platelet therapy is included as an option[19] medical treatment is preferred in some scenarios. Surgery is also usually favoured for unruptured intra-cranial arterio-venous malformation.[20]

Disagreement between decision analyses

The conclusions from different decision analyses may differ. For example for the choice of whether to undergo immediate surgery or watchful waiting for asymptomatic severe carotid stenosis, decision analyses have given different results.[21–22] Sarasin[21] suggested that observation was preferable unless the patient was very risk-tolerant. By this she meant willing to accept short-term mortality and morbidity to decrease future risk of death or chronic disability due to stroke. This attitude can be measured and care individualised. However Cronenwett,[22] concluded that surgery usually increased quality adjusted life expectancy. Naturally we should be cautious when this happens since if they really are considering the same question they cannot both be right. However, the advantage of decision analysis is that in contrast to traditional implicit medical decision-making, the assumptions underlying the model are explicit so that readers can judge for themselves which applies to their own practice. The explanation for the difference above was that Cronenwett[22] used different baseline data from a recent large trial and a slightly different method for structuring the decision,

Other areas subjected to decision analysis

These include the place of anterior temporal lobectomy for intractable temporal lobe epilepsy,[23] surgery for small acoustic neuroma.[24] Both are well worthwhile when quality of life is taken into account. In contrast, arranging autologous blood transfusion to minimise the risk of viral infections after elective surgery[25] provides very little expected health benefit, given the improved safety of allogenic transfusions today.

When should decision analysis be used?

Although all decisions require weighing of risks and benefits and could be affected by individual preferences, decision analysis is not always appropriate. At the very least it takes up intellectual resources, and for many poorly structured problems traditional intuitive thinking is still best. Intuition is most suited to decisions where there are many information cues available but no available organising principle. However, decisions made this way are resistant to criticism, as their bases are not visible to the observer or even the decision-maker. Intuition is ill suited to analysis of probabilistic information because the way people estimate probability subjectively leads to predictable biases. They tend to overestimate the probability of situations that can be easily visualised. They tend to judge the likelihood of things happening by how much they resemble typical examples of the event. This can lead to serious errors if people neglect base rates, especially at low risks. Finally, if people have any idea of the probability of an event they tend to revise this in the light of new information by making an adjustment. If the initial estimate was wrong the new estimate will be wrong. Even if the original estimate was correct, adjustments from anchored values are typically insufficient, leading to predictable biases. This is why, when we have time, and a complex but well structured choice, decision analysis should be used. It spells out the bases of decisions and facilitates criticism by exposing underlying assumptions. As gynaecology becomes more evidence based and as people want the underlying assumptions of decisions to be open, it will be increasingly used. For difficult problems there are good reasons to believe that it will result in decisions that accord better with patient preferences than intuitive methods.

REFERENCES

1. Weinstein MC, Fineberg HV, (1980) Clinical decision analysis. WB Saunders, Philadelphia.
2. Pauker SG, Kassirer JP. Decision analysis. *New Engl J Med* 1987; **316**: 250–258.
3. Thornton JG, Lilford RJ, Johnson N. Decision analysis in Medicine. *Br Med J* 1992; **304**: 1099–1103.
4. Tversky A, Kahnemann D. Judgement under uncertainty: heuristics and biases. *Science* 1974; **185**: 1124–1131.
5. Birkmeyer JD, Birkmeyer NO. Decision analysis in surgery. *Surgery* 1996; **120**: 7–15.
6. Birkmeyer JD, Welch HG. A reader's guide to surgical decision analysis. *J Am Coll Surg* 1997; **184**: 589–595.
7. Johnson N, Lilford RJ, Jones SE, McKenzie L, Billinzly P, Songane F. Using decision analysis to calculate the optimum treatment for microinvasive cervical cancer. *Br J Cancer* 1992; **65**: 717–722.
8. Speroff T, Dawson NV, Speroff L, Haber RJ. A risk-benefit analysis of elective bilateral oophorectomy: effect of changes in compliance with estrogen therapy on outcome. *Am J Obstet Gynecol* 1991; **164**: 165–174.
9. Schrag D, Kuntz KM, Garber JE, Weeks JC. Decision analysis-effects of prophylactic mastectomy and oophorectomy on life expectancy among women with BRCA1 or BRCA2 mutations. *New Engl J Med* 1997; **336**: 1465–1471.
10. Grann VR, Panageas KS, Whang W, Antman KH, Neugut AI. Decision analysis of prophylactic mastectomy and oophorectomy in BRCA1–positive or BRCA2–positive patients. *J Clin Oncol* 1998; **1**: 979–985.
11. Grover CM, Kuppermann M, Kahn JG, Washington AE. Concurrent hysterectomy at bilateral salpingo-oophorectomy: benefits, risks, and costs. *Obstet Gynecol* 1996; **88**: 907–913.
12. Johnson N, Sutton J, Thornton JG, Lilford RJ, Johnson VA, Peel KR. Decision analysis for best management of mildly dyskaryotic smear. *Lancet* 1993; **34**: 91–96.
13. Fung HY, Cheung LP, Rogers MS, To KF. The treatment of cervical intraepithelial neoplasia: when could we 'see and loop'. *Eur J Obstet Gynecol Reprod Biol* 1997; **7**: 99–204.
14. Kovac SR, Christie SJ, Bindbeutel GA. Abdominal versus vaginal hysterectomy: a statistical model for determining physician decision making and patient outcome. *Medical Decision Making* 1998; **11**: 19–28.
15. Fleming C, Wasson JH, Albertsen PC, Barry MJ, Wennberg JE. A decision analysis of alternative treatment strategies for clinically localized prostate cancer. *JAMA* 1993; **269**: 2650–2658.
16. Beck JR, Kattan MW, Miles BJ. A critique of the decision analysis for clinically localized prostate cancer. *J Urol* 1994; **152**: 1894–1899.

17. van Crevel H, Habbema JD, Braakman R. Decision analysis of the management of incidental intracranial saccular aneurysms. *Neurology* 1986; **36**: 1335–1339

18. Leblanc R, Worsley KJ, Melanson D. Tampieri D Angiographic screening and elective surgery of familial cerebral aneurysms: a decision analysis. *Neurosurgery* 1994; **35**: 9–18.

19. Dippel DW, Vermeulen M, Braakman R, Habbema JD. Transient ischemic attacks, carotid stenosis, and an incidental intracranial aneurysm. A decision analysis. *Neurosurgery* 1994; **34**: 449–457.

20. Auger RG, Wiebers DO. Management of unruptured intracranial arteriovenous malformations: a decision analysis. *Neurosurgery* 1992; **30**: 561–569.

21. Sarasin FP, Bounameaux H, Bogousslavsky J. Asymptomatic severe carotid stenosis: immediate surgery or watchful waiting? A decision analysis. *Neurology* 1995; **4**: 2147–2153.

22. Cronenwett JL, Birkmeyer JD, Nackman GB, Fillinger MF, Bech FR, Zwolak RM, Walsh DB. Cost-effectiveness of carotid endarterectomy in asymptomatic patients. *J Vasc Surg* 1997; **25**: 298–309.

23. King JT Jr, Sperling MR, Justice AC, O'Connor MJ. A cost-effectiveness analysis of anterior temporal lobectomy for intractable temporal lobe epilepsy. *J Neurosurg* 1997; **87**: 20–28.

24. Telian SA. Management of the small acoustic neuroma: a decision analysis. *Am J Oto*l 1994; **15**: 358–365.

25. Etchason J, Petz L, Keeler E, Calhoun L, Kleinman S, Snider C, Fink A, Brook R. The cost effectiveness of preoperative autologous blood donations. *New Engl J Med* **332**: 719–724.

4

Current Advances in Surgery for Stress Incontinence

L. Cardozo
J. Bidmead

Introduction

Over the last 50 years the surgical management of female incontinence has undergone a number of significant changes with greater understanding of the mechanism of female incontinence and its surgical treatment. Increased knowledge of the morbidity and long-term results of the great variety of surgical procedures described for treating female incontinence has led to the continuing development of new and alternative procedures.

The aims of any new surgical treatment are to maximise the chances of a successful outcome, while minimising the surgical morbidity and reducing the cost to society and the individual, both of the procedure itself and subsequent convalescence. The cost of any repeat surgery needs to be included. Considerable interest has focused on the financial aspects of medical treatments and interest is developing in methods of measuring surgical outcomes in terms of those that improve the quality of life of the woman concerned, as well as using objective measurements of success.

Whilst there is tremendous enthusiasm for new procedures, appearing to offer a greater chance of success with reduced morbidity, it is important to critically assess the claims made for these procedures.

This chapter outlines those new techniques that appear most promising and evaluates their place in current practice in the light of historical experience.

Established surgical treatment for female stress incontinence

In order to understand and evaluate new procedures it is useful to examine the development of surgery for female genuine stress incontinence (GSI) as there are many lessons which can be learnt from this.

Genuine stress incontinence is defined as the involuntary loss of urine when the intravesical pressure exceeds the intraurethral pressure in the absence of detrusor activity.[1] Over 150 different surgical procedures have been described for the treatment of GSI, and this number continues to increase. While many of these are simply variations on existing techniques, nevertheless there is a huge array of potential operations from which to choose.

Very few of these procedures have been evaluated in prospective, randomised controlled trials. Many authors have published results of their procedures enthusiastically, while on closer examination outcomes are often given as subjective evaluations with very few studies showing objective evidence of success. When Pereyra published the results of his needle suspension technique in 1959, he quoted a 90% continence rate after 14 months follow-up.[2] When Stamey published his variation on this technique in 1969,[3] he reported a 100% success rate although notably this was on subjective criteria only. Marshall, Marachetti and Krantz describing their retropubic procedure in 1949,[4] reported subjective cure rates of 89% but made no mention of the relatively common surgical complication of osteitis pubis which is now known to occur in 2.5–7% of women undergoing this procedure.[5] Burch[6] when describing his retropubic colposuspension reported a 90% success rate but made no mention of the 15% incidence of de-novo detrusor instability which is now known to occur following this procedure.[7] The early results of needle suspension procedures such as the Stamey, Raz or Pereyra, while initially very good in the short term are now well known to have extremely poor results on long-term follow-up.[8] The long-term results of these surgical procedures for GSI have become clear only with the passage of time.

All of these examples illustrate that the initial success rates from any new procedure, particularly when performed by enthusiasts, expressed in subjective outcome measures, are much higher than when the procedure is used more widely by a variety of practitioners. It is also clear that time is needed to assess the long-term results of any new procedure together with any long-term complications that may occur. As with needle bladder neck suspension procedures, the early results may appear promising however, on longer-term examination they may be extremely disappointing. In addition, there is difficulty evaluating one procedure against another as very few comparative randomised controlled trials are published in the literature.

Recently two meta-analyses of procedures for stress incontinence have been published (Jarvis in 1994,[5] Black and Downes in 1996[9]). Both of these studies give useful information as to which procedures offer the most likely chance of objective cure of stress incontinence. Both publications highlight the much higher objective cure rates for a first operation with retropubic suspension procedures, such as Burch colposuspension or Marshall-Marachetti-Krantz, or with sub-urethral sling techniques.

The Marshall-Marachetti-Krantz procedure is complicated by a relatively high incidence of osteitis pubis[4] and for this reason has fallen out of favour. Therefore the modified Burch colposuspension or a sub-urethral sling procedure would currently be regarded as the procedure of choice as a primary continence procedure (**Table 4.1**).

The American Urological Association also published a report on surgical management of female stress urinary incontinence.[10] This reinforces the results of the studies by Jarvis and Black. Retropubic suspensions and slings appear to give better success rates compared to anterior vaginal repair and needle suspension procedures. The results of this report are summarised (**Table 4.2**).

Given that both a modified Burch colposuspension or sub-urethral sling procedure have the potential to give a very high objective cure rate, why then is there a need to search for new surgical techniques?

While the Burch colposuspension is undoubtedly a very successful operation, it is nevertheless a major surgical procedure with significant concomitant surgical morbidity, necessitating a relatively long hospital stay and a prolonged convalescence of 6–8 weeks.

The Burch colposuspension also has two associated long-term problems, the first of which is the obstructive nature of the procedure, (Hilton and Stanton[11]) with a small but significant number of voiding difficulties occurring post-operatively.[12] The second problem associated with Burch colposuspension is post-operative de-novo detrusor instability. This occurs in some 12–15% of women.[13,7] The cause of de-novo detrusor instability is not thought to be due to obstruction and the mechanism remains unknown, however, it seems likely that a proportion of these patients had pre-operative detrusor instability undetected at cystometry and it may be that more stringent pre-operative investigation may reduce this.[14]

Modified Burch colposuspension is associated with post-operative formation of an enterocele or rectocele, the incidence of post-operative rectocele is between 7.6% and 17% of cases.[15]

Sling procedures also have drawbacks. The disadvantage of using autologous sling materials such as rectus sheath or fascia lata is that a second surgical incision needs to be made, which increases the morbidity of the procedure. In addition, it seems increasingly likely that those women suffering from stress incontinence have an inherent defect in collagen biochemistry[16,17] and the use of autologous connective tissue may lead to medium-term failure of the procedure due to collagen deficiency in the sling material.

The use of synthetic slings has been widely described. Mercilene®, Marlex® and Gortex® have been employed and the infection rate appears no greater than with autologous slings. However, urethral erosion has been reported following the use of synthetic material.[10] In addition Hilton[18] has shown that sub-urethral sling procedures increase outflow resistance significantly, and long-term voiding dif-

Table 4.1 Results of surgical treatment of GSI from Jarvis 1994[5]

Procedure	First procedure Mean (%)	Recurrent incontinence Mean (%)
Bladder buttress	67.8	ND
Marshall-Marchetti-Krantz	89.5	ND
Burch Colposuspension	89.8	82.5
Bladder neck suspension	86.7	86.4
Sling	93.9	86.1
Injectables	45.5	57.8

ND – No results reported

Table 4.2 Results of AUA Clinical Guidelines Panel[10]

Procedure	Cure rate at 24–47 months (%)	Cure at over 48 months (%)	De-novo postoperative urgency (%)	Voiding difficulties (%)
Retropubic Suspension	84%	84%	11%	5%
Transvaginal Suspension	65%	67%	5%	5%
Anterior Repair	85%	61%	NA	NA
Sling Procedures	82%	83%	8%	8%

ND – No results reported

ficulty, which may be more common with synthetic sling material is an additional complication of sling procedures.

The development of new continence procedures

A number of factors need to be considered when any new continence procedure is proposed. The first of these is the age and physical activity of the woman concerned. For an older patient who is less physically active a procedure with a lower objective cure rate but high subjective cure rate with minimal morbidity may be more suitable. Whereas, in a younger woman with a more active lifestyle a higher initial morbidity may be acceptable provided it offers the likelihood of longer-term objective cure.

Previous treatment needs also to be considered. It has been shown that women who have had previous failed continence procedures have a much higher failure rate for secondary procedures and a higher operative morbidity.[19] In this situation, a procedure with a lower initial complication rate but slightly lower chance of objective cure may be more acceptable than in a woman undergoing a primary continence operation.

The presence or absence of concurrent pathology also needs to be considered. A lower objective cure rate may be acceptable in women with concurrent pathology such as detrusor instability if the overall effects results in an enhancement of a woman's quality of life.

To complicate all of these factors, a woman's health and expectation of successful treatment also needs to be taken into consideration. We are currently entering an era with an expanding growth in the elderly population. The proportion of elderly people within society is rapidly increasing with an 18% increase in the over 75 year olds, and a 38% rise in the over 85 year olds anticipated in the next 20 years.[20] Improvements in the prevention and management of pelvic floor dysfunction are therefore imperative.

Elderly women need not necessarily expect to have sub-optimal treatment simply on the grounds of their age alone. Indeed age should be no bar to surgery. In general patients' expectations of successful outcome have increased and women are less likely to tolerate any procedure which offers a sub-optimal outcome.

Economic considerations also apply in the current climate of the National Health Service. The cost-benefit relationship of any procedure needs to be taken closely into account before a new operation is adopted. A number of factors come into play; the cost of disposable equipment versus the re-sterilization costs is a particular area of interest in relation to minimal access surgery. Operating time is also expensive and long procedures may not be economically justifiable. The increased costs of hospital inpatient treatment also act strongly in favour of procedures with a minimal inpatient stay. The economic impact of any treatment to society in terms of the length of time that a woman is unable to work or look after her family following operative treatment is also an important consideration. However the cost of unsuccessful continence surgery to society in terms of a woman's reduced capacity to work or look after her family as well as the cost of continence pads and not least the effect of reduced quality of life on a woman's family and relationships should not be forgotten. Lastly, the cost of any necessary further treatment, medical or surgical, which results from failure or complications of a new procedure needs to be taken into account.

Characteristics of an "ideal" continence procedure

The ideal operation would be one which achieved a cure, both objectively and subjectively, as close to 100% as possible. It would be an easy technique, able to be used successfully by any gynaecologist or urologist with an interest in continence surgery and not solely in tertiary referral centres. This surgery would offer minimal morbidity with a short inpatient stay and rapid return to normal activity.

The ideal continence procedure would also produce few long-term complications due to suture failure, erosion of synthetic material into the bladder or urethra, and mechanical failure of any synthetic or autologous material used.

Urethral obstruction and *de-novo* detrusor instability should also be minimal. In effect this means that the ideal technique would restore continence without producing any urethral obstruction or increased voiding pressure.

The effects should also be long lasting, as the peak incidence of GSI is in the 40s and the life expectancy of a woman today is 80, an ideal operation would last forty years.

Lastly, as no surgical procedure can reasonably be expected to have a limitless life-span, the ideal operation would have a minimal effect on any subsequent surgical procedures. Scarring produced at a primary procedure that may hinder a secondary operation should be minimal, any synthetic material used should be easily removed and post-operative scar tissue and adhesion formation should be minimal consistent with producing a reasonably long term cure.

From a technical point of view if any procedure is

to be widely accepted and universally employed it should have a relatively short learning curve and not require the purchase of high capital-cost equipment.

One of the difficulties of assessing any continence procedure has been the choice of a suitable outcome measure. Obtaining data on objective cure rates require invasive investigations such as urodynamics which are impractical in the majority of women having undergone routine surgery. However subjective cure rates may not give an accurate picture of the efficacy of a particular technique. A recent epidemiological study by Black *et al*[21] highlights the discrepancy between surgeons and patients views on the outcomes of surgical treatment. A useful method of assessing outcome which has recently gained some popularity is in measuring the effect of any procedure on quality of life before and after incontinence surgery with the means of validated and disease-specific quality of life questionnaires.[22]

New operative techniques for genuine stress incontinence currently under evaluation

Peri-urethral injectables

The use of injectable peri-urethral bulking agents is gaining popularity both in Europe and in North America although the technique was first described by Murless[23] as long ago as 1938. Two main types of pathologies are thought to contribute to genuine stress incontinence; namely urethral hypermobility and intrinsic sphincter deficiency.[24] Both conditions may exist in the same woman.[25] In those women with urethral hypermobility, raised intra-abdominal pressure leads to descent of the urethra and bladder neck with less effective transmission of pressure to the bladder neck and proximal urethra. In this situation operations which re-position the bladder neck will have a high success rate.[15] In women with mainly intrinsic sphincter deficiency the defect is not in urethral pressure transmission but due to poor urethral closure which results from scarring from previous surgery, childbirth or neurological injury. Maximal urethral closure pressure may be low.[26] It has been suggested that in these patients operations to re-position the bladder neck have a higher failure rate. Whilst low maximal urethral closure pressure has been shown to give a higher probability of failure in bladder neck re-positioning surgery this is not absolute.[27]

As peri-urethral injectables appear to act by co-apting the urethral mucosa and increasing urethral closure pressure, it has been suggested that they would be particularly suitable for women with stress incontinence due to intrinsic sphincter deficiency.[28] Although peri-urethral injectables as a primary procedure are popular in North America in our experience it is unusual to find women with low maximum urethral closure pressure due to intrinsic sphincter deficiency presenting for a primary continence procedure. (**Figure 4.1**).

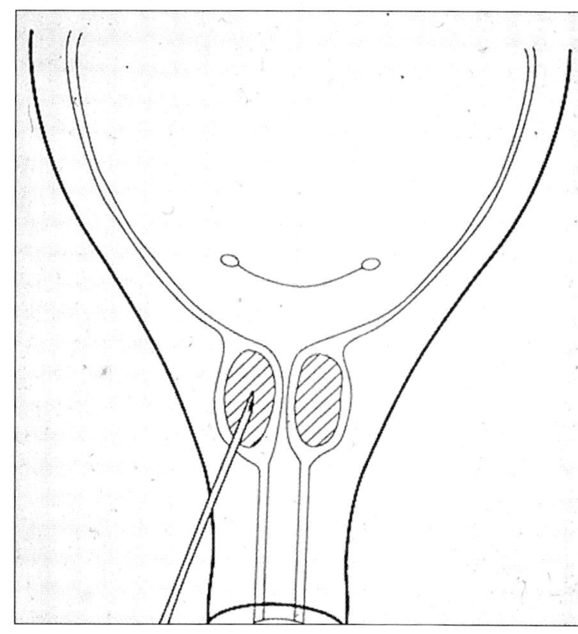

Figure 4.1 Periurethral implants positioned at bladder neck.

Materials used for peri-urethral injections

A number of materials have been used for peri-urethral injection. Ideally these would be completely inert, cheap, easy to inject and free from long-term complications yet provide long-lasting results.

Teflon

Teflon was the first widely used peri-urethral injectable material. Lopez *et al* [29] reported a series of 128 women treated over 27 years with cure rates of up to 61%. Teflon was found to produce dense, fibrous tissue and a granulomatous reaction leading to urinary obstruction, urethral erosion and severe problems with any subsequent surgery. Teflon has also been shown to migrate from the injection site to local lymph nodes, lung and brain in post-mortem studies.[29,30] As a result of these problems Teflon is now rarely used due to concern over particle migration and local tissue response. However the encouraging initial results have led to the use of alternative materials.

Autologous fat

The use of autologous fat has been reported as a urethral bulking agent. It has the advantage of being cheap and easy to obtain. However fat is rapidly phagocytosed and while initial results may be reasonable, longer term results are disappointing and this technique is now little used.

GAX collagen

One of the most common materials used currently is gluteraldehyde cross-linked bovine collagen (GAX collagen, BARD, Crawley UK). This has not been shown to have any side effects due to migration but does produce a local inflammatory response in which injected collagen is replaced with endogenous collagen.[31] Due to the inflammatory response produced by GAX collagen and the resorption of this material repeated injections may be necessary to sustain continence.[32] Cure rates in published case series vary from 7%[33] to 83% (**Table 4.3**).[34] However most studies report cures in the region of 40–60%[35,36] (**Figure 4.2**).

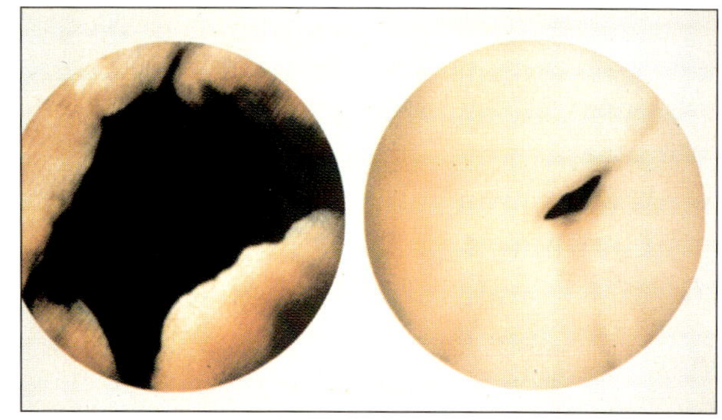

Figure 4.2 Closure of the bladder neck achieved with GAX collagen.

Silicone

The most recently developed injectable material consists of micronised silicone rubber particles suspended in a non-silicone carrier gel.[36] This is currently marketed as Macroplastique (Uroplasty, Reading UK). The larger particle size of this material makes migration and displacement less likely, and in addition, the inert nature of the material makes a local inflammatory reaction less problematic. The silicone particles are designed to act as a bulking agent with a local inflammatory response removing the carrier gel, encapsulating the silicon in fibrin and replacing the gel with collagen fibres. Cure rates reported with Macroplastique are similar to those with GAX.[37] Only one non-randomised trial to compare GAX with Macroplastique has been published.[38]

In general the efficacy of peri-urethral injection of either GAX collagen or Macroplastique appears equivalent, however randomised controlled trials are currently in progress to assess differences between the two.[38,39]

Implantable microballoons

A recent innovation in urethral bulking agents is the use of silicon balloons inflated after positioning in the peri-urethral tissues. The containment of the bulking agent within a silicon capsule should in theory eliminate the problems of particle migration and macrophage phagocytosis of injected material and improve long-term results. At present this technique is in the early stage of development.

Preliminary results by Pycha *et al*[10] show good results in women with intrinsic sphincter deficiency and, interestingly, poor results in women with urethral hypermobility only.

Other peri-urethral injectable materials are currently under development including the use of alternative extracts of bovine collagen, carbon coated silicon particles, bone and ceramic materials, however there is insufficient data at present to compare the use of these new materials.

The mechanism of continence achieved after peri-urethral injection is not well defined. It is thought that peri-urethral bulking achieves a better apposition of urethral mucosa without an increase in obstruction although some authors report obstructive features following peri-urethral injection.

Complications

Complications from peri-urethral injection are uncommon. Urinary infection may occur in some 20% of women (Contigen data sheet). Some studies report that post-operative *de-novo* detrusor instability is rare while others report a rate of 39%.[35]

The lack of long-term data on the use of Macroplastique means that the long-term effects of peri-urethral injection with this material cannot be assessed. GAX collagen has the complication of hyper-sensitivity to bovine collagen which appears to occur in approximately 3% of women.[41]

Cost

Both materials are expensive, however the short inpatient stay and convalescent period required reduces the cost initially in comparison to open surgery although the need for subsequent re-injection dramatically increases the expense of these techniques.

Route of injection

Injections may be made either trans-urethrally via a cystoscope or peri-urethrally under cystoscopic control. A number of small studies published in abstract form have attempted to determine the best route but in general either technique seems to give equivalent results and the route of injection is governed by the surgeons preference.[42]

Conclusions

Peri-urethral bulking agents are undoubtedly useful in the treatment of genuine stress incontinence and may be particularly beneficial in the treatment of intrinsic sphincter deficiency. They are invaluable in the treatment of secondary incontinence in women who have undergone multiple failed procedures or after radiotherapy where the urethra is fixed and scarred – a group of patients for whom other techniques have high morbidity and poor results.

However, as a primary treatment, in view of their relatively low initial objective cure rates and poorer long-term performance, they are more suitable for elderly patients in whom low operative morbidity is a consideration and longer-term objective cure less important.

Minimal access techniques

Laparoscopic colposuspension

The modified Burch colposuspension has become the "gold standard" procedure for correction of

Table 4.3 Short to medium term results of GAX collagen injection

Authors	Objective cure at 3 years (%)	Objective cure at 12 months (%)	Objective cure at 2 years (%)
Monga & Stanton[32]	61	54	48
Swami & Batista[73]	NA	NA	25
Khullar & Cardozo[37]	58	52	48

NA – Results not available

primary stress incontinence. Although this procedure gives a high (85%) objective cure rate with very good long-term results, it is a major abdominal procedure which carries with it significant operative morbidity, requiring a relatively long inpatient stay and a long period of convalescence. Despite this the procedure is well-tolerated even in fit elderly patients.

In recent years interest has grown in attempting to replicate the high objective cure rate and good long-term results of the open colposuspension with the use of minimal access surgery. This was first proposed by Vancaillie and Schuessler[43] in 1991.

A number of series have been published regarding this technique and a wide variety of surgical methods using either a trans-peritoneal or extra-peritoneal approach have been recorded. The extraperitoneal route reduces the risk of visceral injury although establishing a plane of dissection may be more difficult and this technique restricts operating space (**Figures 4.3A & 4.3B**). The transperitoneal approach increases the risk of visceral injury and bladder injury may be commoner when opening the supravesical peritoneal fold. This approach does allow more operating space and allows concomitant pelvic surgery such as hysterectomy to be performed.

A variety of methods for re-positioning the bladder neck have also been used involving absorbable and non-absorbable sutures, staples and synthetic meshes and tissue glue. This variety of techniques makes comparison of different studies difficult.

In general the use of laparoscopic surgery compared with an open Burch colposuspension offers reduced inpatient stay and post-operative convalescence. However the longer-term objective cure results are lower, and the operative time for laparoscopic colposuspension is longer. This is undoubtedly a function of the surgeon's experience and may well reduce, although it is likely that this will always be greater than an open colposuspension.

One of the major advantages cited for minimal

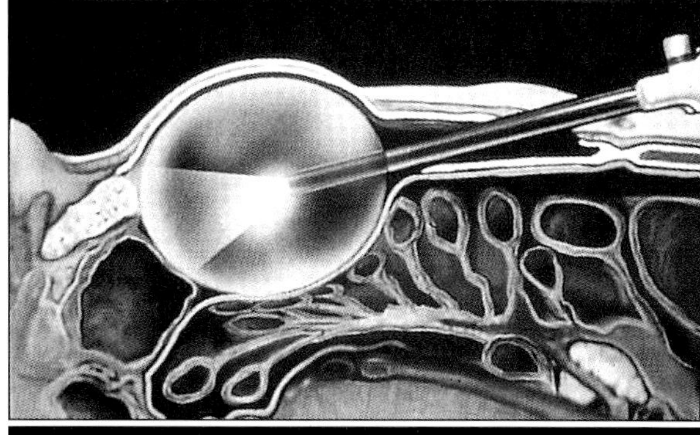

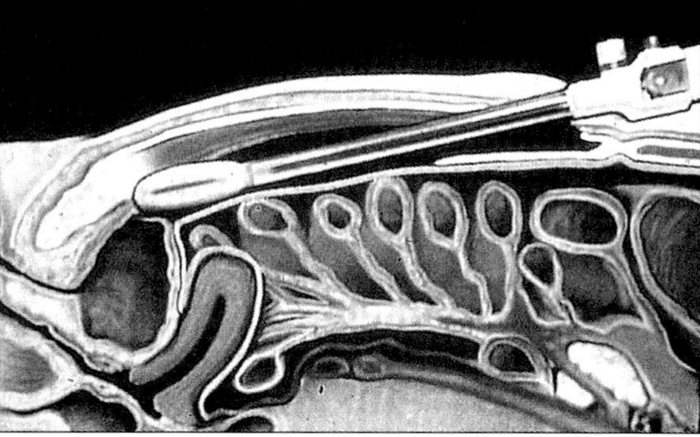

Figure 4.3A & 4.3B Extraperitoneal approaches to laparoscopic colposuspension with balloon tissue expander.

access techniques is the lack of subsequent fibrosis and scarring, which is particularly useful in procedures designed to restore or maintain fertility. The decline in objective cure following minimal access surgery parallels that seen with needle suspension techniques that also produce minimal fibrosis and scarring. It may well be that minimal access techniques are disadvantageous where permanent fibrosis and anatomical repositioning are required.

The incidence of urinary tract injury appears to be higher with the laparoscopic approach. Published series are few but two reports of ureteric injury, (a very unusual occurrence at open surgery – only 15 cases reported in the literature),[44] suggest that the risk of lower urinary tract injury may be much greater with a laparoscopic approach.[45,46]

However, this may change in the future as more experience is gained with the laparoscopic approach.

The cost of laparoscopic procedures in terms of increased use of theatre time and the considerable cost of disposable instruments used also needs to be taken into account. Khol *et al*[47] found that, despite a shorter in-patient stay, costs of laparoscopic procedures were higher than a traditional approach.

Operative morbidity has been extensively studied, intra-operative blood loss appears similar although febrile morbidity and length of hospital stay are both higher in the open colposuspension group.[48] Few reports give details of intra and post-operative morbidity.

Results of laparoscopic surgery

Only two randomised controlled trials exist comparing laparoscopic colposuspension with open colposuspension. Both of these studies show that operating time is considerably longer but recovery time from the surgery is shorter, however in Burton's study successful cure of stress incontinence was only 60% at 36 months compared with 93% following an open surgical approach (**Table 4.4**). Lobel and Sand[50] show a cure rate of 89% at 3 months, 86% at 1 year and 69% at 2 years.

Liu[51] reports the most extensive series of laparoscopic procedures and describes a return to normal activity within a week of surgery. The major drawback of minimal access techniques is the relatively long learning curve taken to gain proficiency in minimal access surgery in order to be able to offer a minimal access approach for laparoscopic Burch colposuspension.

A urogynaecologist needs to be experienced in both urogynaecological techniques and in those used in minimal access surgery. While laparoscopic colposuspension offers some promise for reducing operative morbidity it is yet to be shown that it offers an acceptable alternative to an open procedure and further evaluation with the register of surgeons performing the technique has been proposed recently.[52]

As more surgeons with previous experience in incontinence surgery are adopting a laparoscopic approach, objective cure rates appear to improve, suggesting that the skills required are those of both an experienced laparoscopic surgeon together with experience of open incontinence procedures.

At the time of writing a large multi-centre randomised trial of laparoscopic and open colposuspension funded by the MRC is underway. This will provide definitive evidence of the role of laparoscopic surgery in this area.

Bladder neck stabilisation procedures using bone anchoring techniques

A number of authors have described variations on techniques for achieving bladder neck elevation using long needle suspension techniques in particular Raz,[58] Gittes,[53] Pereyra,[59] and Stamey.[53] It has become clear with long-term follow-up that these techniques have relatively low operative morbidity and rapid recovery from surgery. The early objective success rate of these procedures is comparable with that of an open colposuspension procedure, however, the longer-term results of these procedures have in a number of studies been shown to be extremely disappointing.

Mills *et al*[54] reported a 10-year follow up of 46 patients who had undergone a Stamey procedure; only 25% remained totally dry but overall 80% of those reviewed remained at least subjectively improved.

O'Sullivan *et al*[55] conducted a questionnaire based survey at intervals following surgery. Immediately postoperatively 70% were dry and 15% much improved, after 1 year these figures were 31% and 28% respectively but after 5 years only 18% were dry. However the largest study to date is that of Keveligham *et al.*[56] In a study of 259 patients who underwent the Stamey procedure at St. James' Hospital, Leeds from 1985 to 1995, life table analysis was used to assess long-term results.The subjective cure rates were 45% at 2 years, 18% at 4 years and only 6% at 10 years.

Table 4.4 Short to medium term results of laparoscopic colposuspension

Authors	Cure at 3 months (%)	Cure at 12 months(%)	Cure at over 2 years(%)
Lobel & Sand[50]	89	86	69
Ross[73]	98	93	89
Burton[53]	73	NA	60
Su[49A]	80	NA	NA

NA – results not available

There are three main theories to explain why the longer-term results of these procedures are so poor. The suspending sutures are inserted with the use of a long needle and cause little surgical scarring or permanent fibrosis. Therefore maintaining suspension of the bladder neck relies upon the integrity of the tissue in the para-vaginal fascia and in the rectus fascia anchoring the suture at either end, and also on the integrity of the suture itself. It is not surprising that in women with poorer collagen status suffering from stress incontinence, the strength of the anchoring tissues is less and hence the sutures tend to pull through either at the vaginal fascia or through the rectus sheath. Most of these techniques use monofilament sutures which may fail with repeated stress over time.

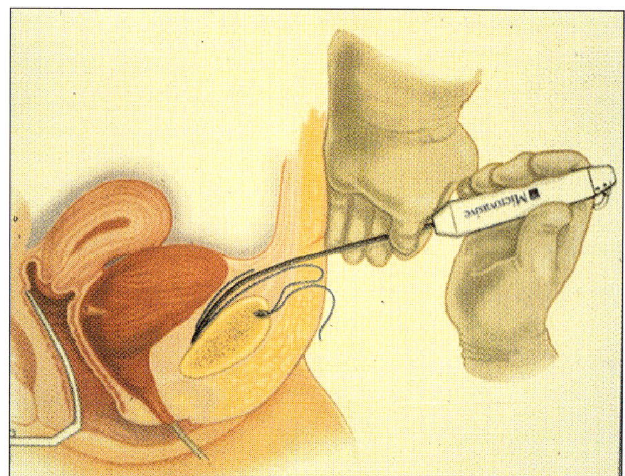

Figure 4.4 Vesica® bone anchoring system. Sutures anchored to pubic bone and passed beneath pubic arch.

In order to avoid these weak points bone anchoring techniques have been suggested to anchor the abdominal end of the suture. (**Figures 4.4 and 4.5**).

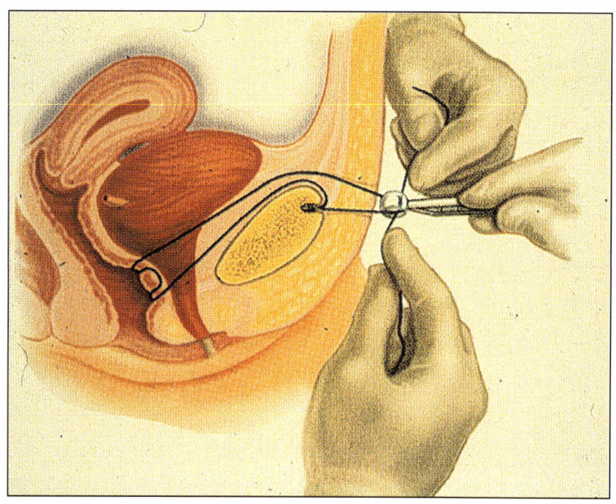

Figure 4.5 Vesica® bone anchoring system. Completed suture anchored to paravaginal tissue and tied.

A number of commercial kits for performing bone anchored bladder neck suspension procedures are available. Published studies on their use are limited and mostly cover relatively short-term follow-up.

The Vesica® technique marketed by Boston Medical consists of a device used to anchor the abdominal end of the sutures into the pubic bone. A vaginal epithelial patch is used to buttress the vaginal end of the suture. Appell *et al* report 94% cure at 12 months using this technique[57] although in a series of 77 women one required re-operation for an infected bone anchor. The advantage of these techniques is that like a traditional needle suspension procedure they have a relatively low surgical morbidity and a faster recovery with very good short-term results. However the high cost of some of the commercially available kits obviates any economic advantage.

While bone anchoring may increase the strength of the abdominal end of the suture attachment, the use of a vaginal epithelial patch is not dissimilar to the techniques used by Raz[58] and Peyrera[59] and this remains a potential weak spot. In addition, the suture material used is still subject to sudden stress-related failure.

Whether the use of bone anchoring will improve the very poor long-term results of the traditional needle suspension techniques remains to be seen, although examination of the surgical principles involved suggests that they may not. Some longer term reports are now being published showing medium-term failure rates similar to those of the needle suspensions.[59] Although no randomised trials comparing the use of bone anchors exist, over 32,000 kits have been sold in the USA. Long-term follow-up will reveal whether these techniques live up to their initial promise.

Other authors have taken a different approach to improving the long-term efficacy of needle suspension. Staskin[65] suggests the use of a Gore-Tex® suture to reduce the risk of suture failure with monofilament materials. A Gore-Tex® patch is used to support the paravaginal tissues. This may reduce the tendency of the sutures to cut out of the paravaginal tissue but introduces the theoretical possibility of urethral erosion. Results to date have been good with few complications reported.

Vaginal sling plasty (TVT procedure)

Most current procedures for the treatment of GSI involve anatomical repositioning of the bladder neck in order to improve pressure transmission to the proximal urethra or the use of bulking agents injected periurethrally to increase urethral closure pressure. In a departure from this, a new technique known as the "Tension-free Vaginal Tape" (TVT) aims to correct stress incontinence using an alternative mechanism. This is based on the premise that stress incontinence results from failure of the pubourethral ligaments in the mid-urethra.[61–63] The failure of pubo-urethral support has also been proposed by other authors, notably Delancey.[64]

The TVT procedure uses a prolene mesh tape placed at the ***mid*** urethra with the aim of encouraging fibrosis and the formation of "neo-pubo-urethral ligaments". The tape is inserted via a small vaginal incision using two 6 mm trocars.

Due to the weave of the tape, which has no salvage edge, the free ends of the weave interlock with the tissues and the tape is self-retaining (**Figure 4.6**).

As the incision is small and the procedure relatively minimally invasive, this can be performed under local anaesthesia with light intravenous sedation. This allows the position of the tape to be adjusted in a conscious patient with a full bladder during a series of coughs. The aim is to have the tape lying free at rest (hence "tension-free") and to only exhort sufficient pressure on the urethra during a cough to prevent leakage of urine.[65] The exact mechanism of action remains unknown.

Short-term results for this procedure have been reported by Ulmsten.[66] These demonstrated an 84% cure rate with no long-term voiding difficulties or de-novo detrusor instability. Although these results are impressive, not all women underwent postoperative urodynamic testing and the results so far relate to the first 2 postoperative years. Other

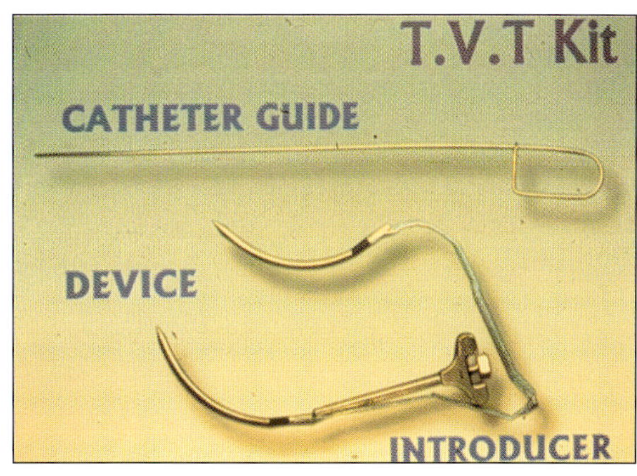

Figure 4.6 TVT instruments and tape.

groups using this device have also begun to report their results with similar outcomes but a relatively high rate (8%) of bladder injury.[67]

Longer-term studies of this procedure are awaited and while the initial results appear promising some concerns remain over the long-term results. In particular the American Urological Association report demonstrated a small but significant incidence of urethral erosion with synthetic slings.

The fact that this tape is made of prolene which produces less tissue reaction than other synthetic materials and that it is not under tension will hopefully prevent the occurrence of this potentially devastating complication. Currently large scale randomised trials comparing the TVT and open colposuspension are underway in the UK and Europe. The results of these trials should be awaited before widespread adoption of this new procedure.

Conclusions

In recent years a greater understanding of the efficacy of surgical treatments for stress incontinence has developed. Retropubic operations such as the Burch colposuspension and sling procedures have been shown to be the gold standard against which new techniques must be judged.[68] A number of new techniques have been developed which appear to offer acceptable results with reduced morbidity. A range of procedures is emerging which allow treatment to be tailored to suit the individual woman. Depending on lifestyle, age and physical fitness women can now be offered a choice of treatment.

However, it is important that before being adopted enthusiastically any new technique is subjected to rigorous scrutiny. The morbidity, long-term results, effect on quality of life and economics of a new treatment should be scientifically evaluated before it is put into widespread clinical use.

REFERENCES

1. Abrams P, Blaivas JG, Stanton SL, Andersen JT. Standardisation of terminology of lower urinary tract function. *Br J Obstet Gynaecol* 1990; **97**(6 Supp):1–16.

2. Pereyra AJ. A simplified surgical procedure for the correction of stress incontinence in women. *West J of Surg* 1959; **67**: 223.

3. Stamey TA. Endoscopic suspension of the vesical neck for urinary incontinence. *Surg Gynaecol Obstet* 1973; **136**: 547–554.

4. Marshal Marachetti AA, Krantz KE. The correction of stress incontinence by simple vesico-urethral suspension. *Surg Gynecol & Obstet* 1949; **88**: 509–518.

5. Jarvis GJ. Surgery for stress incontinence. *Br J Obstet Gynaecol* 1994; **101**: 371–374.

6 Burch JC. Urethrovesical fixation to Coopers ligament for correction of stress incontinence, cystocele and prolapse. *Am J Obstet Gynecol* 1961; **81**: 281–290.

7. Cardozo LD, Stanton SL, Williams JE. Detrusor instability following surgery for genuine stress incontinence. *Br J Urol* 1979; **58**: 138–142.

8. Hilton P, Maine C. The Stamey endoscopic bladder neck suspension: a clinical and urodynamic investigation, including actuarial follow-up over four years. *Br J Obstet Gynaecol* 1991; **98**: 1141–1149.

9 Black NA, Downes SH. The effectiveness of surgery for stress incontinence in women: A systematic review. *Br J Urol* 1996; **78**: 497–510.

10. Dmochowski R, Appell R, Blaivas J, Hadley R *et al.* Female stress urinary incontinence guidelines. Panel summary report on surgical management of female stress urinary incontinence. *J Urol* 1997; **158**: 875–880.

11. Hilton P, Stanton SL. Clinical and urodynamic assessment of the Burch colposuspension for genuine stress incontinence. *Br J Obstet Gynaecol* 1983; **90**: 934–939.

12. Cardozo LD, Cutner A. Surgical management of incontinence. Contemp. *Reviews Obstet & Gynaecol* 1992; **4**: 36–41.

13. Carlay M, Monga A, Stanton SL. Burch colpo-suspension: a ten to twenty year follow-up. *Br J Obstet & Gynaecol* 1995; **102**: 740–745.

14. Khullar V *et al.* Ambulatory urodynamics: a predictor of dei-novo detrusor instability after colposuspension. *Neuro Urol Urodynam* 1994; **13**: 443–444.

15. Stanton SL, Williams JE, Ritchie B. The colposuspension operation for urinary incontinence. *Br J Obstet Gynaecol* 1976; **83**: 890–895.

16. Ulmsten U, Ekman G, Giertz G, Malstrom A. Different biochemical composition of connective tissue incontinent and stress incontinent women. *Acta Obstet Gynnecol Scand* 1987; **66**: 455–457.

17. Landon CR, Smith ARB, Crofts CE, Trowbridge EA. Biomechanical properties of connective tissue in women with stress incontinence of urine. *Neurourol Urodyn* 1989; **8**: 369–370.

18. Hilton P. A. Clinical and urodynamic study comparing the Stamey bladder neck suspension and suburethral sling procedures in the treatment of genuine stress incontinence. *Br J Obstet & Gynaecol* 1989; **96**: 213–220.

19. Cardozo L, Hextall A, Bailey J, Boos K. Colposuspension after previous failed continence surgery. A prospective observational study. RSM Section of Obstetrics and Gynaecology 1998 Prize meeting.

20. Brocklehurst JC. Urinary incontinence in the community – analysis of a MORI poll. *BMJ* 1993; **306**: 8324.

21. Black N, Griffiths J, Pope C, Bowling A *et al. BMJ* 1997; **315**: 1493–1498.

22. Kelleher CJ, Cardozo L D, Khullar V, Salvatore S A. New questionnaire to asses the quality of life of urinary incontinent women. *Br J Obstet Gynecol* 1997; **104**: 1374–1379.

23. Murless BC. The injection treatment of stress incontinence. *J Obstet Gynecol Br Emp* 1938; **45**: 67–73.

24. Chaliha C, Williams G. Peri-urethral injection therapy for the treatment of stress incontinence. *Br J Urol* 1995; **76**: 151–155.

25. Nitti VW, Combs AJ. Correlation of valsalva leak point pressure with subjective degree of stress urinary incontinence in women. *J Urol* 1996; **155**: 281–285.

26. Stanton SL, Williams JE, Ritchie D. The colposuspension operation for urinary incontinence. *Br J Obstet & Gynaecol* 1976; **83**: 890–895.

27. McGuire EJ *et al.* Clinical assessment of urethral sphincter function. *J Urol* 1993; **150**: 1452–1454.

28. Sand PK, Bowen LW, Panganiban R, Ostergaard DR. The low pressure urethra as a factor in failed retropubic urethropexy. *Obstet Gynecol* 1987; **69**: 399–402.

29. Lopez EA, Padron FO, Patsias G, Polytarno VA.Trans-urethral polytetrafluraethylene in female patients with urinary incontinence. *J Urol* 1993; **150**: 856–858.

30. Ferro MA, Smith JH, Smith PJ. Peri-urethral granuloma: unusual complication of Teflon peri-urethral injection. *Urol* 1988; **31**: 422–423.

31. Kligman AM, Armstrong RC. Histological response to intra-dermal zyderm and zyplasy (gluteraldehyde cross-linked) collagen in humans. *J of Dermat Surg Oncol* 1986; **12**: 351–357.

32. Monga AK, Robinson D, Stanton SL. Peri-urethral collagen injections for genuine stress incontinence: a two year follow-up. *Br J Urol* 1995; **76**: 156–160.

33. Homer Y, Kawabe K, Kageyamas *et al.* Injection of gluteraldehyde cross-linked collagen for urinary incontinence. Two year efficacy by self-assessment. *Int J Urol* 1996; **3**: 124–127.

34. Faerber GJ. Endoscopic collagen injection therapy in elderly women with type one stress urinary incontinence. *J Urol;* 1996: **155**: 512–514.

35. Eckford SD, Abrams P. Para-urethral collagen implantation for female stress incontinence. *Br J Urol* 1991; **68**: 586–589.

36. Khullar V, Cardozo LD, Abbott D, Anders K. GAX collagen in the treatment of urinary incontinence in elderly women: a two year follow-up. *Br J Obstet & Gynaecol* 1997; **104**: 96–99.

37. Macroplastique Implants Technical Overview. Maastricht, The Netherlands: Uroplasty BV, 1995.

38. Adile B *et al.* Macroplastique implant for the treatment of type three urinary stress incontinence: one year follow-up. Presented at the Int Urogync. Assoc Meeting: Kuala Lumpur, Malaysia 1995.

39. Fischer M, Szabo N, Durer A. Endoscopic implantation of collagen or microparticulate silicone for the treatment of female urinary incontinence. Presented at the ICS Meeting, Australia 1995.

40. Pycha A, Klinger C, Haitel A, Heinz-Peer G *et al.* Implantable microballoons: An attractive alternative in the management of intrinsic sphincter deficiency. *Eur Urol* 1998; **3**: 469–475.

41. Monga AK, Robinson D, Stanton SL. Peri-urethral collagen injections for genuine stress incontinence: a two year follow-up. *Br J Urol* 1995; **76**: 156–160.

42. Appel RA. Collagen injection therapy for urinary incontinence. *Urol Clin North Am* 1994; **21**: 177–182.

43. Vancaillie TG, Schuessler W. Laparoscopic bladderneck suspension. *J Laparoendoscopic Surg* 1991; **3**: 169–173.

44. Virtanen HS *et al.* Ureteral injuries in conjunction with Burch Colposuspension. *Int Urogynecol J* 1995; **6**: 114–118.

45. Aslan P, Woo H. Ureteric injury following laparoscopic colposuspension. *Br J Obstet Gynae* 1997; **104**: 266–268.

46. Deitz HP, Wilson PD, Samalia KP, Walton J, Fentuman G. Ureteric injury following laparoscopic colposuspension. Letter *Br J Obstet Gynaecol* 1997; **10**: 1217.

47. Kohl N. Jacobs PA, Sze EH, Roat TW, Karram MM. Open compared with laparoscopic colposuspension. A cost analysis. *Obstet Gynaecol* 1997; **90**: 411–415.

48. Lyons TL, Winner WK. Clinical outcomes with laparoscopic and open Burch procedures for urinary stress incontinence. *J Am Assoc Gynaecol Laparosc* 1995; **2**: 193–198.

49. Burton G. A three year prospective randomisedurodynamic study comparing open and laparoscopic colposuspension. *Neuro Urol Urodynam* 1997; **16**: 353–354.

49A. Su T, Wang K, Hsu C, Wei H, Hong B. Prospective comparison of laparoscopic and traditional colposuspensions in the treatment of Genuine Stress incontinence. *Acta Obstet Gynecol Scand* 1997; **76**: 576–582.

50. Lobel RW, Sand PK. Long-term results of laparoscopic Burch colposuspension. *Neuro Urol Urodynam* 1996; **15**: 398–399.

51. Liu CY. Laparoscopic retropubic colposuspension (Burch procedure). *J Repro Med* 1993; **38**: 526–530.

52. Smith ARB, Stanton SL. *Br J Obstet Gynaecol* 1998; **105**: 383–384.

53. Gittes RF, Loughlin KR. No incision pubovaginal suspension for stress incontinence. *J Urol* 1987; **138**: 568–570.

54. Mills R, Persad R, Handley-Asken M. Long term follow up of the Stamey operation for stress incontinence of urine. *Br J Urol* 1996; **77**: 86–88.

55. O'Sullivan DC, Chilton CP, Munson KW. Should Stamey colposuspension be our primary surgery for stress incontinence. *Br J Urol* 1995; **75**: 457–460.

56. Kevelighan E, Aagaard J, Jarvis GJ. The Stamey endoscopic bladder neck suspension – a 10 year follow up. ICS Annual meeting 1997.

57. Appell RA, Rackley RR, Dmochowski RR. Vesica percutaneous bladder neck stabiliation. *J Endourol* 1996; **10**: 221–225.

58. Raz S. Modified bladder neck suspension for female stress incontinence. *Urology* 1981; **17**: 82–84.

59. Pereyra AJ. A simplified surgical procedure for the correction of stress incontinence in women. *West J Surg* 1959; **67**: 223–226.

60. Schultheiss D, Hofner K, Oelke M, Grunewald V *et al.* Percutaneous bladder neck suspension with bone anchors: an improvement in the therapy of Female stress urinary incontinence. *Neurourol Urodyn* 1998; **17**: 457–458.

61. Norris JP, Breslin DS, Staskin DR. Use of synthetic material in sling surgery: a minimally invasive approach. *J Endourol* 1996; **10**: 227–230.

62. Petros P, Ulmsten U. An integral theory on female urinary incontinence. Experimental and clinical considerations. *Acta Obstet Gynecol Scand* 1990; **69** (suppl): 153.

63. Petros P, Ulmsten U. An integral theory and its method for the diagnosis and management of female urinary incontinence. *Scand J Urol Nephrol* 1993; **151**: 1–93.

64. DeLancey JO. The structural support of the urethra as it relates to Stress Urinary incontinence: the hammock hypothesis. *Obstet Gynecol* 1994; **170**: 1713–1723.

65. Petros P, Ulmsten U. Intravaginal slingplasty. An ambulatory surgical proceedure for treatment of female urinary stress incontinence. *Scand J Urol Nephrol* 1995; **29**: 75–82.

66. Ulmsten U, Henriksson L, Johnson P, Varhos G. An ambulatory surgical procedure under local anaesthesia for treatment of female urinary incontinence. *Int Urogynecol J* 1996; **7**: 81–86.

67. Riva D *et al.* Tension free vaginal tape for the therapy of SUI: early results and urodynamic analysis. *Neurourol Urodyn* 1998; **17**: 351–352.

68. Ross JW. Multichannel urodynamic evaluation of laparoscopic Burch colposuspension for GSI. *Obstet Gynecol* 1998; **9**: 55–59.

5

Vaginal Surgery

What can't we do?

S. S. Sheth

"Surgery is the first and highest division of the healing art, pure in itself, perpetual in its applicability and a worthy product of heaven."
- Susruta -

Introduction

Minimal access surgery has revolutionised our treatments for women, but perhaps one of the unexpected benefits of the introduction of these techniques has been the resurgence of interest in vaginal hysterectomy (VH), a route which increasing numbers of gynaecologists now feel also deserves the title of minimal access. There is an adage that "a surgeon's best teachers are his patients" which has been very true for this author. This chapter begins by relating some experiences with patients, to demonstrate how these experiences can alter one's practice.

The first case was a 45-year-old woman,[1] who had had an eventful obstetric history, including a ruptured uterus, previous caesarean sections and repair of an incisional hernia. She complained of severe menorrhagia, resistant to medical treatment, and was referred to the author as a last resort, after being advised by others that she would require an abdominal hysterectomy. She desperately wanted to avoid abdominal surgery, even after the risks of attempting a vaginal hysterectomy were explained to her. A compromise was reached: a vaginal hysterectomy would be performed if pelvic findings under anaesthesia permitted. Somewhat surprisingly, there were only a few adhesions to the uterus, and the hysterectomy was completed within 50 mins.

Encouraged by the experience, a vaginal hysterectomy was performed on another patient with traditional contraindications to the vaginal route. This patient had prior history of 2 previous caesarean sections, and a bowel resection with an anastomosis for intestinal tuberculosis. As a precaution, a general surgeon was instructed to be on standby in case of inadvertent damage to the bowel during surgery, but the surgery was in fact completed safely via the vaginal route without laparoscopic assistance or evaluation. The lesson to be learnt from these two cases, is that rather than automatically excluding the vaginal route for a patient because of an apparent "textbook" contraindication, it may often be of benefit to assess the clinical findings under anaesthesia with an open mind, utilising laparoscopy for evaluation if required, and then to proceed with a tentative/trial vaginal hysterectomy. The impetus to extend the advantages of the vaginal route, and to explore its limits, thus came from hands-on experience with patients, many of whom were desperate to avoid having another abdominal incision. One should not just say "no" without at least trying – much is often possible, if one keeps an open mind and tries a little harder!

Reasons for the vaginal route

The vaginal approach has always been the hallmark of the gynaecological surgeon. After all, what is the difference between a gynaecological surgeon who does an abdominal hysterectomy, and a general surgeon, who can remove the uterus through the abdomen just as competently? Historically, the reason gynaecological surgery became a speciality in its own right was its extensive use of the vaginal route. In 1939, the French surgeon Doyen[2] asserted that one merited the label of a gynaecologist only after one had successfully executed a vaginal hysterectomy.

Table 5.1 shows the author's personal series of 5344 vaginal hysterectomies, 4812 (90%) were performed in the absence of prolapse. The author's personal philosophy is that hysterectomy by the vaginal route should be practised in all cases where there is an indication for hysterectomy and no contraindication to the vaginal route. In the author's practice, vaginal hysterectomies constitute 82% of all hysterectomies; the remainder are abdominal hysterectomies, (**Table 5.2**), but unfortunately this is not true in many parts of the world.[3–5]

Table 5.1 Indications for vaginal hysterectomy in 5344 patients

	Indications	Associated conditions
Dysfunction uterine bleeding/adenomyosis	3012	
Uterine fibroids	1480	
Nullipara		368
Severe mental handicap	112	
Previous abdominal surgery		928
Previous vaginal surgery		84
Cervical polp/fibroid	32	
Carcinoma in situ of the cervix	14	
Endometrial cancer	10	
High risk patients		92
Uterine prolapse	532	
Benign adnexal pathology	152	
Total	5344	1472

Table 5.2 Routes taken for hysterectomy

	VH%	AH%
United States	25	75
RCOG (UK)	31	69
Australia (AUS)	19	81
Brown -Frazer (AUS)	79 (276)	21 (73)
Summit (USA)	65	35
Sheth (INDIA)	82 (5334)	18 (1173)

Vaginal surgery allows the surgeon to operate by the least invasive route of all, utilising an anatomical orifice, without having to make any additional openings. Unfortunately, in the absence of any push to develop vaginal surgery until the advent of laparoscopically assisted vaginal hysterectomy (LAVH), most of these skills were disappearing through underuse. Dicker's audit,[6] although published at a time when antibiotic and thromboembolic prophylaxis were not routinely practised, clearly illustrated the intrinsic benefits of the vaginal versus the abdominal approach for hysterectomy. Perhaps, if vaginal surgery was marketed to patients as "scarless" or "minimal access" surgery, it would become much more popular in today's consumer-driven society.

Why is there a reluctance for vaginal surgery?

The question then arises as to why some gynaecologists have become so reluctant to use the vaginal route, in spite of its many advantages? Possible reasons include:

- inadequate residency training, perhaps because teachers/seniors are not comfortable with the vaginal route, this becomes a tradition with a vicious circle;
- inappropriate concern about difficulties with adequate access, often secondary to operator inexperience;
- difficulty in the intraoperative visualisation of

the surgical field and the need to learn new anatomical landmarks.

In contrast, abdominal surgery offers a comfortable, familiar route, and involves little additional learning difficulties. The loss of vaginal surgical skills simply means that patients will be deprived of the benefits which this route offers. This represents a clear gap in our ability to offer women best surgical practice. Gynaecological surgeons have a responsibility both to patients and trainees to promote vaginal hysterectomy. There is an onus on all practising gynaecologists, particularly those working in teaching hospitals, to provide trainees with appropriate, comprehensive training, including vaginal surgery. Residents in training need to see all surgical options in daily practice so that they can select what suits them and hone their skills under close supervision.

One of the main benefits of the vaginal route is that it is universally applicable, since the surgeon needs only standard instruments and sutures to perform vaginal surgery. Unlike conventional "minimally invasive" surgery, it does not need expensive technology, and the equipment is not difficult to maintain. For the 80% of the world's female population who live in the developing world, a skilled vaginal surgeon with basic surgical equipment represents the most effective and economical use of female health care resources.

Resurgence

Data from the UK[7] shows that the proportion of vaginal hysterectomies has doubled in last 5 years to 31% from 16.5%. Similarly in Texas, USA, after introduction of LAVH, the rate of vaginal hysterectomy rose from 27.7% in 1990 to 53.2% in 1996.[8] It is the author's prediction that there will be a much greater renaissance of interest in vaginal surgery in the near future. There are many reasons for this.

- In financial terms, vaginal surgery is more cost effective. Third party payers, such as insurance companies will "encourage" gynaecologists to perform surgery through the vaginal route.
- Patients prefer the vaginal route, and in a consumer-driven healthcare service will opt for experienced vaginal surgeons.
- Lastly, vaginal surgery is likely to become more fashionable, particularly in the wake of "minimal access" surgery.

A good gynaecological surgeon should be able to operate as comfortably in the pelvis through the vagina as a general surgeon using the abdomen.

Surgical operations on the pelvis can be classified as those which can be done through the vagina and those which cannot (for example, microsurgical tuboplasty). However, a better way of looking at it would be to divide operations into those which one should perform through the vagina and those which one should not.

From a practical viewpoint, patients can be divided into three groups.

1. Those in which surgery via the vaginal route should be the first choice;
2. those in which surgery via the vaginal route is technically feasible, but needs more inclination and effort; and
3. those in which surgery can challenge an experienced surgeon's mettle.

Hysterectomy: which route?

Hysterectomy is the most commonly performed major gynaecological operation, and this is the area where most controversy arises. The crux of the question for any particular case is going to be, "by which route should this hysterectomy be performed?" Unfortunately, some gynaecologists have the attitude that all hysterectomies should be abdominal, unless the patient has a uterovaginal prolapse. An increasing number of gynaecologists, however, take a diametrically opposite viewpoint and suggest that all hysterectomies should be vaginal unless otherwise indicated. This is amply shown by the surge in the incidence of VH and the flourishing of workshops in which to learn vaginal hysterectomy techniques. On balance, it is the author's opinion that the order of choice of hysterectomy route should be (i) vaginal, (ii) vaginal with laparoscopic assistance and (iii) abdominal, the outcome of studies such as EVALUATE in the UK being awaited with interest.

One of the paradoxes of the introduction of new surgical techniques such as LAVH is that, for all their novelty, for a good surgical result, the procedure depends to a large extent on how comfortable the individual surgeon is operating vaginally. Hence the new generation of gynaecologists are fortunately being encouraged to become competent in this area. Total laparoscopic hysterectomy is not considered in this chapter as this procedure is perhaps still within the realm of a few specialists and is still largely experimental.

Table 5.3 shows that for most of the indications for hysterectomy, the route should ideally be vaginal. The author's personal view is that the remaining 20–25% of cases, (and never more than 30%), usually require LAVH or abdominal hysterectomy. This should be the target of all gynaecologists.

The vast majority of hysterectomies are performed for uteri whose size is less than 12 weeks – for patients with DUB, adenomyosis and small fibroids. If all or most of these could be performed using the vaginal route, patients would be much better served and the current global data on hysterectomy would change radically. The first step towards achieving a change of this magnitude requires a simple change amongst the entire body of gynaecologists; namely that all hysterectomies should be vaginal unless otherwise indicated.

An examination under anaesthesia (EUA), prior to the start of surgery can provide invaluable information, particularly with regard to uterine descent and mobility, uterine size and adnexal pathology.[9] The most useful time to do the EUA is when investigating the patient for her symptoms (e.g. abnormal uterine bleeding and hysteroscopy/dilatation and currettage). The vital role of an EUA in deciding the hysterectomy route is shown in a flow-chart format **(Table 5.4)**.

Pre-operative ultrasound (U/S) can provide useful clinical information that may be difficult to acquire, especially in the obese patient, by allowing a detailed evaluation of the adnexa and an accurate

Table 5.3 Choice of hysterectomy – indications/associated situations

Conditions/situations	Vaginal	Tentative vaginal	LAVH	ABD
Dysfunctional uterine bleeding	●			
Adenomyosis	●			
Fibroid(s): uterus up to 12 weeks size	●			
Fibroids: uterus up to 16–18 weeks size		■	●	❍
Fibroids: uterus more than 16–18 weeks size				●
Endometrial hyperplasia	●			
Poly: cervical/ endometrial	●			
Nulliparity	●	❍		
Severe mental handicap	●			
Cervical intraepithelial neoplasia	●			
Endometrial malignancy	❍		■	●
Benign adnexal pathology		❍	■	●

● First Choice ■ First Alternative ❍ Second Alternative

Table 5.4

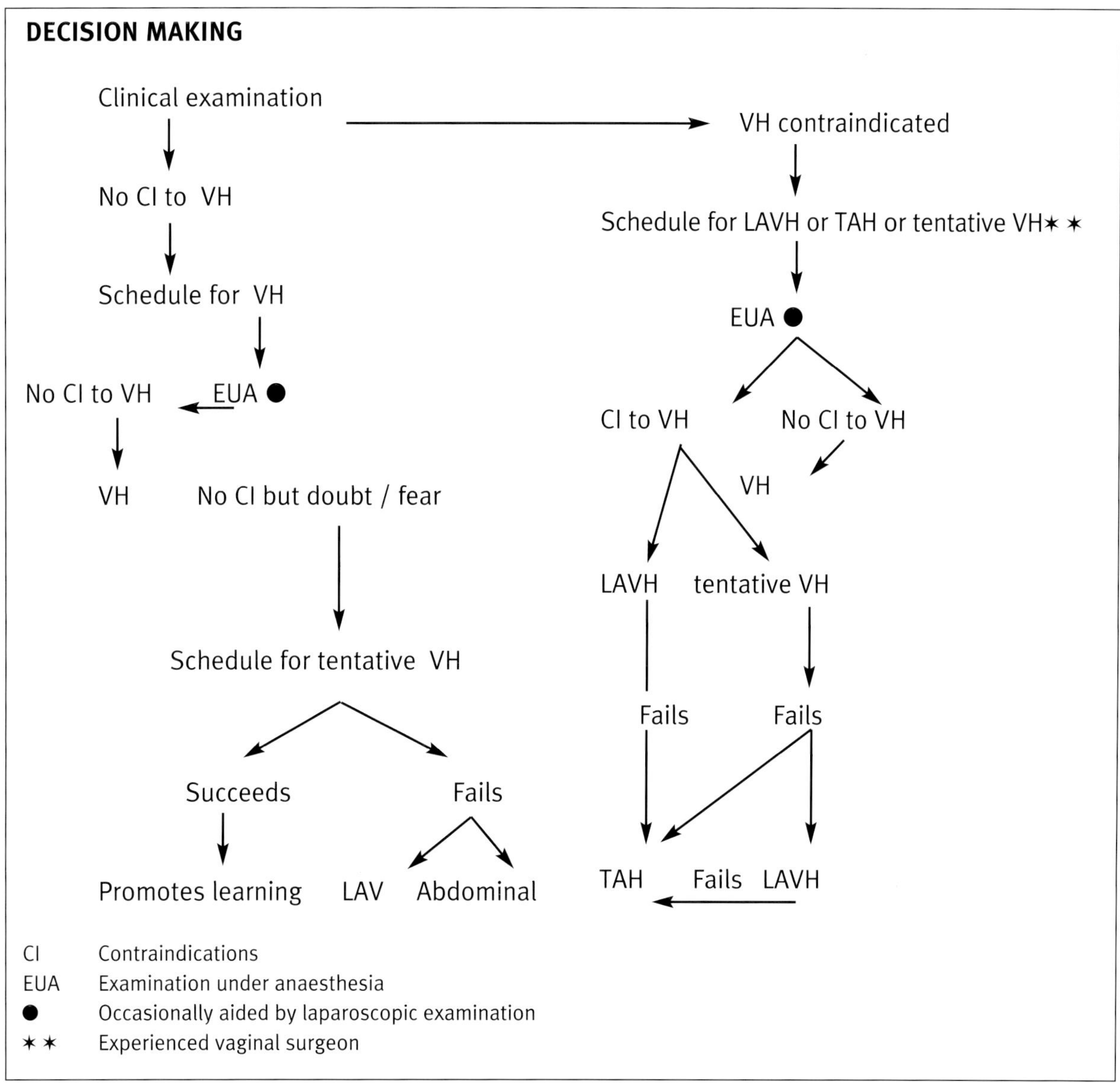

estimation of the uterine size. The normal uterine volume is approximately 80 ml. As shown in **Table 5.5**, if the uterine volume is less than 100 ml, the average gynaecologist should be able to attempt and perform a vaginal hysterectomy in most cases without difficulty. If the volume is between 100–200 ml, a vaginal hysterectomy can still be performed by an experienced surgeon. If the uterine volume is more than 200 ml, then a vaginal hysterectomy may still be technically feasible, but is best performed by a gynaecologist who has considerable expertise. Laparoscopic assistance, or the abdominal route should be considered where the uterine volume is more than 400 ml or the uterine size is greater than a 16 week pregnancy. However, in vaginal surgery there are few absolutes, the author has performed VH without laparoscopic assistance on uteri with volumes of 780 and 960 ml but also failed on uteri between 500–600 ml on three occasions.

Table 5.5

Uterine volume (ml) and VH	
100 or less	Easy: average gynaecologist should be able to do it
101–200	Interested gynaecologist should be able to do it easily
201–400 or more	Best performed by gynaecologists with expertise
300–350 or more	Needs debulking
401–500	Schedule as tentative or trial VH. Needs debulking. Consider availability of LAVH and/or abdominal hysterectomy

"Minimal access" gynaecological surgery has also introduced the use of tissue morcellators into gynaecolgical surgery. Kovac,[10] a dedicated vaginal surgeon, has accomplished a difficult VH by volume reduction using a tissue morcellator for a uterus weighing 163 g. A significant number of larger uteri have been subjected to morcellation in order to expedite their removal and this was reported in a case series (Pelosi, 1997).[11]

Favourable factors for a vaginal hysterectomy are:-

- mobile uterus with normal dimensions
- large pelvis to allow manoeuvrability
- single, large accessible fibroid
- experience
- counselling for a "tentative" VH.

The "tentative" VH or trial of vaginal route for hysterectomy

In the absence of obvious contraindications, but with doubt concerning the route of hysterectomy, gynaecologists should consider scheduling patients for a tentative VH, a situation analogous to obstetricians performing a trial of forceps. For an appropriately consented patient, one can always switch to the abdominal route if needed, which is paradoxically much easier now as most of the pelvic floor supports have been divided. A "trial" of the vaginal route is recommended at any level of experience, as there will always be cases were it is felt that a vaginal hysterectomy is potentially difficult and may be contraindicated, but may conceivably succeed if attempted. Meanwhile, everything should be kept in readiness to switch over to the abdominal route, intraoperatively, if this becomes necessary.

Nullipara

What if the patient is nulliparous or has good pelvic floor support? This is a common pretext for gynaecologists to choose the abdominal route, but it really represents no more than a mental block towards the vaginal route rather than a surgical contraindication. Uterine descent is usually evident in the multiparous women; however, this may not be manifest in the nulliparous patient. Therefore, most surgeons consider nulliparity as a precondition for abdominal hysterectomy. But even in the nulliparous patient, there is often sufficient uterine descent to facilitate a vaginal hysterectomy if the uterus is freely mobile, less than 12 weeks in size and without associated adnexal pathology. Before the advent of LAVH, 90% of hysterectomies in the nulliparous were undertaken using the abdominal route![12] Prolapse is not required in order to perform a VH. The author has performed 332 vaginal hysterectomies in the absence of any prolapse in nulliparous women, with pathology such as fibroids, adenomyosis and DUB. This case series also includes 112 virgins with severe mental handicap[13] Every uterus has a physiological descent[9] and under general anaesthesia this is increased. This illustrates the importance of an adequate examination under anaesthesia. It is possible to start the hysterectomy and as the pelvic supports are progressively divided, the uterus can usually be easily mobilised.

What if anterior adhesions are anticipated?

Kovac[14] suggests using LAVH to gain safer entry through a scarred anterior cul-de-sac. The author recommends creating a surgical window using the uterocervical broad ligament space[15] shown in **Figure 5.1** to enable the competent gynaecologist more vaginal access to the vesico-uterine peritoneum and depend less on LAVH.

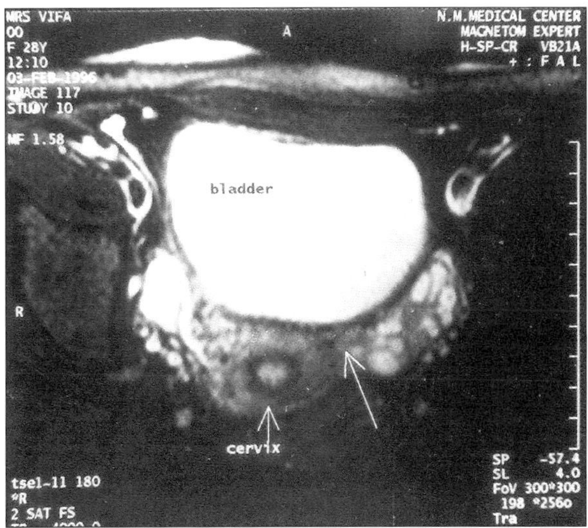

Figure 5.1 Surgical window demonstrated on MRI studies.

Monaghan[16] finds this space increasingly of interest in vaginal surgery. On average, 20% of women undergoing VH have a history of previous abdomino-pelvic surgery[12] and with the increase in Caesarean sections, familiarity with this surgical window will reduce the dependance on LAVH, as well as decreasing the risk of bladder trauma. **Table 5.6** gives a guide to selection of the type of hysterectomy where there is a history of abdomino-pelvic surgery. However, as always, operator experience and inclination will be the deciding factors.

Surgical technique

What is required is the ability to gain access to both pouches and have sufficient experience and familiarity with the key anatomical "landmarks." It is not necessary to open the peritoneum at the beginning of the operation, providing that the bladder and rectum are adequately protected. It is also worth learning the clampless technique[17] for performing a VH, since this is particularly useful when space is at a premium. Using specially designed fibreoptic illuminated retractors[18] can also help.

The techniques for coring or debulking uteri in order to remove a large uterus vaginally are often scorned as being 'surgical gymnastics.' However, there are surgical steps which allow the surgeon to remove bulky uteri through the vagina. It is the author's opinion that a uterine size of 14 to 16 weeks gestation should not be a limiting factor if this equipment is available. Debulking is usually performed when no further uterine descent is possible and all the lateral accessible tissues have been cut around the enlarged uterus. Despite this, often in these cases, the top of the uterine fundus still cannot be reached by the surgeon's fingers passed either behind or in front of the uterus, due to the uterine size.

Prophylactic oophorectomy

In stark contrast, prophylactic oophorectomy is performed in only 10% of all VH compared with more than 60% of abdominal hysterectomies.[19] Davies *et al* [20] were able to perform oophorectomy successfully in 39 out of 40 cases scheduled for VH and bilateral salpingo-oophorectomy, without laparoscopic assistance. The author's published series of 740 VH had a 95% success rate of oophorectomy[21] and this is now 96.8%, (of 1224 women undergoing VH, 1186 had a successful oophorectomy or salpingo-oophorectomy). For successful oophorectomy at VH, the use of specific techniques[22] and instruments helps to simplify the procedure. These include:

1. clamping and cutting the round ligaments separately;
2. using a special ovarian clamp (**Figures 5.2 & 5.3**);

Table 5.6 Routine surgery on the genital organs in the past

	Routine VH	Needs extra care at VH	tentative VH	LAVH	TAH
ABDOMINAL					
UTERINE					
Previous caesarean	●				
Myomectomy	●				
Caesarean + myomectomy	●				
Hysterectomy	●				
Metroplasty	●				
Sling operation			❍	●	
Ventrofixation			❍	●	❍
TUBES AND OVARIES					
Tubal sterilisation	●				
Salpingectomy	●				
Tubal microsurgery	●				
Ovarian cystectomy	●				
Oophorectomy	●				
Salpingo-oophorectomy	●				
VAGINAL					
CERVIX					
Internal os tightening	●				
Amputation					●
Conisation		●			
Anterior colporrhaphy		●			
Posterior colpoperineorrhaphy	●				
Colpotomy-tubal sterilisation		●			
Fothergill's					●
Shirodkar's		●			
Bartholin's abscess	●				
SURGERY ON EXTRA-GENITAL ORGANS					
BLADDER					
VVF repair					●
Cystotomy					●
Bladder neck repair		●			
RECTUM					
RVF repair\abscess		●			❍
Piles	●				
ABDOMINAL CONTENTS					
Appendicectomy	●				
Intestinal	●				
Cholecystectomy	●				

● First Choice
❍ Second Choice

3. better exposure; and
4. using speculum and bladder retractors with incorporated fibreoptic light sources (**Figure 5.4**).

Where should we now define the boundaries of vaginal surgery? This is not easy, and is always fluid, depending upon the patient's problem and the surgeon's skills. Thus, the traditional, standard text book approach of removing a dermoid cyst would be a laparotomy. In the current climate, laparoscopic removal seems to be the vogue. In fact, Reich[23] managed an ovarian dermoid cyst laparoscopically, but then removed the cyst wall via a posterior colpotomy. However, the author would counter that if the dermoid cyst is being removed through a colpo-

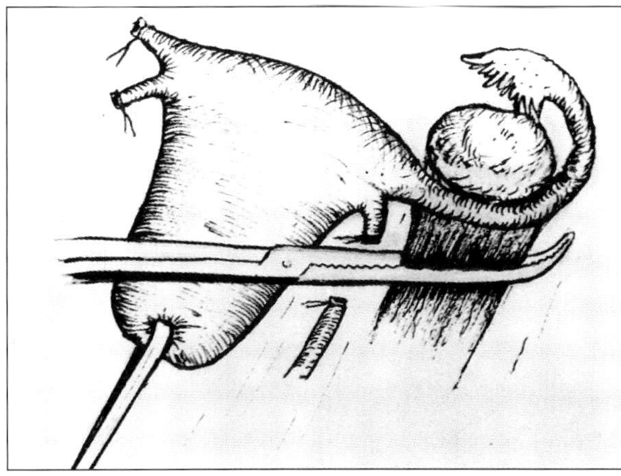

Figure 5.2 Ovarian clamp on infundibulo-pelvic ligament after round ligament is cut separately.

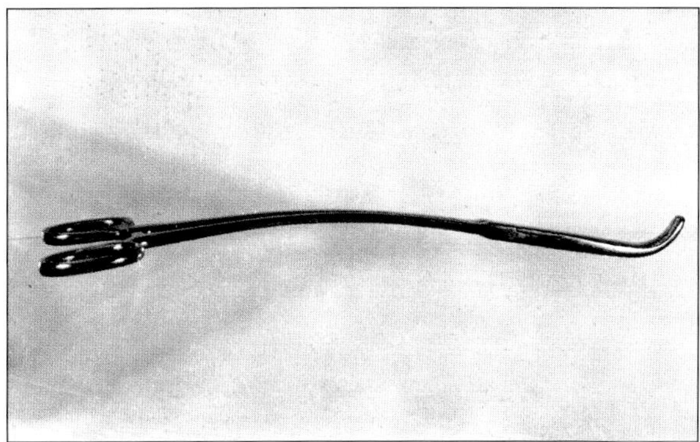

Figure 5.3 Ovarian clamp with curve designed to accommodate ovary or infundibulo-pelvic ligament.

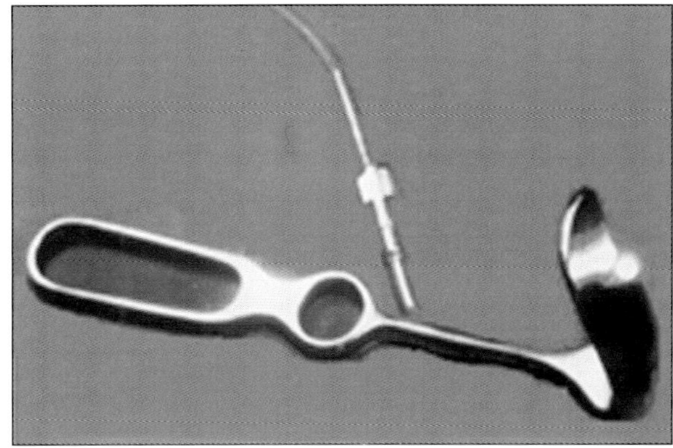

Figure 5.4: Bladder retractor with fibre-optic light facility.

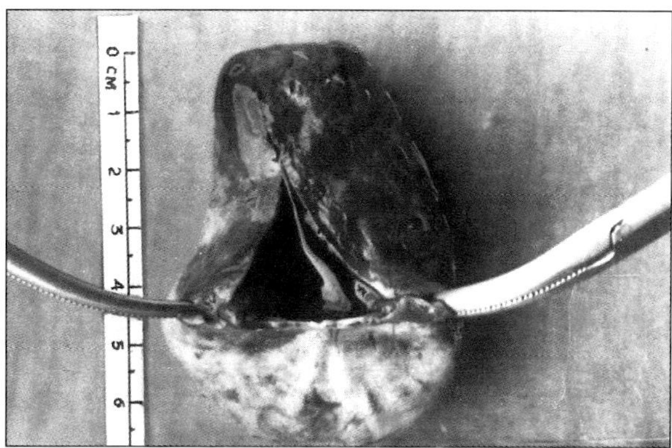

Figure 5.5 Dermoid cyst removed via posterior colpotomy, 11 x 7cms preoperatively.

tomy incision, then why not remove the entire dermoid through the vaginal route? Thus, the vaginal route should be strongly considered for removing a single dermoid cyst which can be initially drained to debulk if necessary, particularly in multiparous women (**Figure 5.5**).

The same logic applies to all benign ovarian cysts. In fact, size should never be a limiting factor, since this can always be reduced. If a colpotomy incision is to be made, then laparoscopic punctures should be avoided, other than one for pelvic evaluation if this is felt to be necessary. When all factors favour the exclusion of malignancy and the necessary preoperative counselling has been given, the vaginal route can be attempted in most parous women. It is essential that the cyst is freely mobile and close to the Pouch of Douglas. The author has managed 22 cases of ovarian cysts, via a posterior colpotomy incision without laparoscopic operative assistance and has only resorted to laparoscopic evaluation in eight cases. There is some variation on this principle in the literature: Parkar[24] recommends the laparoscopic removal of clinically benign ovarian cysts, and Teng[25] cautions that before a transvaginal approach, a laparoscopy is necessary. In the author's practice, when adnexal pathology has been encountered performing a VH (whether anticipated or unexpected) this can invariably be tackled without laparoscopic assistance or opening the abdomen.

Table 5.7 Details of ovarian cyst

	At hysterectomy	With hysterectomy
Dermoid.....	4	10
Pseudomucinous.....	3	–
Simple serous.....	16	8
Simple.....	6	–
Follicular.....	4	–
Endometrial....	45	4
	78	22

The role of LAVH?

There is little doubt that the 1980s will be remembered as the era of minimally invasive surgery. Some of our colleagues have taken this concept to extremes especially when attention was turned towards the uterus. Since it was technically very difficult to remove the entire uterus through the tiny laparoscopic incisions, the operation of laparoscopically assisted vaginal hysterectomy (LAVH) was developed.[26] The question still remains however – how is this a significant improvement on the old fashioned simple vaginal hysterectomy? The results of the UK EVALUATE study are awaited with interest.

Simple logic dictates that surgical trauma vaginally *and* abdominally cannot be better than trauma confined to the vagina. LAVH seems to provide additional "assistance" in the form of increased profits to the instrument manufacturers and to surgeons who can charge separately for the individual components of the operation.[27]

Another interesting phenomenon has been the glut of recent papers claiming that laparoscopic subtotal hysterectomy is better for the patient than a conventional total hysterectomy. This appears to the author to be an ingenious way of converting the disadvantage of having to conserve the cervix into an apparent advantage.[27] Subtotal hysterectomy, if required, can be done vaginally with adequate skill and experience, to minimise access and morbidity. As Morrow[28] rightly questions, "is the conventional wisdom that teaches that the cervix be removed with the uterus to be discarded for technology, cost savings and reduced recovery time?"

On other hand LAVH has a definite role when VH is not possible unless the contraindications can be overcome by using a laparoscope. For example, LAVH to facilitate adhesiolysis or excision of an endometrial cyst, can make a VH possible. Paradoxically, it is the increasing popularity of LAVH which has convinced many more surgeons to learn and perform VH. The author was invited to watch an operation recently in the Far East, where the patient was scheduled for a LAVH, since she had a pre-operative diagnosis of endometriosis. However, EUA suggested that the uterus was freely mobile, and that the vaginal route would be feasible. However, the surgeon was diffident and the laparoscope was inserted. This confirmed the EUA findings that there were no adhesions or adnexal masses. Instead of proceeding with LAVH, he switched to VH instead and completed the surgery uneventfully. The intra-operative laparoscopy provided the necessary confidence to proceed as described. It is initially easier to perform a VH after laparoscopy, with the scope providing guidance for the vaginal surgeon. However, as confidence grows, surgeons usually become less dependent on the laparoscope.

Transcervical resection of the endometrium (TCRE)

What about the role of the other popular operations to manage abnormal uterine bleeding – namely, transcervical resection of the endometrium? TCRE was introduced with a lot of fanfare as a potentially superior alternative to hysterectomy and it soon become the vogue. Every doctor wanted to be the "first" to do this surgery – and this was then followed by competition. However, it is only now that potential problems with TCRE are becoming evident. Cases of cryptic endometrial cancer after endometrial ablation are already being reported.[29] An even bigger problem in the future may be the number of patients who present with cancer of the cervix after TCRE, which might have been prevented if they had undergone a conventional hysterectomy. This is going to be more common in developing countries, where few women have a chance to get 'Pap' smear performed.

There are times when an operator is understandably reluctant to advise hysterectomy and is looking for a treatment which can provide symptomatic relief. The introduction of the levo-norgestrol intra-uterine system (Mirena™) may provide an effective treatment for these women.

Excuses for not performing VH

In summary, many gynaecologists will convince their patients (and themselves) that the abdominal route is preferable for one of the following reasons.[12]

- The patient is nulliparous.
- There is no uterine descent.
- The uterus is large.
- There may be adnexal adhesions or endometriosis.
- There is an adnexal mass.
- There is a fibroid in the uterus.
- The patient needs an oophorectomy.
- Inspection of the abdominal organs, particularly the appendix, is essential.

Actually, none of these are contra-indications to the vaginal route – they either act as a mental block or they are simply ways of justifying the abdominal route by gynaecologists who may lack the necessary vaginal surgical skills.

In these progressive days of minimally invasive surgery, it is mandatory for every gynaecologist to think of the vaginal route and use it in the best interests of our patients. When performing pelvic surgery, this should be the first choice and when dealing with abdominal or abdomino-pelvic surgery, the vaginal route can also be considered. The following situations should be considered as potential areas where a vaginal route can be used.

(1) Tubal sterilisation via posterior colpotomy
This can be combined as part of any operation where the vaginal route is indicated, for example, excision of benign ovarian cysts through a posterior colpotomy or with an anterior or posterior colporrhaphy (or Kelly's repair) for genuine urinary stress incontinence. The author has also used this method as a combined procedure for spontaneous or induced abortion as a family planning method.[30]

(2) Oophorectomy via the Pouch of Douglas
In women with metastatic carcinoma of breast, if oophorectomy is recommended,[31] despite tamoxifen, oophorectomy via a posterior colpotomy will spare an abdominal incision.

(3) Benign ovarian cyst via a posterior colpotomy (vide supra).

(4) Myomectomy
A single low-placed, posterior wall fibroid, either cervical or low in the uterine corpus, almost invites myomectomy via a posterior colpotomy. Although other gynaecologists have removed a greater number of fibroids by laparoscopically assisted vaginal myomectomy (LAVM), the author has removed fibroids of between 3–8 cm in diameter from four patients via a posterior colpotomy without laparoscopic assistance.

(5) Removal of cervical stump
In view of the increasing number of subtotal hysterectomies, the number of cervical stumps requiring resection will rise. This is of increased importance in those geographical areas where there is no cervical screening programme. Careful dissection to separate the bladder and rectum with bisection of the cervix guides the excision as achieved in five cases by the author with advantages of minimal access.

(6) Vaginal pneumoperitoneum
Although the transabdominal route is the most widely accepted for creating a pneumoperitoneum,

there are occasions, for example, in scarred abdomens or morbidly obese patients, when one can resort to this route to enable laparoscopy to take place. The author has used this on more than 210 occasions, including 24 at mass sterilisation camps.[32,33]

(7) Tapping of ascites

Similarly, scarred abdomens or morbidly obese patients pose a risk for abdominal paracentesis, and the author reports that the vaginal route allows the procedure to be undertaken more quickly, and in theory, more safely even with mild/minimal ascites. Simultaneous diagnostic laparoscopy can also be performed.[34]

(8) Intra-uterine contraceptive device (IUCD) retrieval via a posterior colpotomy

This can occasionally be indicated when facilities for laparoscopy are unavailable, or laparoscopy is unable to extricate an IUCD lodged in the omentum. Laparoscopic-guided vaginal retrieval should have priority over opening the abdomen as reported in five cases by the author.[35]

Unfortunately, the problem of under-utilisation of the vaginal route is not restricted to hysterectomies alone. Many patients with simple ovarian cysts could have their cysts removed through a small posterior colpotomy incision, rather than have their abdomen scarred by the multiple punctures required for laparoscopic access.

Fortunately, there does seem to be a resurgence of interest in exploring the vaginal route in other areas. Many urologists now realise that their results for the surgical correction of urinary stress incontinence may be improved through the use of the vaginal route.

Gynaecological oncologists are also rediscovering Schauta's radical vaginal hysterectomy[36] for the treatment of selected cases of cervical cancer (FIGO stage I and II), especially when combined

VAGINAL SURGERY: WHAT CAN WE DO?

- VH:
  1. If hysterectomy indicated and no CI to VH
  2. Advanced vaginal surgery: debulking, enucleation, morcellation, bisection, coring and schauta's radical hysterectomy
- Oophorectomy or salpingo-oophorectomy at vaginalhysterectomy

• Benign ovarian cyst	Via posterior colpotomy
• Oophorectomy for breast CA	Via posterior colpotomy
• Tubal sterilisation	Via posterior colpotomy
• IUCD retrieval	Via posterior colpotomy + laparoscopic assistance
• Myomectomy	Via posterior colpotomy
• Creating pneumoperitoneum	Via posterior colpopuncture
• Tapping of ascites	Via posterior colpopuncture
• Excision of cervical stump	Vaginal

with a laparoscopic pelvic lymphadenectomy, since it is possible to remove much more of the parametrium, paracervical tissues and a larger vaginal cuff through the vaginal route. This is more inviting and less morbid than radical abdominal surgery.

The real tragedy of vaginal surgery – and vaginal surgeons – has been a lack of progress, in terms of new techniques, innovations or operations over the last 50 years. The question is why – especially when other surgical fields have made dramatic advances, using new technology such as computers, lasers, sonography, endoscopes and fibreoptics. For example, the author uses fibreoptic retractors and speculums to improve the illumination of the surgical field during vaginal surgery. Similarly, the use of morcellators, originally designed to debulk a large uterus to assist in LAVH, have a place in the armamenterium of the experienced vaginal surgeon. Why not use head-mounted cameras to teach residents vaginal surgery? These suggestions are based on the personal experience of the author.

Have we accomplished everything we can through the vaginal route? This is highly unlikely, and it is going to be the challenge for the gynaecologists of the 21st century to optomise the surgical use of women's natural anatomy in order to benefit them most.

"If you give a man more than he can do
he'll do it
If you only give him what he can do
he'll do nothing."
- Kipling, R. -

REFERENCES

1. Sheth SS. Vaginal hysterectomy following previous caesarean section. *Int J Gynaecol Obstet* 1996; **52**(2): 167–171.
2. Doyen V, Cited in Green-Armytage VB. Vaginal hysterectomy: new technique – follow-up of 500 consecutive operation for haemorrhage. *J Obstet Gynecol Br Empire* 1939; **46**: 848–856.
3. Brown DA, Frazer MI. Hysterectomy revisited J. Aust NZ *Obstet Gynecol* 1991; **31**: 148.
4. Summitt RL, Stovall TG, Lipscomb GH, *et al.* Randomized comparison of laparoscopy assisted vaginal hysterectomy with standard Vaginal Hysterectomy in an out patient setting. *J Obstet Gynecol* 1992; **80**: 895.
5. Wilcox LS, Koonin LM, Pokras R, Strauss LT, Xiaz, Peterson HB. Hysterectomy in the United States 1988–90. *Obstet-Gynecol* 1994; **83**: 549–555.
6. Dicker RC, Greenspan JR, Strauss LT *et al.* Complications of abdominal and vaginal hysterectomy among women of reproductive age in the US. *Am J Obstet Gynecol* 1982; **144**(7): 841–848.
7. Davies AE, Hefni MA. Vaginal endoscopic oophorectomy with vaginal hysterectomy: A simple minimal access surgery technique. *Br J Obstet Gynecol* 1997; **104**: 621–622.
8. Bost BW. Assessing the impact of introducing laparoscopically assisted vaginal hysterectomy into a community based gynecology practice. *J Gynecol Surg* 1995; **11**: 171–178.
9. Sheth SS. Vaginal hysterectomy: In progress in *Obstetrics and Gynecology* -10th Ex. – John Studd: London, Churchill Livingston: 1993; 317–340.
10. Kovac SR. Guidelines to determine the route of hysterectomy. *Obstet Gynecol* 1995; **85**: 18–23.
11. Pelosi MA, Pelosi MA III. A comprehensive approach to morcellation of the large uterus. *Contemporary Ob/Gyn* 1997; 106–125.
12. Chapron C, Dubuisson JB. Total hysterectomy by laparoscopy: Advantage for the patient or only a surgical gimmick? *Gynecologic surgery* 1996; **12**: 76–77.
13. Sheth SS, Malpani A. Vaginal hysterectomy for the management of menstruation in mentally retarded women. *Int J Gynecol Obstet* 1997; **35**: 319–321.
14. Kovac SR, Cruikshank SH, Retto HF. Laparoscopy assisted vaginal hysterectomy. *J Gynecol Surg* 1996; 85–88.
15. Sheth SS: An approach to vesico-uterine peritoneum, through a new surgical space. *J Gynecol Surg* 1996; **12**(2): 135–140.
16. Monaghan JM; A personal Communication: 1994.
17. Halban, J Gynakolosche operations. Lehre, Veinna, UR Bau & Schwarzcnberg, 1932.
18. Sheth SS. Fiberoptic light for oophorectomy at vaginal hysterectomy. *J Gynecol Surgery* under publication.

19. Kammerer-Doak DN, Magrina JF, Weaver A *et al.* Vaginal hysterectomy with and without oophorectomy: The Mayo Clinic experience. *J Pelvic Surgery* 1996; **2**(6): 304–309.

20. Davies A, O'Connor H, Magos AL. A Prospective study to evaluate oophorectomy at the time of VH. *Brit J Obstet Gynecol* 1996; **103**: 915–920.

21. Sheth SS. The place of oophorectomy at vaginal hysterectomy. *Bri J Obst Gynec* 1991; **98**: 662–666.

22. Sheth SS, Malpani A. Technique of vaginal oophorectomy during vaginal hysterectomy. *J Gynecol Surg* 1994; **10**: 197.

23. Reich H. Laparoscopic oophorectomy and salpingo-oophorectomy in the treatment of benign tubo-ovarian discases. *Int J Fertil* 1987; **32**: 233.

24. Parker WH. Management of adnexal masses by operative laparoscopy. Selection criteria. *J Reprod Med* 1992; **37**: 603–606.

25. Teng F Y, Muzsnai D, Perez R *et al.* A comparative study of laparoscopy and colpotomy for the removal of ovarian Dermoid cysts. *Obstet Gynecol* 1996; **87**: 1009–1013.

26. Sheth SS, Malpani AM. Inappropriate use of new technology: Impact on womens health. *Int Jr Gynec Obstet* 1997; **58**: 159–165.

27. Baggish MS. The most expensive hysterectomy. *J Gynecol Surgery* 1992; **8**: 57–58.

28. Morrow CP, Mishell DR, Kirschbaum RH, Morrow CP. Operative Gynecology In 1994 year book of *Obstet. Gynecol.* Cap 11 257–283 Mosby St. Louis. USA.

29. Cooperman AB, DeCherney AH, Olive DL. A case of endometrial ablation for dysfunctional uterine bleeding. *Obstet Gynecol* 1993; **82**: 640–642.

30. Sheth SS, Kothari ML, Munshi VR. Post aborted posterior colpotomy and sterilisation. *J Obstet Gynecol* of Br Commonwealth 1973; **80**: 274–275.

31. Sheth SS. Vaginal oophorectomy for breast cancer. *J Ob Gynec* 1989; **9**: 36–238.

32. Sheth SS. Laparoscopic Female Sterilisation Camps. *Lancet* 1988; **625**: 1415–1416.

33. Sheth SS. Transvaginal induction of Pneumo Peritoneum prior to Laparoscopy. *Asian Jr Obst Gynec* 1976; 50–53.

34. Sheth SS. Ascitic tapping by the vaginal route. Brief communication. *J Gynecol Obst* 1997; **56**: 65–66.

35. Sheth SS. Removal of extra uterine IUDs - Advances in Contraception. 1988; **4**: 213–216.

36. Laparoscopic assisted radical vaginal hysterectomy, modified according to Schauta – Stoecke. *Obst-Gynecol* 1996; **88**: 10576.

6

Laparoscopic Colposuspension

S. Pringle
R. Hawthorn

Introduction

Rapid technological developments in the field of laparoscopic surgery in recent years have coincided with a critical re-appraisal of the outcomes of continence surgery. It is widely recognised that the results of primary procedures for genuine stress incontinence (GSI) are superior to those of subsequent attempts. Furthermore, of the host of procedures described in the literature, few have been subject to proper scientific assessment. The literature is particularly deficient in terms of comparative effectiveness of different procedures and their long-term outcomes.[1]

In spite of these problems, there is an emerging consensus that colposuspension is the 'gold standard' operation in the management of GSI. Burch in 1967 reported a 93% success rate with this procedure.[2] He also reported the development of enterocoeles in 7% of women. Other studies have confirmed this finding as well as postoperative voiding difficulties[3] and new detrusor instability in up to 19% of cases.[4] The Burch procedure is clearly superior to anterior colporrhaphy[1] and a number of series have demonstrated its long-term effectiveness,[5,6] Earlier 'minimally invasive' operations for GSI such as the Stamey procedure have proved particularly disappointing by this latter measure. It is against this background that we have to consider the development of laparoscopic approaches to colposuspension.

History

In 1990, Liu was pioneering laparoscopic colposuspension while Vancaillie[7] described a laparoscopic version of the Marshall-Marchetti-Krantz as well as the Burch procedure. These early reports used a variety of techniques as individual surgeons experimented to overcome the undoubted technical difficulties of the procedure. By 1993, Liu[8] was able to report 107 cases with a 97% success rate, a figure that no-one has been able to match since.

Clearly, laparoscopic colposuspension was a technically viable procedure. But how did it compare with its 'open' counterpart? The earliest reports used either historical or contemporary controls, in non-randomised studies with all their weaknesses.[9] Again, laparoscopic colposuspension seemed to give acceptable short-term results with additional benefits such as reduced hospital stay and earlier return to normal bladder function. At the same time, a number of groups, ourselves included, embarked upon prospective, randomised controlled trials comparing laparoscopic with traditional Burch colposuspension.

Pre- and post-operative counselling

The following discussions apply only to women with a diagnosis of GSI after thorough clinical evaluation. In 1994, Liu gave a list of indications for more detailed pre-operative urodynamic assessment. We feel that no woman should undergo continence surgery without having uroflowmetry and filling and voiding cystometry as a minimum. Pre-operative counselling is also important as patients should still be advised that there is a small potential risk of voiding difficulty with the need to learn intermittent self-catheterisation, although this has not been described following laparoscopic surgery.

Operative techniques

As yet, there is no universally accepted technique for performing laparoscopic colposuspension. At each step of the operation a number of different methods have been employed and it is typically the personal experience of the surgeon than any objective measure that has guided technical developments. In many instances there has been an aversion to laparoscopic suturing and this largely accounts for the variations in technique. Thus it is difficult to assess the outcomes of laparoscopic colposuspension when performed by different groups. Consequently we will discuss the various options in turn with their advantages and disadvantages.

Access to the retropubic space

Extra-peritoneal approach

We prefer a completely extra-peritoneal approach like the traditional Burch procedure. A Veress needle is inserted through the rectus sheath in the midline 2 cm above the pubic symphysis, below any previous transverse lower abdominal incisions. The space is then insufflated with CO_2. Through an umbilical incision the laparoscope is inserted into the extra-peritoneal space using an optical viewing trocar (Visiport®) which allows the sheath to be incised under direct vision. Blunt dissection with the telescope then brings the anatomical landmarks of the space into view. There is space to insert 2 or 3 additional ports and bladder injury is rare. The advantages are summarised in **Table 6.1**. An alternative method of dissecting this space is to use an inflatable balloon[11] inserted through the rectus sheath suprapubically. This is said to have the advantage of speed but we have found the method described above to take a matter of minutes in the vast majority of cases.

Trans-peritoneal approach

Insertion of the laparoscope through the umbilicus into the peritoneal cavity has the obvious advantage of familiarity. Access to the retropubic space involves grasping the peritoneum overlying the superior surface of the bladder on the anterior abdominal wall and dissecting the space between these structures. Bladder injury may occur at this stage. With dissection of the retropubic space complete there is plenty of room to manipulate the instruments for suture placement. The advantages and disadvantages are summarised in **Table 6.2**. Kadar proposes a quite different method.[12] Since the paravaginal fascia and Cooper's ligament which are being opposed lie in the paravesical space rather than in the cave of Retzius, he recommends a trans-peritoneal dissection of this space. The umbilical ligament is used as a landmark, avoiding the risk of bladder injury whilst giving excellent exposure of Cooper's ligament.

Clearly there are a number of different methods, which can successfully be used to expose the operative field. There are few studies, none of them randomised, which compare the two main approaches (*vide infra*). Different circumstances will dictate which is most appropriate in each case and we believe that surgeons undertaking these procedures should be able to operate both trans- and extra-peritoneally.

Suturing methods and materials

Whichever approach is used, the bladder neck can be easily visualised and is mobilised in virtually the same technique as with open colposuspension. A combination of a finger in the vagina and a pledget or scissors are used to displace the bladder neck

Table 6.1 Features of the extra-peritoneal approach

Advantages	Disadvantages
Less risk of bladder injury	Unfamiliar approach
Quicker to perform	Confined space to use instruments
Mimics open method	

Table 6.2 Features of the trans-peritoneal approach

Advantages	Disadvantages
Familiar method and anatomy	More risk of bladder injury
More space to manipulate instruments	Takes more time
Allows other surgery to be performed simultaneously	

medially and expose the paravaginal fascia. Typically the view is superior and there is less bleeding than at the open procedure. Disposable or reusable pledgets are adequate for this purpose. Most of the variations surrounding laparoscopic colposuspension are in the methods used to oppose the paravaginal fascia to the iliopectineal ligament.

Suturing methods

We have attempted to copy the standard methods for open colposuspension using a laparoscopic approach. For this reason we use 2 Ethibond® sutures on each side but find a straight needle easier to manipulate. Each suture is placed and tied in turn before proceeding to the other side rather than tying all the sutures once they are placed as in the open procedure (**Figures 6.1, 6.2 and 6.3**). A finger in the vagina may be used to support the tissues during tying.

Other groups use curved needles or absorbable materials such as polyglycolic acid.[13] Su *et al*[14] describe taking a double bite through the vagina prior to suturing the ligament, but often found there was no room for a second suture.

Laparoscopic sutures may be tied intra- or extracorporeally. The tension under which they are placed is controversial with a number of authors warning against excessive tension[10] but poorer elevation of the bladder neck during stress is said to be a marker of a lower cure rate.[14] There is no doubt that it is possible to achieve the same degree of elevation as with open surgery; we currently prefer a lesser degree of tension in the hope of avoiding failure of the suture and voiding problems.

The difficulties of laparoscopic suturing have resulted in a variety of other methods of suture placement particularly to the ligament. These include the use of suture/staple combinations,[15] an Endo-Stitch® device[16] and bone anchors.[17] Pelosi's technique is to dissect the retropubic space laparoscopically and use a Stamey needle passed under direct vision through the iliopectineal ligament then through

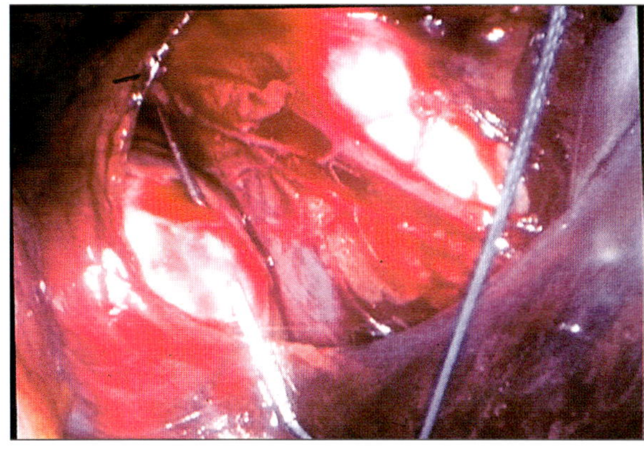

Figure 6.1 Laparoscopic suturing: first needle passes through the vagina, the ilio-pectineal ligament having been previously exposed.

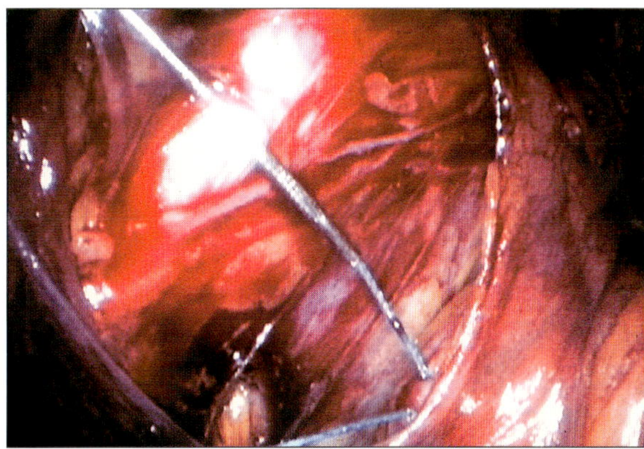

Figure 6.2 The needle then passes through the ilio-pectineal ligament.

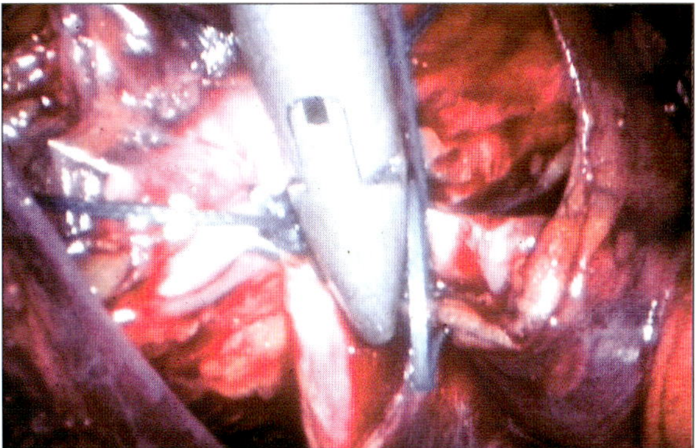

Figure 6.3 Having tied and cut the first suture the needle then passes through the remaining 'dog-ear' of the vagina before passing through the ilio-pectineal ligament again.

the vagina and back.[18] Breda takes the opposite approach and describes a vaginal suturing method.[19] Finally, the use of special laparoscopic suturing equipment can be avoided altogether by gasless 'laparoscopy' using the Laparolift® device.[20]

Stapling methods

As stated above, laparoscopic suture placement can be technically demanding and several groups advocate the use of staples and polypropylene (Prolene) mesh familiar to general surgeons for hernia repair. Typically, the bladder neck is mobilised as above and a strip of mesh is stapled first to the vagina then to the ilio-pectineal ligament with any excess being trimmed. The stapler may then be used to close the peritoneum if it is felt necessary. Satisfactory bladder neck elevation and short-term results have been reported.[21, 22] Ross[23] carried out a randomised controlled trial (RCT) to compare the staple/mesh method with standard suturing. This is the only RCT so far to compare the various techniques of laparoscopic colposuspension; others are necessary.

Fibrin glue

Volz[24] and Kiilholma[25] have reported the application of fibrin glue between the mobilised paravaginal fascia and the ilio-pectineal ligament with limited follow-up information.

Post-operative care

Catheters and drains

Following open colposuspension, a suprapubic catheter is typically inserted for a few days until normal voiding is restored and suction drainage of the retropubic space is routinely employed.

Certainly this was our initial approach but it has become clear with experience that there is usually very little bleeding either during or after laparoscopic colposuspension so that a drain is rarely required.

Similarly, the return to normal voiding with the laparoscopic approach is usually much quicker than with open cases. Although we still prefer to insert a suprapubic catheter under direct vision at the end of the operation, others simply remove the Foley catheter immediately and reinsert a urethral catheter temporarily if the patient fails to void.[16] In Ross' study,[23] only one patient failed to void within 24 h. Thus, different approaches to catheter management are needed to match the very short hospital stays and rapid recovery of the typical patient and her bladder!

Discharge advice

One of the advantages cited for minimally invasive surgery is the rapid return to normal (especially economic) activities. Does this apply to laparoscopic colposuspension? Whilst it is plain that patients leave hospital and are physically more active following laparoscopic surgery, it is not clear what effect this has on the success of the operation. Some believe it may be detrimental[26] but there are no data on which to base an opinion. We arbitrarily advise women not to rush back to normal activities and allow some time for the healing process to be completed.

Laparoscopic colposuspension in complex cases

Previous continence surgery

Most of the studies of laparoscopic colposuspension have excluded women who have had previous surgery for stress incontinence. A scarred anterior vaginal wall with reduced bladder neck mobility contraindicates colposuspension by whichever route and fibrosis of the retropubic space leads to a tedious dissection.

Von Theobald *et al*[27] describe their experience of using the laparoscope to investigate cases of failed open colposuspension. The retropubic space was dissected in all five cases with only one bladder injury. In some cases it was clear why the operation had failed: failure of the suture or inadequate bladder neck elevation. In these cases they recommended repeat colposuspension. Foote and Lam[27] report a small series of patients who underwent laparoscopic colposuspension following previous failed continence surgery with 100% subjective success.[28]

Complex pelvic floor defects and other surgery
Many reports in the literature describe laparoscopic colposuspension being carried out at the same time as other pelvic surgery such as laparoscopic hysterectomy. This is one of the indications for the trans-peritoneal approach.

More controversial is the best way to tackle complex pelvic floor defects. The debate is not new; Burch long recognised the occurrence of posterior defects following his procedure and advocated simultaneous obliteration of the cul-de-sac. Even so, there was a 7% incidence of enterocoele. Liu followed his example and recommended a laparoscopic Moschowitz procedure using one or more purse-string sutures at the time of colposuspension.[10] In another study, two-thirds of the women undergoing colposuspension had simultaneous correction of other defects - McCall culdoplasties, sacrocolpopexy or posterior vaginal repairs.[23] Whilst the concept of total pelvic floor reconstruction is attractive, there is very little information about the results of such procedures.

Effectiveness of laparoscopic colposuspension - assessing the literature

We have already discussed some of the difficulties in assessing the literature on laparoscopic colposuspension. In preparing this review we identified relevant publications by searching Medline and the Cochrane library using 'laparoscopic, colposuspension and continence surgery' as search terms. Other publications were sought from references in the papers identified from Medline as well as personal contacts. It quickly became apparent that much of the published material consists of personal series of cases which may include the author's initial experience of the technique, i.e. the whole learning curve. Most authorities agree that this is a significant issue with laparoscopic colposuspension. In general however better results are reported in retrospective series than can be repeated in prospective (especially randomised) studies. Another problem is that there is no uniform method of reporting outcomes. Ideally there would be objective tests of cure of GSI at set times post-operatively but much more commonly we find patient-reported success with median follow-ups and ranges from a few months to a few years. Perhaps the biggest problem is that the longest reported follow-up to date is only 3 years, so any evaluation of the procedure must be regarded with caution at this stage. The literature on complications of the procedure are also scanty. For these reasons this chapter should not be regarded as a systematic review of the literature but a critique of the minority of studies where the outcomes are well described. **Table 6.3** summarises the publications reviewed.

Effectiveness of laparoscopic colposuspension
The overall short-term success rate of laparoscopic colposuspension judging from these series of cases is impressive. However, the results from the laparoscopic arms of the RCTs are rather less so, perhaps in part due to the use of objective measures of cure in these trials. It also raises a question mark as to whether or not the results reported by expert laparoscopic surgeons can be widely replicated.

Laparoscopic versus open colposuspension
There are three randomised trials comparing the laparoscopic and open methods.[14, 29, 30] In addition, two other non-randomised studies provide data on outcomes,[9,31] the trials together include some 300 women. As discussed earlier, direct comparisons between these studies are inappropriate given that the surgical techniques employed are so variable. Success rates range from 60-94% for laparoscopic compared with 70-93% for open colposuspension.

Much larger studies will be required to demonstrate conclusively even a 10% difference between

Table 6.3 Published reports of laparoscopic colposuspension

Study type	Authors (Ref.)	Numbers	Success rate %
Case series	Liu[8]	107	97
	Ross[32]	48	89
	Von Theobald[33]	37	86
	O'Shea[34]	58	98
	Wallwiener[35]	20	92
	Papasakelariou[41]	32	91
	Laparoscopic versus open	(lap:open)	
RCT	Burton[29]	60	73:97 (1y) 60:93 (3y)
	Su[14]	96	80:96
	Hawthorn[30]	70	94:91
Comparative studies	Ross[31]	62	93:90
	Polascik[9]	22	83:70
	Trans- versus extra-peritoneal	(trans:extra)	
	Shwayder[39]	40	100:100
	O'Shea[40]	59	97:100
	Sutures versus staples/mesh	(sutures/staples)	
RCT	Ross[23]	69	91:94

cure rates. The main concern of those who are sceptical about minimally invasive surgery for GSI is that success rates will decline with time. Obviously, it will be several years before this question can be resolved, given that the operation has barely existed for a decade. Burton reported a decline in cure rate from 86% at 6 months to 73% and 60 % at 1 and 3 years respectively.[29] Our experience in this respect[30] is closer to that of Ross, who describes cure rates at 6 weeks, 12 and 24 months of 98, 93, and 89%, respectively.[32] It is essential that the pioneers in this field continue to follow-up and publish their findings so that its true value can be assessed.

Cost

The relative costs of laparoscopic and traditional surgery have now been reported in three studies.[36-38] This is a reflection of the importance attached to economic evaluation of new healthcare procedures but it also implies, perhaps prematurely, that laparoscopic colposuspension is a 'proven' procedure. The studies give conflicting results; whereas Kohli found that laparoscopic surgery was more expensive, primarily due to the theatre expenses.[36] the Australian study found that the shorter hospital stay more than compensated for this.[37] Kung agreed with this finding and because the outcomes of the two methods were similar, claimed that laparoscopic colposuspension was the more cost-effective approach.[38] Clearly, the relative costs of disposable laparoscopic equipment and a hospital bed will vary from one institution to another.

Trans- versus extra-peritoneal surgery

Two studies have compared the trans- and extra-peritoneal approaches to the bladder neck although neither were randomised.[39, 40] Shwayder reported a study of 40 women undergoing laparoscopic colposuspension, with 20 patients in each group, but the choice of operation depended in part on whether or not laparoscopic hysterectomy was to be performed at the same time. In this small study, the clinical outcomes were similar and all patients were reported to be continent, but the operating time and costs were less in the extraperitoneal group.[39] Again, the two groups in O'Shea's study were not strictly comparable, however, all but one of the patients became continent post-operatively. Hospital stay was longer in the extraperitoneal group.[40] Thus, there is no clear evidence of superiority for either approach and the surgeon must decide on the best method for individual patients.

Suturing versus stapled colposuspension
As discussed earlier, Ross's randomised trial of sutured versus stapled colposuspension is the only RCT which evaluates any of the variations between these operations.[23] Thirty-five women were allocated to the suturing group and 34 to staples and mesh. At 1 year, the objective cure rates were 91 and 94% respectively. Of the five failures, two were true failures with continuing GSI and hypermobility of the urethrovesical junction, two had detrusor instability, (3%) and one was thought to be due to intrinsic sphincter deficiency. The clinical and urodynamic outcomes for both groups were therefore similar, but Ross, clearly an accomplished laparoscopic surgeon, reported the stapled cases to be much easier to perform. Notably, all those who underwent laparoscopic colposuspension alone were discharged in less than 24 hs and only one incidence of voiding difficulty arose.

Complications

For obvious reasons, new reports of surgical techniques fail to dwell on the difficulties and complications that might arise. There is comparatively little written about this aspect of laparoscopic colposuspension. Is this because there are fewer problems than with the open procedure? Although it is clear that short-term morbidity is reduced, the frequency of other problems remains uncertain at present and we can only look at some of the complications that have been described. As far as the overall rate is concerned, Liu[10] and Su[14] both report an incidence of about 10% when minor problems such as haematuria and urinary tract infections are included.

Laparoconversion

The vast majority of colposuspensions can be successfully completed laparoscopically. Reports of the need to convert to laparotomy often include the learning curve of the operator(s) and the figures of 3.6-11.5%[42,43] seem to us to be unduly high.

Injury to urinary tract

Many series have reported injuries to the bladder dome of up to 9%.[43] Typically, these occur when the retropubic space is opened trans-peritoneally. Either an extraperitoneal approach or Kadar's method of exposure[12] may reduce this risk, while previous continence surgery increases it. Small cystotomies rarely pose a significant problem however, they may be repaired laparoscopically or allowed to close with catheter drainage. Prolonged drainage seems to be unnecessary.[23]

Injury to the ureter is much more serious but apparently uncommon. Liu[10] and Aslan[44] have reported cases that were corrected by releasing the suspension sutures by laparoscopic and open surgery respectively. Mobilising the bladder too medially seems to increase this possibility[45] and this should be suspected if unilateral loin pain develops after surgery.

Injuries to inferior epigastric vessels

While this can occur with any laparoscopic procedure the position of the ports may increase the possibility of injury at colposuspension. Abdominal wall haematomas can cause substantial morbidity and may require evacuation.[46] On occasion, a laparotomy may be required to arrest the bleeding.[43,47]

Port hernias

While this has not been described after laparoscopic colposuspension, closure of lateral ports over 5 mm is good practice. These last two complications are not features of the extraperitoneal approach described but are most likely with transperitoneal surgery.

Voiding difficulty

One of the great benefits of the laparoscopic method is the rapid return to normal voiding even within 24 hs.[23,30] The explanation for this is unclear, but the possibilities include reduced postoperative pain and trauma to the autonomic nerves in the retropubic space. Interestingly, in Su's study, several of the patients undergoing laparoscopic colposuspension then immediately underwent laparotomy for another gynaecological procedure. This group of women also voided earlier than their open counterparts.[14] While patients requiring catheter drainage for up to 10 days have been described[10] there are no reports of long-term voiding problems requiring self-catheterisation.

Detrusor instability

As with open colposuspension, detrusor instability can arise *de novo*. Its reported incidence varies from 2.3–8 %.[10,43] It is not clear whether or not one procedure differs from the other in this respect. Most reported cases have responded well to conservative management.

Prolapse

Again there is a paucity of information on which to make any judgement. We and others[43] have encountered postoperative enterocoeles and as stated above, prophylactic culdoplasty has its advocates. Ross found no significant prolapse in 48 patients 2 years postoperatively.[32] Long-term results will be needed before any true assessment can be made of the frequency of this complication.

Conclusions

In 10 years, great strides have been made in overcoming the technical difficulties of laparoscopic colposuspension, and as we have seen, surgical variations abound. What can we expect of the next decade? Undoubtedly, instrumentation will continue to improve. Robot assistance[48] and 3-D laparoscopy[49] have already been applied to bladder neck surgery. The trend towards early hospital discharge may have reached its limit; certainly on this side of the Atlantic, few patients are likely to be sent home after 5 hs and 30 min.[50] At present, it is unclear which of the methods described above will stand the test of time, and become the standard method of laparoscopic colposuspension.

Surgeons in every speciality have a poor reputation for introducing new operations without proper evaluation of their efficacy. It is to the credit of laparoscopic surgeons and urogynaecologists that laparoscopic colposuspension has passed from introductory reports and small case series to comparative and randomised trials within less than a decade. Good quality clinical data are now emerging to guide our decision making and patient counselling. Although there remain many sceptics who will be satisfied only when five year (or longer) follow-up statistics are available, in our view laparoscopic colposuspension is close to having an established place in the management of GSI.

REFERENCES

1. Jarvis GJ. Surgery for genuine stress incontinence. *Br J Obstet Gynaecol* 1994; **101**: 371–374.
2. Burch JC. Cooper's ligament urethrovesical suspension for stress incontinence, cystocoele and prolapse. *Am J Obstet Gynecol* 1968; **100**: 764–774.
3. Kiilholma P, Makinen J, Chancellor MB *et al.* Modified Burch colposuspension for stress urinary incontinence in females. *Surg Gynaecol Obst* 1993; **176**: 111–115.
4. Cardozo LD, Stanton SL, Williams JE. Detrusor instability following surgery for genuine stress incontinence. *Br J Urol* 1979; **51**: 204–207.
5. Feyereisl J, Dreher E, Haenggi W, Zikmund J, Schneider H. Long-term results after Burch colposuspension. *Am J Obstet Gynecol* 1994; **171**: 647–652.

6. Alcalay M, Monga A Stanton SL. Burch colposuspension – how long does it cure stress incontinence? *Neurourol Urodyn* 1994; **13**: 495–496.

7. Vancaillie TG, Schuessler W. Laparoscopic bladder neck suspension. *J Laparoendo Surg* 1991; **1**: 169–173.

8. Liu CY, Paek W. Laparoscopic retropubic colposuspension (Burch procedure). *J Am Assoc Gynecol Laparosc* 1993; **1**: 31–35.

9. Polascik TJ, Moore RG, Rosenberg MT, Kavoussi LR. Comparison of laparoscopic and open retropubic urethropexy for treatment of stress urinary incontinence. *Urology* 1995; **45**: 647–652.

10. Liu CY. Laparoscopic treatment for genuine urinary stress incontinence. Bailliéres Clin *Obstet Gynaecol* 1994; **8**: 789–798.

11. O'Shea RT, Seman E, Taylor J. Different Approaches to Laparoscopic Burch Colposuspension. *J Am Assoc Gynecol Laparosc* 1995; **2**(4 Suppl): S38.

12. Kadar N. Avoiding the Space of Retzius during the Laparoscopic Burch Procedure. *J Am Assoc Gynecol Laparosc* 1996; **3**(4 Suppl): S20.

13. Burton G A. Randomised comparison of laparoscopic and open colposuspension. *Neurourol Urodyn* 1994; **13**: 497–498.

14. Su TH, Wang KG, Hsu CY, Wei HJ, Hong BK. Prospective comparison of laparoscopic and traditional colposuspensions in the treatment of genuine stress incontinence. *Acta Obstet Gynecol Scand* 1997; **76**: 576–582.

15. Lyons TL, Winer WK. Clinical outcomes with laparoscopic approaches and open Burch procedures for urinary stress incontinence. *J Am Assoc Gynecol Laparosc* 1995; **2**: 193–198.

16. Gill F, Enzelsberger H. A new surgical aid – the "endo-stitch disposable suture device" – for pelviscopic pre-peritoneal Burch incontinence operation. A pilot study. *Gynakol Geburtshilfliche Rundsch* 1996; **36**: 75–78.

17. Das S, Palmer JK. Laparoscopic colposuspension. *J Urol* 1995; **154**: 1119–1121.

18. Pelosi MA 3rd, Pelosi MA. Laparoscopic-Assisted Transpectineal Needle Suspension of the Bladder Neck. *J Am Assoc Gynecol Laparosc* 1998; **5**: 39–46.

19. Breda G, Silvestre P, Gherardi L, Xausa D, Tamai A, Giunta A. Correction of stress urinary incontinence: laparoscopy combined with vaginal suturing. *J Endourol* 1996; **10**: 251–253.

20. Davila GW. Gasless Laparoscopic Burch Colposuspension. *J Am Assoc Gynecol Laparosc* 1995; **2**(4 Suppl): S12.

21. Ou CS, Presthus J, Beadle E. Laparoscopic bladder neck suspension using hernia mesh and surgical staples. *J Laparoendosc Surg* 1993; **3**: 563–566.

22. Birken RA, Leggett PL. Laparoscopic colposuspension using mesh reinforcement. *Surg Endosc* 1997; **11**: 1111–1114.

23. Ross J. Two techniques of laparoscopic Burch repair for stress incontinence: a prospective, randomized study. *J Am Assoc Gynecol Laparosc* 1996; **3**: 351–357.

24. Volz J, Strittmatter H, Koster S, Wischnik A, Melchert F. Endoscopy of the preperitoneal interstitium – a new approach for colposuspension. *Zentralbl Gynakol* 1993; **115**: 488–491.

25. Kiilholma P, Haarala M, Polvi H, Makinen J, Chancellor MB. Sutureless endoscopic colposuspension with fibrin sealant. *Tech Urol* 1995; **1**: 81–83.

26. Burton G. Personal communication. 1997.

27. Von Theobald P, Barjot P, Levy G. Feasibility of and interest in laparoscopic assessment in recurrent urinary stress incontinence after Burch procedure performed by laparotomy. *Surg Endosc* 1997; **11**: 468–471.

28. Foote AJ, Lam A. Laparoscopic colposuspension in women with previously failed anti-incontinence surgery. *J Obstet Gynaecol Res* 1997; **23**: 313–317.

29. Burton G. A three year prospective randomised urodynamic study comparing open & laparoscopic colposuspension. *Neurourol Urodyn* 1997; **16**: 353–354.

30. Hawthorn RJS, Donaldson KF, Ramsay I. Randomised trial of laparoscopic extra-peritoneal colposuspension versus open colposuspension (submitted for publication) 1999.

31. Ross JW. Laparoscopic Burch Repair Compared With Laparotomy Burch to Cure Urinary Stress Incontinence. *J Am Assoc Gynecol Laparosc* 1995; **2** (4 Suppl): S47–S48.

32. Ross JW. Multichannel urodynamic evaluation of laparoscopic Burch colposuspension for genuine stress incontinence. *Obstet Gynecol* 1998; **91**: 55–59.

33. Von Theobald P, Guillaumin D, Levy G. Laparoscopic preperitoneal colposuspension for stress incontinence in women. Technique and

results of 37 procedures. *Surg Endosc* 1995; **9**: 1189–1192.

34. O'Shea RT, Seman E, Taylor J. Laparoscopic Burch Colposuspension for Urinary Stress Incontinence. *J Am Assoc Gynecol Laparosc* 1996; **3** (4 Suppl): S36.

35. Wallwiener D, Grischke EM, Rimbach S, Maleika A, Bastert G. Endoscopic retropubic colposuspension:"Retziusscopy"versus laparoscopy - a reasonable enlargement of the operative spectrum in the management of recurrent stress incontinence? *Endosc Surg Allied Technol* 1995; **3**: 115–118.

36. Kohli N, Jacobs PA, Sze EH, Roat TW, Karram MM. Open compared with laparoscopic approach to Burch colposuspension: a cost analysis. *Obstet Gynecol* 1997; **90**: 411–415.

37. Loveridge K, Malouf A, Kennedy C, Edgington A, Lam A. Laparoscopic colposuspension. Is it cost-effective? *Surg Endosc* 1997; **11**: 762–765.

38. Kung RC, Lie K, Lee P, Drutz HP. The cost-effectiveness of laparoscopic versus abdominal Burch procedures in women with urinary stress incontinence. *J Am Assoc Gynecol Laparosc* 1996; **3**: 537–544.

39. Shwayder JM. Laparoscopic Burch Cystourethropexy Compared with the Transperitoneal and Extraperitoneal Approaches. *J Am Assoc Gynecol Laparosc* 1996; **3**(4 Suppl): S46–S47.

40. O'Shea RT, Seman E, Taylor J. Laparoscopic Burch Colposuspension for Urinary Stress Incontinence. *J Am Assoc Gynecol Laparosc* 1996; **3** (4 Suppl): S36.

41. Papasakelariou C. Laparoscopic Bladder Neck Suspension. *J Am Assoc Gynecol Laparosc* 1995; **2**(4 Suppl): S40.

42. Grossmann T, Darai E, Deval B, Benifla JL, Sebban E, Renolleau C, Madelenat P. Role of endoscopy in surgery for urinary incontinence. *Ann Chir* 1996; **50**: 896–905.

43. Cooper MJ, Cario G, Lam A, Carlton M. A review of results in a series of 113 laparoscopic colposuspensions. *Aust N Z J Obstet Gynaecol* 1996; **36**: 44–48.

44. Aslan P, Woo HH. Ureteric injury following laparoscopic colposuspension. *Br J Obstet Gynaecol* 1997; **104**: 266–268.

45. Mostwin JL, Genadry R, Sanders R, Yang A. Anatomic goals in the correction of female stress urinary incontinence. *J Endourol* 1996; **10**: 207–212.

46. Smith AR. Laparoscopic and needle colposuspension. *Baillieres Clin Obstet Gynaecol* 1995; **9**: 757–767.

47. Lam AM, Jenkins GJ, Hyslop RS. Laparoscopic Burch colposuspension for stress incontinence: preliminary results. *Med J Aust* 1995; **162**: 18–21.

48. Partin AW, Adams JB, Moore RG, Kavoussi LR. Complete robot-assisted laparoscopic urologic surgery: a preliminary report. *J Am Coll Surg* 1995; **181**: 552–557.

49. Koster S, Volz J, Melchert F. Indications for 3D laparoscopy in gynaecology. *Geburtshilfe Frauenheilkd* 1996; **56**: 431–433.

50. Taylor RH. Outpatient Laparoscopic Hysterectomy with discharge in 4 to 6 hours. *J Am Assoc Gynecol Laparosc* 1994; **1** (4, Part 2): S35.

7

Vault Prolapse

Can it be prevented?

D. A. Johns

Introduction

The recorded history of pelvic organ prolapse dates to 2000 BC.[1] The subsequent decades have been littered with descriptions of techniques designed to treat and/or prevent this malady. Many of these procedures still carry the name of their inventor and most are unquestionably effective in treating prolapse disorders. None, however, have been subjected to long-term study to determine if they do, indeed, prevent anything. During their years of training, most gynaecological surgeons are taught to routinely incorporate one of these prophylactic measures during hysterectomy, but the choice of procedure is largely based on our teacher's experience and training. Then, as now, no data exist concerning the efficacy of these procedures.

Although every gynaecologist commonly encounters the group of disorders described as 'pelvic relaxation', pure vaginal vault prolapse or vaginal vault eversion is extremely uncommon. The true incidence of vaginal vault prolapse following hysterectomy is unknown, but available data would suggest that it occurs in less than 1% of post-hysterectomy patients.[2–4] Most often, the patient with 'pelvic relaxation' has several identifiable pelvic floor defects, and descent of the vaginal apex represents only one component of this dilemma.[5] Pure vaginal vault prolapse not associated with any other pelvic floor defect is exceedingly rare.

This fact, along with decades of individual physician bias, has prevented the development of a reproducible reliable descriptive classification system for pelvic floor defects. As a result, virtually all published data on the treatment of this plethora of anatomic abnormalities reflects the experience of individual physicians or institutions, making comparative studies almost impossible.

Our literature is replete with reports describing the treatment of vaginal vault prolapse. Virtually every conceivable approach (vaginal, abdominal, and laparoscopic) has been proposed. The vagina has been sewn, meshed, spiked, and glued to most every available pelvic structure. These reports, however, all address treatment of an existing problem, not its prevention. Can this obviously difficult surgical problem be prevented by a procedure performed at the time of hysterectomy?

Pelvic floor defects (cystocele, cystourethrocele, rectocele, enterocele and vaginal vault prolapse) are seen by gynaecologists many times every day during routine pelvic examinations. Most patients are not symptomatic and do not require surgical intervention. Most (but not all) of these patients are parous; some have undergone hysterectomy. Are these defects related to prior surgery, injury, childbirth, or unavoidable consequences of the individual patient's tissues? Is a patient 'destined' to prolapse her vaginal vault after hysterectomy because of her genetic makeup or can this problem be delayed or avoided?

Based on current data, these questions are unanswerable, but a review of the pathogenesis and surgical treatment of vaginal vault prolapse may be revealing.

Anatomy and pathophysiology

The upper portion of the vagina and cervix are supported by the uterosacral-cardinal 'ligaments.' These structures are not ligaments, but a condensation of fibroelastic tissue, smooth muscle fibres, vessels, lymphatics, and nerves comprising what is known as the endopelvic fascia. The 'pelvic diaphragm' and 'urogenital diaphragm', along with the pubourethral ligaments, complete the structures supporting the vagina and cervix.

These anatomical concepts were largely unknown in the 1930s and 40s. As a result, patients suffering from uterine and vaginal prolapse were likely to undergo ventral fixation of the uterus or cervix, a procedure fraught with problems.[6] Fortunately, the last two decades have brought a better understanding of the anatomic support of the cervix and vagina, resulting in better and more effective reconstructive procedures.

Current knowledge suggests that the uterus is not a factor in vaginal vault support. It will, however, prolapse along with the vagina when support structures are damaged. Uterine descensus is the result, but not the cause, of vaginal vault prolapse. Surgical correction of this defect, therefore, does not involve the uterus or mandate its removal.

Modern surgical procedures designed to correct pelvic floor defects, including vaginal vault prolapse, rely on reconstructing those structures normally supporting the vagina. This is usually accomplished by:

- identifying and reapproximating the endopelvic fascia;
- reattaching remnants of the uterosacral ligaments to the vagina; or
- securing the vaginal vault to other pelvic structures with various types of mesh or permanent suture material.

The last of these options simply represents our best effort at rebuilding support structures that have been destroyed or are no longer identifiable.

The cause of female genital prolapse is unknown, but there are undoubtedly many contributing factors. Congenital anomalies of these 'ligaments', trauma from pregnancy or delivery, denervation from neurological disease or trauma, and chronic diseases resulting in increased intra-abdominal pressure (obesity, COPD, ascites, etc.) could all contribute to loss of support and subsequent vaginal vault prolapse.

Our patients will continue to become pregnant (hopefully), therefore trauma to pelvic support structures from pregnancy or delivery cannot be avoided or prevented. Similarly, chronic disease states that may contribute to these problems are not likely to be avoided. If vaginal vault prolapse is avoidable, we can only hope to influence those iatrogenic factors that might predispose our patients to this condition.

Although none have been proven or even extensively studied, several iatrogenic factors potentially leading to prolapse of the vaginal vault have been proposed. These include:

- poor surgical technique resulting in excessive damage to vessels and nerves in the endopelvic fascia;
- failure to 'adequately' support the vaginal apex after removal of the cervix;
- excessive shortening of the vagina with loss of the normal support of the upper one-third of the vagina;
- failure to employ a 'prophylactic' step prior to closure of the vaginal cuff;
- removal of a normal cervix along with the uterus;
- failure to recognize and repair subtle pelvic floor defects during hysterectomy.

Do any of these intraoperative factors truly affect the incidence of vault prolapse? Does attention to any of these alter the ultimate outcome? Could, possibly, attempts at 'reattaching' support structures to the vaginal apex actually *increase* the likelihood of subsequent prolapse? There are few answers, but many educated guesses.

The role of supracervical hysterectomy in prevention of vaginal vault prolapse

Supracervical hysterectomy originated in the pre-antibiotic era as a method to minimize contamination of the peritoneal cavity with vaginal flora. In those times, peritonitis following hysterectomy was common and often fatal. A technique avoiding this inoculum was readily accepted. With the discovery and widespread use of antibiotics, supracervical hysterectomy was just as readily abandoned.

As originally described,[7] supracervical hysterectomy involved removal of the uterus abdominally followed by excision of the endocervical canal. The remaining portion of the cervix was left intact. This was accomplished by excising a conical shaped 'plug' (consisting of the entire endocervical canal) from the cervix. The remaining edges of the upper cervix (from which the uterus had been amputated) were approximated with sutures. This technique preserved most of the blood and nerve supply to the cervical stump, uterosacral ligaments, and endopelvic fascia.

Today, proponents of supracervical hysterectomy argue that the procedure offers many advantages over total hysterectomy, one being better postoperative support of the vaginal cuff (implying less chance of subsequent prolapse). Today's techniques, however, differ from the original. When compared to the traditional abdominal approach, 'modern' laparoscopic supracervical hysterectomy techniques[8–10] describe a different approach to the upper cervix. A larger portion of the cervix is removed, potentially compromising the vascular supply to the cervical stump and weakening those structures supporting the cervix and upper vagina.

One proponent of supracervical hysterectomy[11] recommends performing a 'high McCall procedure' routinely in all cases to provide posterior vaginal vault support. Obviously, it is his belief that simply leaving the cervix in place is not adequate to provide long-term support.

If supracervical hysterectomy truly preserves vaginal cuff support, vaginal vault prolapse should occur less frequently among patients who have undergone this procedure as compared to those undergoing total hysterectomy. Unfortunately, no data have been published confirming (or denying) this proposed benefit of supracervical hysterectomy. Until studies have answered the question, the role of supracervical hysterectomy in preventing subsequent vaginal vault prolapse is, at best, mere conjecture.

Surgical technique

Although the use of meticulous surgical technique during vaginal or abdominal hysterectomy is the goal of every gynaecological surgeon, there is no objective evidence that it will influence the subsequent development of pelvic floor defects, including vault prolapse. Most authors discussing reparative techniques for vault prolapse cite 'poor surgical technique' as a probable aetiology for the problem. None, however, cite any evidence (other than their opinion) supporting this assumption.

Dissection techniques, clamp placement, choice of suture material, methods for haemostasis, and operative 'skill' are as individualized and varied as the surgeons' personalities. Worldwide, millions of hysterectomies are performed every year utilizing an infinite variety of techniques, instruments, and sutures. Given this enormous diversity of technique, instrumentation and skill, it is unlikely that variations in these parameters will ever be studied in adequate detail to determine if any are related to subsequent prolapse of the vaginal vault.

With a combination of this diversity and the relative rarity of post-hysterectomy vaginal vault prolapse, it could be argued that surgical technique is of little (at best) or no (at worst) importance if one is concerned about subsequent vault prolapse.

'Preventative' measures

Between 1912 and 1970, Moschowitz,[12] McCall,[13] and others described surgical procedures for the correction of pelvic floor defects. These techniques invariably involved obliteration of the cul-de-sac, plication of the uterosacral ligaments, denuding of peritoneal surfaces, or suturing the uterosacral-cardinal ligament complex to one structure or another. All were proposed as measures to correct existing defects.

Over the past 20–30 years, some of these procedures have been incorporated into routine hysterectomies performed in patients without identifiable pelvic floor defects. Believing that subsequent enterocele or vault prolapse could be prevented, most of us were taught to utilize one of these techniques (usually a modification of the McCall culdoplasty) after the uterus had been removed.

In a recent unpublished review of operative reports at Harris Methodist Hospital in Fort Worth, Texas, 85% of the gynaecologists described using one of the above-mentioned techniques at the conclusion of their hysterectomies. In their preoperative assessment, none of these patients were reported to have enterocele, rectocele, or any other pelvic floor defect. At least in our facility, these procedures are almost routinely utilized as prophylactic measures. Although no study has evaluated the question, it is likely that some components of the procedures originally described to treat pelvic floor defects have become a routine part of hysterectomy everywhere. Has the incorporation of uterosacral plication, cul-de-sac obliteration, etc. into the routine hysterectomy provided any protective effect?

If these procedures did, in fact, prevent the subsequent development of vaginal vault prolapse, enterocele, or rectocele, and if they were uniformly applied, we should see very few patients with these problems following hysterectomy. One would expect the incidence of vault prolapse to have decreased since McCall first described his procedure in 1957.[13] Unfortunately, there is no data available to support such a conclusion. It could also, however, be argued that the almost routine use of prophylactic procedures (such as the modified McCall culdoplasty) in conjunction with hysterectomy over the past 30–40 years is the very reason vault prolapse following hysterectomy is such a rare occurrence.

Currently, one must conclude that additional steps taken during routine hysterectomy to prevent subsequent vault prolapse are:

- widely utilized; and
- unproven.

It could even be argued that some of these 'prophylactic' procedures might actually increase the risk of subsequent pelvic floor defects by increasing the amount of tissue damage to the very support structures one is trying to reinforce.

We return to the original question: Can vaginal vault prolapse be prevented?

Even with the incorporation of procedures meant to improve 'support' for the vagina after hysterectomy, pelvic floor defects following surgery occur. Is this inevitable? Are we lousy surgeons?

As mentioned earlier, the cardinal-uterosacral ligament complex provides support for the upper vagina. This 'ligament' inserts into the upper vagina and cervix posteriorly and laterally. During routine total hysterectomy, this complex structure is clamped, cut, and ligated. The vagina is not, however, separated from the uterosacral or cardinal ligaments during this process. Most surgeons reinforce this attachment by suturing the uterosacral-cardinal ligament complex to the lateral aspects of the vagina, utilizing the standard 'Richardson' technique.[14]

Whether the cervix is left in place or not, those structures that supported the vagina prior to removal of the uterus remain attached to the vaginal apex. If no defects in this support structure existed prior to hysterectomy, it seems unlikely that these structures become detached from the vagina during surgery.

It has been proposed that damage to the uterosacral-cardinal complex at the time of hysterectomy may be a factor leading to subsequent vaginal vault prolapse. During routine hysterectomy, however, this damage is confined to the most distal portions of these structures (at their attachment to the cervix and extreme upper vagina). The majority of the uterosacral-cardinal ligament complex remains intact and in direct contact with the vaginal 'cuff'. Sutures attaching the *distal* end of this complex to the vaginal apex are very unlikely to damage the more proximal portions of this important support structure.

Conversely, when the uterosacral ligaments are 'plicated', several sutures are placed through the distal 4–5 cm of these structures. The sutures are tied, usually under considerable tension, bringing these ligaments together in the midline. From an anatomic standpoint, it is unclear how pulling these ligaments together in the midline (well away from their attachment to the vagina) could have any positive effect on vaginal support, but this is the prescribed technique. In reality, these sutures could significantly damage the ligaments *proximal* to their critical attachments to the vagina, thereby inhibiting (rather than enhancing) support for the vagina. It is, therefore, possible that the routine use of this technique may *increase* rather than decrease the risk of subsequent vault prolapse.

Similarly, placement of sutures meant to 'obliterate' a normal cul-de-sac or removal of normal peritoneum in order to 'scar' the same area may actually damage vascular or neurologic structures that would have otherwise remained intact. An increased risk of vault prolapse could result.

Data supporting these arguments against the routine use of such 'prophylactic' steps is the same as that supporting these techniques: non-existent.

What should we do?

There is no currently available data suggesting whether prophylactic steps to prevent vault prolapse should or should not be routinely undertaken. In those patients with no identifiable pelvic floor defects, the prophylactic efficacy of these procedures is unknown. Whether or not hysterectomy itself increases the risk of subsequent pelvic floor defects is also unknown. Our understanding of the aetiology of vaginal vault prolapse constitutes little more than 'educated guesses'. Although the intraoperative steps meant to prevent subsequent vault prolapse are commonly taken, it can also be argued that such 'prophylactic' procedures may actually increase intraoperative damage to the very support structures we are desperately trying to preserve.

Defects in the support structures of the vagina occur in a variety of anatomic locations and present different clinical problems in each patient. Virtually every author discussing the surgical treatment of pelvic floor defects (including vaginal vault prolapse) suggests that treatment must be individualized for every patient after careful evaluation of each anatomic defect present.

'Prophylactic' procedures performed at the time of hysterectomy, however, are 'shotgun' approaches to problems that have not yet occurred. All of these techniques address a single component of vaginal support – the uterosacral-cardinal ligament complex. Since vaginal support is dependent on other anatomical structures as well, it seems unlikely that a prophylactic procedure directed at only one of these components will inhibit the development of vault prolapse later in the patient's life.

From our current knowledge of pelvic floor defects, it is likely that these problems develop slowly over a period of years. The patient destined to develop vault prolapse within a few years after hysterectomy probably has identifiable, although subtle, defects in the support structures of the vagina at the time of her surgery. This might be manifested by exaggerated descent of the cervix, defects in the lateral endopelvic fascia with resultant lateral vaginal wall herniation, or a small asymptomatic enterocele. Any or all of these might indicate a predilection towards vaginal vault prolapse or pelvic floor defects later in life. Left untreated, these defects might fulfill that predilection.

Prior to any hysterectomy for benign disease, the surgeon must thoroughly examine the vagina for evidence of defects in vaginal support. These abnormalities should be further evaluated intraoperatively after the uterus has been removed.

Appropriate surgical correction can then be undertaken in conjunction with the hysterectomy.

Although the natural progression of such subtle defects is not well documented or understood, it seems logical that progression to symptomatic defects requiring subsequent surgery is likely if these problems are missed or ignored.

Fortunately, the incidence of post-hysterectomy vaginal vault prolapse is extremely low. Those factors leading to this distressing problem remain unclear, as does the role of 'preventative' measures. It is certain, however, that careful identification and correction of subtle vaginal support defects at the time of routine hysterectomy is more likely to prevent future vault prolapse (and other pelvic floor defects) than any 'prophylactic' procedure.

REFERENCES

1. Emge LA, Durfee RB. Pelvic organ prolapse: Four thousand years of treatment. *Clin Obstet Gynecol* 1996; **9**: 997.
2. Phaneuf LE. Inversion of the vagina and prolapse of the cervix following supracervical hysterectomy and inversion of the vagina following total hysterectomy. *Am J Obstet Gynecol* 1952; 64–739.
3. Symmonds RE, Pratt JH. Vaginal prolapse following hysterectomy. *Am J Obstet Gynecol* 1960; **79**: 899.
4. Birnbaum RE, Pratt JH. Vaginal prolapse following hysterectomy. *Am J Obstet Gynecol* 1973; **115**: 411.
5. Nichols DH. Eversion of the vagina. *Reoperative Gynecologic Surgery*, Mosby Year Book, 1991; 65.
6. Nichols DH. Massive Prolapse. Clinical Problems, Injuries and Complications of Gynecologic Surgery, Williams and Wilkins, 1983; 72.
7. *An Atlas of Pelvic Operations*, Parsons (ed), WB Saunders, 1968; 44–8.
8. Semm K. Hysterectomy via laparotomy or pelviscopy. A new CASH method without colpotomy. *Geburtshilfe Frauenheilkd* 1991; **51**: 996–1003.
9. Lyons TL. Laparoscopic supracervical hysterectomy: A comparison of morbidity and mortality results with laparoscopically assisted vaginal hysterectomy. *J Reprod Med* 1993; **38**: 763–767.
10. Diamond M, Daniell J, Jones H. (ed), *Hysterectomy*. 84–98.
11. Diamond M, Daniell J, Jones H. (ed), *Hysterectomy*. 93.
12. Moschowitz AV. The pathogenesis, anatomy, and cure of prolapse of the rectum. *Surg Gynecol Obstet* 1912; 15–17.
13. McCall ML. Posterior culdoplasty: Surgical correction of enterocele during vaginal hysterectomy, a preliminary report. *Obstet Gynecol* 1957; **10**: 592.
14. *Te Linde's Operative Gynecology*. Edited by John D. Thompson, John A. Rock – 7th edition. 704.

8

Photodynamic Therapy in Gynaecology

M. J. Gannon

Introduction

In 1924, it was observed that certain malignant tumours infected by haemolytic bacteria demonstrated the reddish fluorescence of endogenous porphyrins.[1] The possibility that reproduction of this porphyrin fluorescence might facilitate cancer diagnosis was supported by studies carried out on tumour-bearing mice.[2] Exogenously induced fluorescence was also demonstrated in human studies, which led to the seminal work of Richard Lipson in the 1960s. He reported tumour fluorescence using a mixture of porphyrins known as haematoporphyrin derivative (Hpd).[3] This gave better fluorescence with a lower dose and shorter administration time than the crude haematoporphyrin used in earlier work.

Black light

Near ultraviolet or "black light" was used in early experiments to visualise endofluorescence. The delivery of activating light was refined by using a direct current carbon arc lamp and passing the light through a copper sulphate solution to remove red light. This resulted in an intense beam between wavelengths 400 nm and 407 nm. Tumour fluorescence was viewed through a filter which blocked the activating light. Using this improved methodology it proved possible to induce fluorescence for the identification of certain malignant tumours including carcinomas of the bronchus, oesophagus and cervix.[4]

Diagnosis of cervical neoplasia

Although it was known from previous literature that some eosin dyes could be activated by sunlight, research into porphyrin-induced fluorescence concentrated at this time on its use as a diagnostic aid. Systemically administered Hpd which accumulated in areas of cervical neoplasia fluoresced with a typical salmon pink colour on exposure to activating light. A good correlation between fluorescence and biopsy-proven malignancy was shown in several studies.[5,6]

Porphyria-like effect

In porphyria cutanea tarda and some other porphyrias, overproduction of porphyrins causes generalised cutaneous photosensitivity. The notion that a similar effect could be induced by means of an administered porphyrin was developed by Lipson. He realised that the porphyrin derivatives which induced tissue fluorescence would at the same time make the fluorescent tissue sensitive to light. These porphyrin derivatives were also photosensitisers which could be used, when followed by light delivery at an appropriate wavelength, to kill tumour cells. The first reference to this in the literature is in a short report describing tumour detection studies in breast cancer by Lipson.[7]

First PDT treatment

The patient was a woman with a large ulcerating breast tumour. She received multiple Hpd injections followed by tumour exposure to filtered light from a Xenon arc lamp and it was reported that her tumour responded to this form of treatment. The short abstract failed to stimulate further interest at the time. The lack of clinical studies may have been related to the side-effects of available photosensitisers and the complexity of laser light delivery systems.

Photosensitisers

Early studies were carried out using Hpd, a derivative of porphyrin which is a complex mixture of monomeric porphyrins and oligomeric porphyrin esters and ethers. A more efficient photosensitiser was obtained by partial removal of the monomers, which do not localise in tumour tissue, to yield Photofrin® (QLT PhotoTherapeutics Inc., Vancouver, Canada), a semi-purified proprietary preparation of Hpd.

Newer photosensitisers

Photofrin has specificity for many types of malignant tissue, although it also accumulates in liver,

Table 8.1 Second generation photosensitisers

Porphines	meso-tetra(m-hydroxyphenyl)porphyrin (mTHPP)
Chlorins	meso-tetra(m-hydroxyphenyl)chlorin (mTHPC)
	benzoporphyrin derivative monoacid ring A (BpDMA)
	tin ethyl etiopurpurin (SnET2)
	mono-L-aspartyl chlorin e6 (MACE)
Phthalocyanines	disulphonated zinc phthalocyanine (ZnPcS2)

spleen, kidneys and skin. Its retention in skin necessitates protection of patients from bright lights, especially bright sunlight, for several weeks.[8] There is continuing research into improving the original porphyrin photosensitisers and several new, second generation photosensitising drugs are undergoing Phase I and Phase II clinical trials (**Table 8.1**).

5–aminolaevulinic acid

An alternative approach uses 5–aminolaevulinic acid (ALA) to produce protoporphyrin IX (PpIX), a precursor of haem in most body cells. Administration of excess ALA leads to accumulation of PpIX which acts as an endogenous photosensitiser. Like the other porphyrins, PpIX accumulates preferentially in tumour tissue. Kennedy and Pottier[8] studied the distribution of ALA induced PpIX in normal tissues and found that fluorescence occurred primarily in surface and glandular epithelium of the skin and the lining of hollow organs. Photosensitiser did not tend to accumulate in muscle and connective tissue. This selective uptake in vascular and proliferative tissues is used to target certain tissues, as well as tumours, for destruction. As ALA is a natural body compound which is completely metabolised within 24 h the problem of prolonged skin sensitivity is avoided by its use.

Safety of ALA in man

To simulate the plasma concentration of ALA seen during acute attacks of porphyria a human volunteer was given an oral loading dose of ALA followed by nasogastric instillation over 4 days.[9] There were no detected symptoms or pathophysiological changes in a battery of assays including serum aspartate aminotransferase levels. Temporary skin sensitivity due to ALA has been described only after a very large systemic dose.

Topically applied ALA in doses up to 7 gs was shown to have no influence on the systemic accumulation of porphyrins and porphyrin precursors in a study of 20 patients being treated by PDT for skin cancer.[10]

Mechanism of action

PDT requires a photosensitiser localised with some degree of selectivity in the target tissue and the means for its activation. The latter is generally achieved by visible light derived from a laser and directed to the site by an optical fibre.

Light delivery

At present only large, complex laser systems are capable of delivering sufficient power (up to about 1 W) for effective treatment. A primary pumping laser such as an argon-ion or a copper-vapour laser is coupled to a separate, tunable, dye laser.[11] These laser systems are associated with high capital and maintenance costs which is a limiting factor in the widespread application of PDT. Simpler, more compact and less expensive sources such as diode lasers and filtered arc lamps are being developed for use in PDT (**Figure 8.1**).

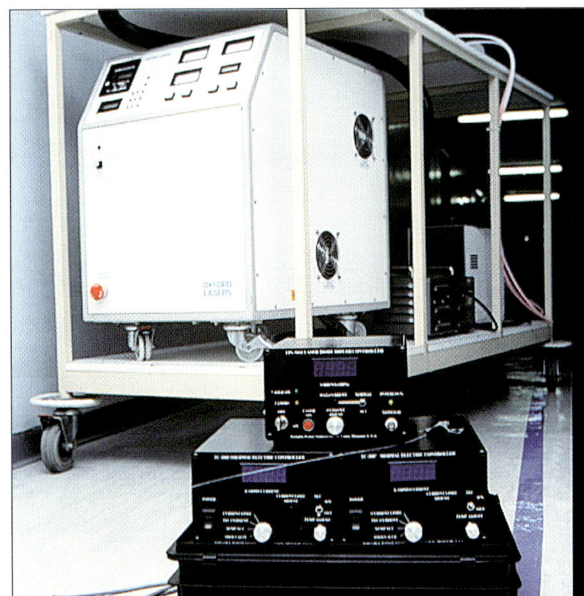

Figure 8.1 Lasers used to deliver red light at 630 nm for photodynamic therapy. Conventional large copper-vapour laser coupled to a tunable dye laser and, in foreground, prototype of new generation diode laser.

Table 8.2

PS + hv	->	$^{1}PS^{*}$
$^{1}PS^{*}$	->	$^{3}PS^{*}$
$^{3}PS^{*} + O_2$	->	$PS + {}^{1}O_2$

Where PS = photosensitiser
hv = light quantum^{1}
PS* = excited singlet state of PS3
PS* = excited triplet state of PS1
O_2 = excited singlet state of oxygen
T = cellular target

Tissue penetration by light

Red light at a wavelength of 630 nm is usually chosen to perform PDT because it has greater tissue penetration than shorter wavelength blue or green light. The limit of about 5 mm is sufficient to allow adequate treatment of skin and epithelial linings by surface illumination. Interstitial light delivery fibres are used for treatment of solid tumours.

Photodynamic effect

In addition to the photosensitiser and light the third element required for successful PDT is molecular oxygen. In the photodynamic process oxygen is converted to the highly toxic activated species termed singlet oxygen.[12] This reaction is described as a type II photochemical reaction (**Table 8.2**).

When light of sufficient energy is absorbed by the sensitiser it triggers the release of singlet oxygen, possibly along with other highly reactive intermediates such as free radicals. The result is an irreversible oxidisation of essential cellular components. The destruction of crucial cell membranes, organelles and vasculature leads to cell necrosis.

This mechanism was demonstrated in experiments in which gynaecological tumour cell lines treated in vitro by ALA PDT were examined using electron microscopy.[13] This demonstrated early mitochondrial damage with injury to membranes and the nucleus and complete loss of intracytoplasmic organisation subsequently.

Development of PDT for cancer therapy

In 1972, two American groups commenced experimental laboratory and animal studies of PDT. Diamond and colleagues reported that the administration of haematoporphyrin followed by light therapy proved lethal to glioma cells in culture and produced massive destruction of porphyrin-containing gliomas transplanted subcutaneously in rats.[14] Dougherty demonstrated eradication of a transplanted mouse mammary tumour using Hpd activated by red light from a filtered xenon arc lamp.[15]

Establishment of PDT

By 1978 there was considerable experience in the use of PDT for the treatment of human cancers. A series of malignant tumours were treated using intravenous Hpd and red laser light.[16] The emphasis in research was on advanced or recurrent cancers unsuitable for curative surgery. The main thrust at this time came from Dougherty who continued to investigate and support PDT for cancer treatment.[12,17] He was instrumental in achieving United States approval for the therapeutic use of Photofrin® in December 1995. Photofrin® is now licensed in a number of countries for treatment of cancer of the lung and oesophagus and for superficial bladder cancer.

Use in gynaecology

The potential use of PDT covers a wide spectrum. Photodynamic therapy may provide an alternative or an adjunctive treatment for gynaecological cancers where other modalities fail. It may also have a place as a less invasive treatment for superficial conditions which are extensive or prove difficult to eradicate. These include pre-malignant lesions such as genital tract intraepithelial neoplasia. Research is now also being directed to benign indications for PDT like endometriosis and menorrhagia.

Treatment of gynaecological malignancy

The early studies in gynaecological PDT were for cancer treatment. Reported patient numbers are small and results variable.

PDT for advanced cancers

To be suitable for PDT, tumours must be accessible for light delivery, such as skin metastases[16,18,19] and vulval,[19,20] vaginal[18,19,21] or vault[22] tumours. In the advanced state these cancers pose a difficult surgical problem yet are well situated for PDT. Treatment by PDT may help to alleviate distressing symptoms of haemorrhage or discharge which are often associated with extensive, surface cancers. As with any new, unproven cancer therapy PDT was initially employed for disease resistant to conventional methods. The first treatment was for an ulcerating tumour.[7] Considerable experience of PDT in advanced gynaecological malignancy has been gained in several centres.[18–23] Direct illumination is used in most cases[21] and for larger tumours access for light delivery is by multiple interstitial fibre placements.[22]

Peritoneal carcinomatosis

Disseminated malignant disease within the peritoneal cavity is a difficult clinical problem usually resistant to therapeutic efforts. Radiotherapy and chemotherapy may benefit some patients but the rate of treatment-related toxic side-effects can be high. PDT is well suited for the treatment of superficial peritoneal cancer deposits due to the relatively easy access throughout the peritoneal cavity via fibreoptic techniques during laparoscopy or laparotomy.[24] The free application of photosensitiser may not be optimal for widely disseminated peritoneal disease and attempts to improve photosensitiser localisation have used carrier systems such as liposomes or antibodies.[25]

PDT as adjunctive treatment

Ovarian carcinomas are frequently large at presentation and surgical debulking is considered an integral part of PDT in the abdominal cavity to reduce tumour volume. The smaller size allows complete penetration of the neoplasm by light to activate the photosensitiser. Preliminary results are available from an ongoing study at the National Cancer Institute (NCI) of the United States.[26] Photofrin® was given intravenously from 48–72 h prior to debulking laparotomy and intraperitoneal 630 nm laser light. Dilute Intralipid® was used as a scattering medium and the limit of tumour treatment was up to 5 mm diameter. Six of 23 patients remained free of disease for up to 18 months. These promising results are also supported by a small study from Austria.[27] The advantage of the ready accessibility of the peritoneal cavity is offset by its geometric complexity, which makes light dosimetry difficult to calculate. Research on the optimum methods of intraperitoneal light delivery continues.

Treatment of pre-malignant conditions

Condyloma acuminatum due to human papillomavirus (HPV) infection are often widespread in the lower female genital tract. Results of treatment are disappointing and relapse is common. Intraepithelial neoplasia may likewise be widespread and extremely difficult to treat. There has been a trend away from CO_2 laser destructive therapy of extensive cervical (CIN) and vulval intraepithelial neoplasia (VIN).

Condyloma acuminatum

It was postulated that selective photosensitiser uptake might occur in condylomatous epithelium, as well as in tumour tissue. This uptake was confirmed for topical ALA-induced PpIX in vulval condylomata.[28] A pilot study of ALA PDT treatment for genital warts in males and females was recently reported.[29] Locally applied 20% ALA in gel was covered by gauze which was in turn occluded under plastic and fixed with tape. After 16 h the area was exposed to 630 nm light in a dose of up to $100\,J.cm^{-2}$. Two thirds of patients in this small study showed a complete response. A major drawback was pain during illumination.

Cervical intraepithelial neoplasia

A modified cervical loop biopsy with a larger diathermy loop is now mainly used to treat CIN by excision of the transformation zone (LLETZ).[30] Because LLETZ is so effective there have been few attempts to develop other techniques. The excisional technique however may be complicated by bleeding, pain and infection. These problems are less likely using PDT, which is also a simpler procedure whose potential was shown by Lipson's early studies.[4]

Research is in progress at a few centres into this application of PDT.[31,32] Typically, the photosensitiser can be applied to the cervix using a device such as a contraceptive cap containing photosensitiser in a viscous hydrogel. This method has been shown to induce selective fluorescence in dysplastic tissues using ALA (**Figures 8.2A & 8.2B**).[31] Attempts have been made to treat CIN using a topical photosensitiser combined with laser light via a purpose-made delivery system. Published results do not match the results of standard treatment methods.[32]

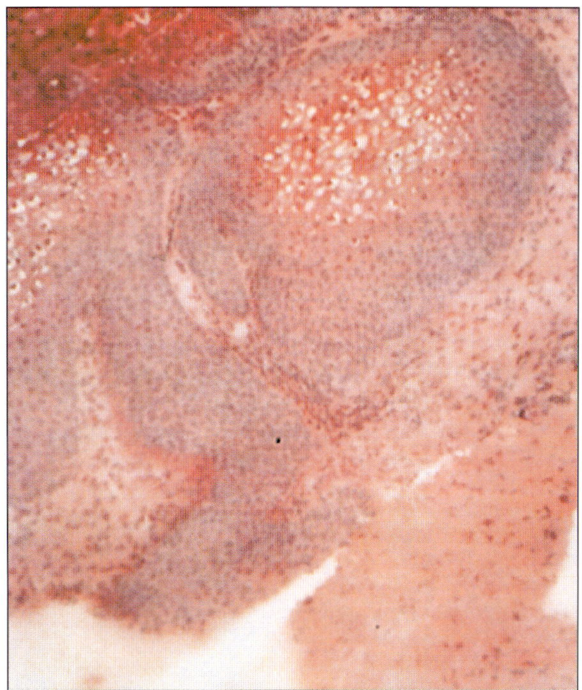

Figure 8.2A Cervical dysplasia seen under H&E microscopy.

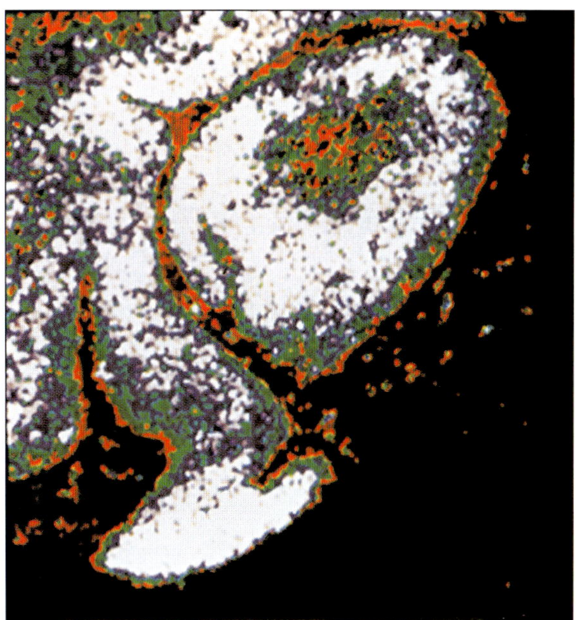

Figure 8.2B Cervical dysplasia seen by quantitative fluorscence.

Vulval intraepithelial neoplasia

The management of VIN presents a more difficult clinical dilemma. Although there is a small risk of progression to invasive disease, this cannot be accurately predicted and the performance of radical procedures offer no guarantee of cure. PDT may offer a simpler and less disfiguring method of treatment with a good success rate. A complete response in over 80% of women after 1–3 treatments was reported in one study.[33] This was not replicated in a more recent clinical series in which less than 40% showed clearance of disease by biopsy at 12 weeks.[32] There are also disparate reports regarding the tolerability of VIN treatment. In one study multiple treatments were well tolerated.[33] The author's unreported findings are in keeping with the experience of others[29] in that vulval treatments can be intensely painful.

PDT in benign gynaecology

The endometrium has enormous regenerative power which is reflected in the clinical challenges of endometriosis and endometrial ablation for menorrhagia. Both of these conditions are the subject of ongoing research in PDT.

Endometriosis

The diagnosis of endometriosis is usually made by visual identification of typical peritoneal lesions. It is often difficult to detect all the affected areas and as a result treatment may be inadequate. Animal studies suggested a role for PDT in both the diagnosis and treatment of endometriosis. Successful photodiagnosis was demonstrated in rabbits with surgically-induced endometriosis[34] and using a model created by intraperitoneal seeding of endometrial cells.[35]

Photosensitising agents, including tetracycline hydrochloride, tamoxifen citrate and clomiphene citrate were shown to elicit variable degrees of fluorescence that were hard to detect with the naked eye and could only be recorded by use of time-lapse photography. The activating light for these compounds (wavelength 350 nm) is strongly absorbed by haemoglobin and results in poor tissue penetration.

Histologic examination of transplants revealed that fluorescence, when it did occur, was localised to transplants with active endometrium and not to those with obliterative fibrosis, suggesting that the concept of fluorescence induction in endometriosis may be valuable for differentiating areas of viable endometriosis from old fibrotic lesions.

Treatment of experimental endometriosis

Studies of endometriosis are restricted because humans and higher primates are the only species in which this disorder occurs naturally. Nearly all surgically-induced animal models of endometriosis have used autotransplantation of uterine or endometrial patches to the peritoneal cavity. Such a model was used in rabbits[36,37] and rats[38] to investigate PDT destruction of endometriosis. Separate studies using Photofrin®,[36] Hpd[37] and ALA[38] have shown a high degree of destruction in endometrial transplants.

Risk of damage to surrounding tissue

Concern has been raised about the risk of damage to surrounding tissue during generalised intraperitoneal exposure to photoactivating light to treat endometriosis. Damage might occur if there was a significant uptake of photosensitiser in normal tissue. This may be the case for Photofrin® thus precluding its use intraperitoneally without directing light onto specific lesions.[39] Selection of an appropriate photosensitiser may give a better differential accumulation. Use of ALA was shown to give fluorescence in rat endometrial implants which was twice as bright as that seen in peritoneum.[38] Whether this is sufficient to enable safe human use is uncertain and no human studies of PDT in endometriosis have been reported to date. Normal tissue surrounding rabbit endometriotic lesions that had been exposed to HpD and to light was unaffected.[37] There is also a lack of reports of ancillary damage during PDT for ovarian malignancy.[26]

Dysfunctional uterine bleeding

Current methods for endometrial ablation generally require anaesthesia and despite meticulous technique about 1 in 5 women subsequently need hysterectomy. PDT is simple to perform and may give better results because of endometrial targeting.

PDT endometrial ablation

Ten years ago, it was shown that the photosensitiser dihematoporphyrin ether (DHE) was preferentially taken up by the endometrial layer of the estrogen-primed rat uterus.[40] Photoradiation of the uterine surface 72 h after DHE administration caused selective coagulation necrosis in the entire endometrium and the inner part of the muscularis of the PDT-treated right uterine horn only.[41]

This report was followed by successful PDT endometrial ablation in rabbits, which also have a double uterus providing a convenient treatment and control uterine horn in each animal.[42] Photofrin® was taken up and retained preferentially by the endometrium, with the greatest concentration observed in the stroma. Despite the rabbit's relatively thin myometrium, full thickness uterine destruction was not seen in any case.

Intrauterine photosensitiser
As a means of minimising photosensitiser-induced skin sensitivity topical administration in rats was investigated. Intrauterine Photofrin® provided better uptake and distribution at lower drug doses than intravenous or intraperitoneal administration.[39] There was selective endometrial fluorescence from intrauterine ALA and light exposure produced endometrial ablation.[43] Some glandular elements resisted treatment, yet no regeneration of endometrium was evident at 10 days. The functional effect was confirmed by demonstrating a profoundly decreased rate of implantation in treated uterine horns.[44]

Further animal studies
Intrauterine benzoporphyrin derivative (BPD)[45] and ALA[46] were used for substantial, persistent endometrial destruction in rats and rabbits.[45,46] The larger rabbit uterine horns required multiple, segmental irradiation resulting in uneven light dosimetry. This may have accounted for the variations in re-epithelialisation which were found after irradiation. Monkeys demonstrated endometrial PpIX fluorescence following ALA administration via a needle into the uterine fundus, transcervically or by intravenous injection[47]. Peak fluorescence occurred 4–5 h after injection and decreased gradually to less than 20% of peak value at 8 h.

First human studies
The author investigated the use of ALA PDT of the endometrium in model systems and in a series of patients.[48] ALA was introduced into the cavities of perfused ex vivo uteri. Measurement demonstrated PpIX formation in the endometrium at ten times the concentration of PpIX in the underlying myometrium. A minimal amount of ALA passed through into the perfusate making systemic photosensitisation unlikely. When ALA was administered to patients scheduled for hysterectomy similar results were found (**Figure 8.3**).

In clinical studies, a customised light delivery system was constructed using a balloon cataheter with the end replaced by a shaped latex balloon (**Figure 8.4**). A silica fibre inside the catheter terminated in a cylindrical diffusing section within the balloon.[49] The 630 nm light was generated by pumping a dye laser with the output from a copper vapour laser (**Figure 8.1**). A prescribed light dose of 50 J.cm^{-2} was delivered at a rate of 30 mW.cm^{-2}, with 2 catheter placements ensuring treatment of the entire endometrial surface in less than 30 min.[50]

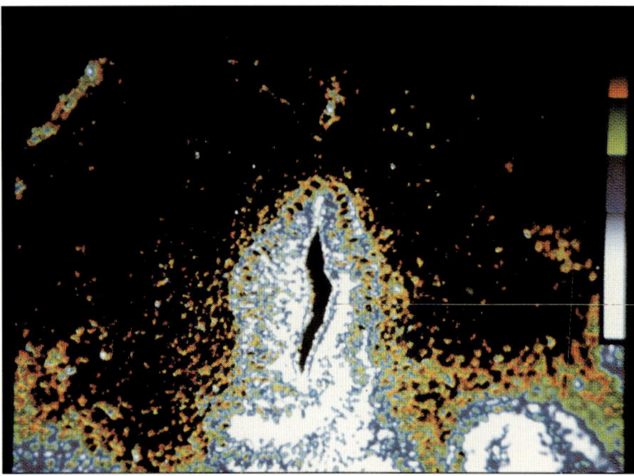

Figure 8.3 Fluorescence microscopy shows an endometrial gland in an ALA treated uterus.

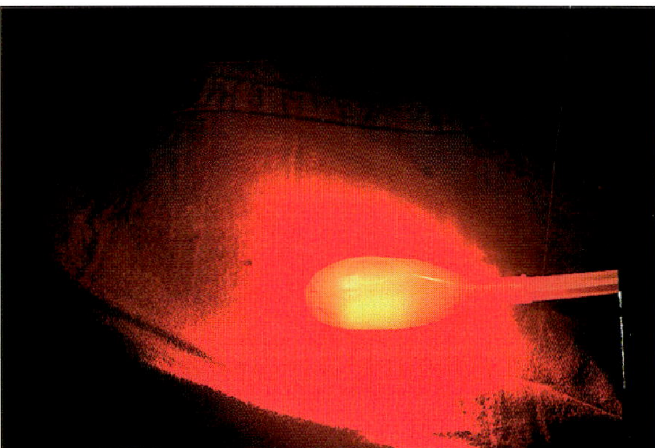

Figure 8.4 Intrauterine balloon laser delivery system for photodynamic therapy.

Summary

Successful PDT depends on the critical interaction of several complex, interrelated factors. These include tissue thickness which determines penetration of both drugs and light. Manipulation of tissue depth may be either medical as for endometrium or surgical as in peritoneal cancer. The choice of photosensitiser, vehicle and route of administration will vary depending on the pathology and site being treated. There has been a trend towards topical photosensitiser administration for accessible lesions. Various purpose-made devices are becoming available for the treatment of the uterine cavity and cervix etc. Perhaps the biggest recent advance which will allow more widespread use of PDT is the development of a new generation of compact diode lasers capable of producing light at more than 600 nm on a narrow wavelength. There is an increased interest in PDT across a wide spectrum of specialties.[51] The technique, which started as a cancer treatment, is now entering a new era in benign gynaecology.

REFERENCES

1. Policard A. Etude sur les aspects offerts par des tumeurs experimentales examinees a la lumiere de Wood. *C R Soc Biol* 1924; **91**: 1423–1424.
2. Figge FHJ, Weiland GS, Manganiello LOJ. Cancer detection and therapy: Affinity of neoplastic, embryonic and traumatised tissues for porphyrins and metalloporphyrins. *Proc Soc Exper Biol & Med* 1948; **68**: 640–641.
3. Lipson RL, Baldes EJ, Olsen AM. The use of derivative of haematoporphyrin in tumor detection. *J Natl Cancer Inst* 1961; **26**: 1–11.
4. Lipson RL, Pratt JH, Baldes EJ, Dockerty MB. Hematoporphyrin derivative for detection of cervical cancer. *Obstet Gynecol* 1964; **24**: 78–84.
5. Gray MJ, Lipson RL, Van S Maeck J, Parker L, Romeyn D. Use of hematoporphyrin derivative in detection and management of cervical cancer. A preliminary report. *Am J Obstet Gynecol* 1967; **99**: 766–771.
6. Kyriazis GA, Balin H, Lipson RL. Haematoporphyrin-derivative-fluorescence test colposcopy and colpophotography in the diagnosis of atypical metaplasia, dysplasia, and carcinoma in situ of the cervix uteri. *Am J Obstet Gynecol* 1973; **117**: 375–380.
7. Lipson RL, Gray MJ, Baldes EJ. Haematoporphyria derivative for detectionand management of cancer. *Proc 9th Int Cancer Congr* 1966; 393.
8. Kennedy JG, Pottier RH. Endogenous protoporphyrin IX, a clinically useful photosensitizer for photodynamic therapy. *J Photochem Photobiol B: Biol* 1992; **14**: 275–292.
9. Mustajoki P, Timonen K, Gorchein A, Seppalainen AM, Matikainen E, Tenhunen R. Sustained high plasma 5–aminolaevulinic acidconcentration in a volunteer: no porphyric symptoms. *Euro J Clin Invest* 1992; **22**: 407–411.

10. Fritsch C, Verwohlt B, Bolsen K, Ruzicka T, Goerz G. Influence of topical photodynamic therapy with 5–aminolevulinic acid on porphyrin metabolism. *Arch Dermatol Res* 1996; **288**: 517–521.

11. Fehr MK, Madsen SJ, Svaasand LO et al. Intrauterine light delivery for photodynamic therapy of the human endometrium. *Hum Reprod* 1995; **10**: 3067–3072.

12. Dougherty TJ. Photodynamic therapy (PDT) of malignant tumours. *Crit Rev Oncol Hematol* 1984; **2**: 83–116.

13. Rossi FM, Campbell DL, Pottier RH, Kennedy JC, Dickson EF. In vitro studies on the use of 5–aminolaevulinic acid-mediated photodynamic therapy for gynaecological tumours. *Br J Cancer* 1996; **74**: 881–887.

14. Diamond I, McDonagh AF, Wilson CB, Granelli SG, Nielsen S, Jaenicke R. Photodynamic therapy of malignant tumours. *Lancet* 1972; **ii**: 1175–1177.

15. Dougherty TJ. Activated dyes as anti-tumor agents. *J Natl Cancer Inst* 1974; **51**: 1333–1336.

16. Dougherty TJ, Kaufman JE, Goldfarb A, Weishaupt KR, Boyle D, Mittleman A. Photoradiation therapy for the treatment of malignant tumors. *Cancer Res* 1978; **38**: 2628–2635.

17. Dougherty TJ. Photosensitization of malignant tumors. *Sem Surg Oncol* 1986; **2**: 24–37.

18. Rettenmaier MA, Berman ML, DiSaia PJ, Burns RG, Berns MW. Photoradiation therapy of gynecologic malignancies. *Gynecol Oncol* 1984; **17**: 200–206.

19. Lobraico RV, Waldow SM, Harris DM, Shuber S. Photodynamic therapy for cancer of the lower female genital tract. *Colposcopy Gynecol Laser Surg* 1986; **2**: 185–199.

20. Dahlman A, Wile AG, Burns RG, Mason GR, Johnson FM, Berns MW. Laser photoradiation therapy of cancer. *Cancer Res* 1983; **43**: 430–434.

21. Soma H, Akiya K, Nutahara S, Kato H, Hayata Y. Treatment of vaginal carcinoma with laserphotoirradiation following administration of haematoporphyrin derivative. *Ann Chir Gynaecol* 1982; **71**: 133–136.

22. Ward BG, Forbes IJ, Cowled PA, McEvoy MM, Cox LW. The treatment of vaginal recurrences of gynecologic malignancy with phototherapy following hematoporphyrin derivative pretreatment. *Am J Obstet Gynecol* 1982; **142**: 356–357.

23. McCaughan JS, Schellhas HF, Lomano J. Photodynamic therapy of gynaecologic neoplasia after presensitization with hematoporphyrin derivative. *Lasers Surg Med* 1985; **5**: 491–498.

24. Tochner Z, Mitchell JB, Harrington FS, Smith P, Russo DT, Russo A. Treatment of murine intraperitoneal ovarian ascitic tumor with haematoporphyrin derivative and laser light. *Cancer Res* 1985; **45**: 2983–2987.

25. Goff BA, Hermanto U, Rumbaugh J, Blake J, Bamberg M, Hasan T. Photoimmunotherapy and biodistribution with an OC125–chlorinimmunoconjugate in an in vivo murine ovarian cancer model. *Br J Cancer* 1994; **70**: 474–480.

26. Sindelar WF, DeLaney TF, Tochner Z et al. Technique of photodynamic therapy for disseminated intraperitoneal malignant neoplasms. Phase I study. *Arch Surg* 1991; **126**: 318–324.

27. Wierrani F, Fiedler D, Grin W et al. Clinical effect of meso-tetrahydroxyphenylchlorine based photodynamic therapy in recurrent carcinoma of the ovary: preliminary results. *Br J Obstet Gynaecol* 1997; **104**: 376–378.

28. Fehr MK, Chapman CF, Krasieva T et al. Selective photosensitizer distribution in vulvar condyloma acuminatum after topical application of 5–aminolevulinic acid. *Am J Obstet Gynecol* 1996; **174**: 951–957.

29. Frank RGJ, Bos JD, vd Meulen FW, Sterenborg HJCM. Photodynamic therapy for condylomata acuminata with local application of 5 aminolevulinic acid. *Genitourin Med* 1996; **72**: 70–71.

30. Prendeville W, Cullimore J, Norman S. Large loop excision of transformation zone (LLETZ): a new method of management for women with cervical intraepithelial neoplasia. *Br J Obstet Gynaecol* 1989; **96**: 1054–1060.

31. Haller JC, Roberts DJH, Lane G, Brown SB, Cairnduff F. Distribution of ALA-induced PpIX in cervical intra-epithelial neoplasia (CIN). *Proc 7th Int Photodynamic Ass Congr* 1998; 110.

32. Martin-Hirsch PL, Whitehurst C, Buckley CH, Moore JV, Kitchener HC. Photodynamic treatment for lower genital tract intraepithelial neoplasia. *Lancet* 1998; **351**: 1403.

33. Lobraico RV, Grossweiner LI. Thermal lasers and photodynamic therapy in gynaecology. In: Spinelli P, Dal Fante M, Marchesini R, eds. Photodynamic therapy and biomedical lasers, Amsterdam, *Elsevier Science*, 1992; 37–41.

34. Vancaille TG, Hill RH, Riehl RM, Gilstad D, Schenken RS. Laser-induced fluorescence of ectopic endometrium in rabbits. *Obstet Gynecol* 1989; **74**: 225–230.

35. Manyak MJ, Nelson LM, Solomon D, DeGraff W, Stillman RJ, Russo A. Fluorescent detection of rabbit endometrial implants resulting from monodispersed viable cell suspensions. *Fertil Steril* 1990; **54**: 356–359.

36. Manyak MJ, Nelson LM, Solomon D, Russo A,Thomas GF, Stillman RJ. Photodynamic therapy of rabbit endometrial transplants: a model for treatment of endometriosis. *Fertil Steril* 1989; **52**: 140–145.

37. Petrucco OM, Sathenanden M, Petrucco MF et al. Ablation of endometriotic implants in rabbits by hematoporphyrin derivative photoradiation therapy using the gold vapor laser. *Laser Surg Med* 1990; **10**: 344–348.

38. Yang JZ, Van Dijk-Smith JP, Van Vugt DA, Kennedy JC, Reid RL. Fluorescence and photosensitization of experimental endometriosis in the rat after systemic 5–aminolevulinic acid administration: A potential new approach to the diagnosis and treatment endometriosis. *Am J Obstet Gynecol* 1996; **174**: 154–160.

39. Chapman JA, Tadir Y, Tromberg BJ et al. Effect of administration route and estrogen manipulation on endometrial uptake of Photofrin porfimer sodium. *Am J Obstet Gynecol* 1993; **168**: 685–692

40. Schneider DF, Schellhas HF, Wesseler TA, Chen I-W, Moulton BC. Haematoporphyrin derivative uptake in uteri of estrogen-treated ovariectomized rats. *Colposcopy Gynecol Laser Surg* 1988; **4**: 67–72.

41. Schneider DF, Schellhas HF, Wesseler TA, Moulton BC. Endometrial ablation by DHE photoradiation therapy in estrogen-treated ovariectomized rats. *Colposcopy Gynecol Laser Surg* 1988; **4**: 73–77.

42. Bhatta N, Anderson RR, Flotte T, Schiff I, Hasan T, Nishioka NS. Endometrial ablation by means of photodynamic therapy with photofrin II. *Am J Obstet Gynecol* 1992; **167**: 1856–1863.

43. Yang JZ, Van Vugt DA, Kennedy JC, Reid RL. Intrauterine 5–aminolevulinic acid induces selective fluorescence and photodynamic ablation of the rat endometrium. *Photochem Photobiol* 1993; **57**: 803–807.

44. Yang JZ, Van Vugt DA, Kennedy JC, Reid RL. Evidence of lasting functional destruction of the rat endometrium after 5–aminolevulinic acid-induced photodynamic ablation: Prevention of implantation. *Am J Obstet Gynecol* 1993; **168**: 995–1001.

45. Wyss P, Tadir Y, Tromberg BJ et al. Benzoporphyrin derivative (BPD): a potent photosensitizer for photodynamic destruction of the rabbit endometrium. *Obstet Gynecol* 1994; **84**: 409–414.

46. Wyss P, Tromberg BJ, Wyss MT et al. Photodynamic destruction of endometrial tissue with topical 5–aminolevulinic acid in rats and rabbits. *Am J Obstet Gynecol* 1994; **171**: 1176–1183.

47. Yang JZ, Van Vugt DA, Roy BN, Kennedy JC, Foster WG, Reid RL. Intrauterine 5–aminolaevulinic acid induces selective endometrial fluorescence in the rhesus and cynomolgus monkey. *J Soc Gynecol Invest* 1996; **3**: 152–157.

48. Gannon MJ, Johnson N, Roberts DJH et al. Photosensitization of the endometrium with topical 5–aminolevulinic acid. *Am J Obstet Gynecol* 1995; **173**: 1826–1828.

49. Stringer MR, Hudson EJ, Dunkley CP, Boyce JC,Gannon MJ, Smith MA. Light delivery schemes for uterine photodynamic therapy. In: Jori G, Moan J, Star WM, eds. *Photodynamic therapy of cancer, Proc SPIE* 1994; **2078**: 41–49.

50. Gannon MJ, Vernon DI, Holroyd JA, Stringer M, Johnson N, Brown SB. PDT of the endometrium using ALA. *Proc SPIE* 1997; **2972**: 2–13.

51. Rowe PM. Photodynamic therapy begins to shine. (Feature) *Lancet* 1998; **351**: 1496.

9

Virtual Reality Surgery

N. McClure
A. G. Gallagher
J. McGuigan

Introduction

Many surgeons think that virtual reality surgery is simply gynaecology by a different name. This, of course, is not so. Pinciroli and Valenza defined virtual reality as "an effective simulation of complex environmental aspects related to both interaction-dependent and higher risk operations, where mistakes will lead to unacceptable consequences."[1] Whilst some might argue that the world's religions provided the first virtual reality scenarios, the first recognised description of a virtual reality system comes from the 1600s in Leibniz's "Palace of the Fates."[2] Here, he presented an organised system of virtual worlds available for human perceptual exploration along with an interface for exploring them. Virtual reality has only become a reality in itself, though, with the development of high-powered, sophisticated computers and software. The potential roles for virtual reality in surgery will be explored in this chapter both in training and surgical practice. Clearly, the main advantage of virtual reality in skills acquisition is that it provides a safe and simulated environment where no patient can be damaged. Thus, operator flexibility and performance during actual surgical procedures can be rehearsed and improved.

The virtual reality world and the operator can interface in three ways.[3] The commonest uses a computer desktop environment. Here, the operator watches a computer screen and interacts with the environment he sees thereon. Alternatively, a visual head mounted display can be used which isolates the operator from the surrounding environment. This, then, imposes unnatural social and physical constraints on the user. Thirdly, it is possible to synthesise real and virtual realities within a life-size environment. This has the advantage that the simulator is not isolationist and the operator can truly interact with his virtual environment. In effect, this third group often represents a mixture of virtual reality and simulation.

Many other professions have already embraced virtual reality. For example, flight simulators are a major part of the training of airline pilots. These simulators produce a life-size environment. Thus, they are extremely expensive but, nonetheless, extremely realistic. It is possible to programme in the characteristics of any individual aeroplane, and from the cockpit, to give a visual display of the runways of any individual airport. Environmental factors can be adjusted and emergencies artificially simulated. Fire fighters, similarly, can use virtual reality systems to learn spatial navigation. For example, 35 fighters from Madison County, Alabama, were randomised to receive conventional blueprint training, no training and virtual reality training for navigation through the Administrative Science Building.[4] They were then tasked to retrieve a mock baby from the building. Those trained in the virtual reality and blueprint groups made significantly fewer wrong turns and reached their target significantly faster than the untrained group.

Within medicine, virtual reality extends from the creation of virtual humans through to the creation of relatively simple computer surgical training tasks. However, all virtual reality systems are limited by the computer power. In the USA, army medical services now utilise remote sensors, intelligent systems, telepresence surgery and virtual reality simulations as routine parts of training and field work in combat casualty care.[5] Scarborough *et al* have produced a 3–dimensional virtual reality image of the embryonic heart from computerised tomography and magnetic resonance imaging scans.[6] This has been utilised for both training and the study of heart development.

Virtual reconstruction

The virtual reconstruction of body organs for diagnosis from radiological images has also been reported. Merkle *et al* have produced 3–dimensional virtual bladders from helical CT scan data on a graphic computer workstation.[7] They then compared diagnoses made from these images with those obtained by fibre-optic cystoscopy in real time:

results were very similar. Clearly, though, much more extensive evaluation will be necessary before real-time images are replaced with virtual computer graphic images in diagnosis. Wagner *et al* described interventional video tomography.[8] Here, a virtual visualisation of anatomical structures is obtained in 3-dimensions for intraoperative-stereotactic navigation. This is then orthotopically coregistered to the surgical field in a head-mounted display giving the surgeon visual access to nonvisual anatomy. Robb *et al* similarly reported the creation of 3–dimensional medical images from 'fly-through' CT or MRI scans.[9] Black *et al* reported how at Brigham and Women's Hospital Boston, the Brain Tumour Group is using such reconstructions to identify the tumor's proximity to the sagittal and other sinuses as well as the presence of vascular feeders and major vessels.[10] Klaue *et al* reported the application of similar techniques to orthopaedic surgery; preoperative assessment is considerably enhanced and the effects of surgical osteotomies can be predicted.[11] Virtual reality has even been reported in the treatment of males with erectile dysfunction,[12] however, subjects had to be over 18!

Clearly, the reconstruction of body parts into a virtual image can provide satisfactory visual stimuli for diagnosis. However for surgery, auditory, proprioceptive and haptic stimuli must also be provided. In a virtual reality scenario, auditory stimuli are relatively easy to reproduce. Haptic, or tactile feedback can be reproduced but this requires considerable computer power if it is to be generated successfully. Proprioceptive stimuli are the most difficult to reproduce; they depend on information from a variety of sources including the inner ear. If virtual reality systems are to be applied to endoscopic surgery, all of these stimuli must be satisfied. This would require vast amounts of computer power. Thus the concept of virtual humans who require virtual operations in virtual environments is still a long way off. By contrast, computer-augmented surgery is much closer. Troccaz *et al* proposed the use of virtual reality in the design of new surgical approaches, evaluating the downstream effects in a virtual reality environment.[13]

Training and virtual reality

If we are some way from virtual operations then what of virtual reality in training? In the past, surgical training has traditionally been by apprenticeship. Junior doctors travel from hospital to hospital spending up to one year with individual consultants before moving on to a different firm. There are many benefits from such a system; as juniors progress in their training they absorb much of the experience their trainers have acquired in their own professional careers. However, the acquisition of basic core surgical skills is not so well served, as they can only be acquired on living subjects with medical problems requiring treatment. Thus, juniors who are slower to learn or who are attached to a surgeon who is not a good teacher of core skills can find themselves disadvantaged (as are their patients). In response to this problem, the various Surgical Colleges in the United Kingdom have introduced a Basic Surgical Skills Course. This is only of 3 days duration and gives only the broadest overview of core skills. The students are under pressure to perform, as the skills are practised in front of their peers and superiors in open forum. The Royal College of Obstetricians and Gynaecologists has similar plans to produce a Basis Surgical Skills course for gynaecologists.

Much of the training on these courses is in the laboratory, using pieces of animal flesh or plastics of varying kinds designed to simulate parts of the human body. In mainland Europe and the USA it is still possible to learn surgical skills by practising on animals. This, however, is illegal in the United Kingdom. Anaesthetists now have very advanced mannequins which they place in mock operating theatres. The mannequins have heart and breath sounds. There is a full read-out of electronic data simulating that obtained from routine monitoring of patients in theatre. Injections can be given, their nature and volume being determined by a bar-code reader. Thus, a computer can calculate the effect this will have on the patient and induce the necessary changes on the monitor read-outs. This is an excellent system for training but again utilises simulation rather than virtual reality.

In training for endoscopic surgery, pelvic and abdominal simulators have been utilised for some time. These, however, have significant limitations. They are expensive, especially if plastic body parts are used in the training tasks. Diathermy cannot be performed. There is no objective measure of performance quality or success. It is not possible, unless the episode has been video recorded, for a supervisor to review the standard of performance unless the supervisor is with the trainee throughout the procedure. This is intimidating for the trainee.

Virtual reality trainers, by contrast, are based on computer systems. Therefore, training sessions can be recorded, proper targets can be set and performance can be assessed both in terms of accuracy and successful completion of tasks set. However, until recently, the major limiting factor in virtual reality trainers has been limitations imposed by the computer size and power. Surgeons have been reluctant to utilise trainers that did not provide accurate tissue simulation. This is an error. Particularly in endoscopy, surgical practice can be broken down into a series of defined functions, for example, grasping, cutting and the ballistic movements necessary for the application of diathermy. In order to acquire these skills it is not necessary to have tissue simulation. In fact, removing the task from a simulated clinical environment removes distractions for the trainee and they are, therefore, better able to focus on the individual skill.

MIST VR system

A variety of virtual reality training systems have been reported. The Karlsruhe trainer was reported by Kuhnapfel *et al.*[14] Playter and Raibert reported a system for training in endoscopic suturing.[15] Whilst this system is unique in that it provides haptic feedback it is still not commercially available.

The MIST VR system has been developed by Wilson *et al.*[16] This system has removed all traces of tissue simulation. Computer generated images are combined with real-time movement. Two standard instrument handles are supported in a frame. Their movement is replicated exactly on the screen as if the active ends were within the body cavity. Therefore, the fulcrum effect of the body wall on the instruments is captured. The target image is a ball which must initially be grasped. This allows the candidate to practice ballistic movements. Once touched, the ball reappears within a grid. Attached to it are four cubes and these must, in turn, be diathermied off. The tasks are staged and have defined goals which increase in complexity. By the final task trainees must perform all of the hand-eye co-ordination exercises in a recognised sequence. Clearly there is immediate proximal feedback. Thus practice and assessment can be performed anywhere at any time. Further more, the play-back facility allows trainees to visualise their performance and for remote assessment by the training supervisor.

Theoretically, the MIST VR training system should translate to good endoscopic surgical practice. To investigate this, Gallagher *et al* randomly assigned 16 laparoscopically naive trainees to receive either MIST VR or no training.[17] The performance of the subjects was then compared using a basic laparoscopic cutting task. Each candidate was given ten 2-min trials. The performance of the MIST VR group was consistently, significantly better than the untrained group. This study has been subsequently repeated comparing subjects who were randomised to receive no training, standard training and MIST VR training (Gallagher, personal communication).[18] Again, the MIST VR group performed consistently better. More importantly, they spontaneously used both hands whilst operating: those from the other two groups operated almost exclusively with their dominant hand.

Conclusion

In conclusion, virtual reality surgery is some way off. Currently, virtual reality is being applied to the generation of anatomical and pathological images obtained from imaging systems. In surgery its major role is in training. Until much more powerful computers are generated it is unlikely that the role of virtual reality will extend much further.

REFERENCES

1. Pinciroli F, Valenza P. An inventory of computer resources for the medical application of virtual-reality. *Computers in Biology and Medicine*, 1995; **25**: 115.
2. Steinhart E. Leibniz's palace of the fates: Seventeenth-century virtual reality system. *Presence-Teleoperators and Virtual Environments*, 1997; **6**: 133.
3. Traill DM, Bowskill JM, Lawrence PJ. Interactive collaborative media environments. *BT Technology Journal* 1997; **15**: 130.
4. Bliss JP, Tidwell PD, Guest MA. The effectiveness of virtual reality for administering spatial navigation training to firefighters. *Presence-Teleoperators and Virtual Environments* 1997; **6**: 73.
5. Satava RM. Virtual-Reality and Telepresence for Military Medicine. *Computers in Biology and Medicine* 1995; **25**: 229.
6. Scarborough J, Aiton JF, McLachlan JC *et al.* The study of early human embryos using interactive 3–dimensional-computer reconstructions. *Journal of Anatomy* 1997; **191**: 117.
7. Merkle EM, Fleiter T, Wunderlich A *et al.* Virtual cystoscopy based on helical CT scan data: First results. *Rofo-Fortschritte Auf Dem Gebiet DerRontgenstrahlen Und Der Bildgebenden Verfahren* 1996; **165**: 582.
8. Wagner A, Ploder O, Enislidis G *et al.* Image-guided Surgery. *International Journal of Oral and Maxillofacial Surgery* 1996; **25**: 147.
9. Robb RA, Aharon S, Cameron BM. Patient-specific anatomic models from 3-dimensional medical image data for clinical applications in surgery and endoscopy. *Journal of Digital Imaging* 1997; **10**: 31.
10. Black PM. Hormones, radiosurgery and virtual reality: new aspects of meningioma management. *Canadian Journal of Neurological Sciences* 1997; **24**: 302.
11. Klaue K, Bresina S, Guelat P *et al.* Morphological 3–dimensional assessment, pre-operative simulation and rationale of intra-operative navigation in orthopaedic surgery: practical application for re-orienting osteotomies of the hip joint. *Injury International Journal of The Care of The Injured* 1997; **28**: 12.
12. Optale G, Munari A, Nasta A *et al.* Multimedia and virtual reality techniques in the treatment of male erectile disorders. *International Journal of Impotence Research* 1997; **9**: 197.
13. Troccaz J, Lavallee S, Cinquin P. Computer-augmented surgery. *Human Movement Science* 1996; **15**: 445.
14. Kuhnapfel UG, Kuhn C, Hubner M *et al.* The Karlsruhe endoscopic surgery trainer as an example for virtual reality in medical education. *Minimally Invasive Therapy & Allied Technologies* 1997; **6**: 122.
15. Playter R, Raibert M. A virtual surgery simulator using advanced haptic feedback. *Minimally Invasive Therapy & Allied Technologies* 1997; **6**: 117.
16. Wilson MS, Middlebrook A, Sutton C *et al.* MIST VR: a virtual reality trainer for laparoscopic surgery assesses performance. *Annals of The Royal College of Surgeons of England* 1997; **79**: 403.
17. Gallagher AG, McClure N, Crothers I *et al.* MIST VR Training: Faster proprioceptive automation to the fulcrum effect for laparoscopic novices. *Gynaecolological Endoscopy* 1997; **6**: 90.
18. Gallagher AG, McClure N. Personal communication, 1998.

10

New Surgical Techniques for the Treatment of Menorrhagia

N. N. Amso
E. Tsakos

Introduction

Menorrhagia is a common problem and it represents a major component of medical workload. Medical treatment is commonly inadequate and ineffective[1] and a great proportion of women eventually have a hysterectomy for an anatomically healthy uterus. Approximately 22%[2] of women are affected by menorrhagia, which accounts for 12–22% of gynaecology referrals.[3] Additionally, 60% of women referred to the gynaecologist with menorrhagia will have a hysterectomy within 5 years of presentation.[4] By the age of 55, 20% of British women have had a hysterectomy, with menorrhagia being the indication in 35–64% of cases.[5] Hysterectomy for menorrhagia has a primary success of 100% and is associated with patient satisfaction rates of approximately 95%.[6]

Hysterectomy, however, regardless of the route by which it is performed, is a major surgical procedure with significant physical and psychological complications. Mortality rates after hysterectomy for benign disorders are about 6 per 10,000[7] and early morbidity (e.g. infection, haemorrhage) is common, occurring in over 40% of women having an abdominal hysterectomy and about 25% following a vaginal hysterectomy.[8]

Short-term problems such as urinary tract and wound infections are common after hysterectomy and major problems such as haemorrhage, bowel and ureteric injury and thromboembolic phenomena are well recognised. Hysterectomy requires a significant length of hospital stay and a period of convalescence of 2–3 months. Long-term consequences include pelvic floor weakness, urinary and bowel dysfunction and also psychosexual problems.[9]

The economic and health service costs are also significant and becoming more pronounced in the UK with the increasing demand for hysterectomy due to menstrual disorders[4] in combination with the financial restraints of the health service. Many women do not want to have a hysterectomy for an anatomically normal uterus and many gynaecologists feel that hysterectomy is probably excessive surgery when the "diseased" organ is only the endometrium.

In recent years, a number of new surgical techniques that aim to destroy the endometrium have been developed and are currently under evaluation. Although the present place of hysteroscopic surgery is mainly as an alternative to hysterectomy when medical management has failed,[10] there is now growing evidence that early hysteroscopic surgery should be considered by women seeking specialist advice for the first time.[11]

Historical background

The first successful hysteroscopy was reported by Pantaleoni in 1869 when he described the examination of a 60-year-old woman with postmenopausal bleeding. He found an endometrial polyp which he cauterised with silver nitrate.[12] The first destruction of the endometrium was attempted by Baumann in 1948 with the blind insertion of steel ball electrodes.[13] However, it was not until the 70s that optical lenses, light sources and distension media were greatly improved and the initial hesitations of surgeons started to dissipate. This resulted in the establishment of diagnostic hysteroscopy and the development of hysteroscopic surgery. In 1971 Droegemueller *et al*[14,15] used nitrous oxide cryosurgery for endometrial ablation. Goldrath[16] published the first endometrial ablation under direct vision with the use of Neodymium: Yttrium Aluminium Garnet (Nd: YAG) laser photovaporisation. Electrosurgical resection techniques were first described by DeCherney and Polan in 1983[17] and the following year the same group[18] reported the use of the resectoscope to ablate the endometrium. Lin[19] and Vaincaillie[20] were the first to describe a hysteroscopic method of ablating the endometrium with the rollerball. Radiofrequency-induced hyperthermia was later reported by Phipps in 1990.[21]

Hysteroscopic techniques of endometrial destruction aim to destroy tissue to the level of the basal glands which are invariably present within the myometrium and thus resection should therefore include 2–3 mm of myometrium as well. This will result in fibrosis and produce a "therapeutic" Asherman's syndrome[22] within the endometrial cavity resulting in amelioration of menstrual symptoms. These techniques were initially employed by pioneers in specialised centres but are now carried out by a large number of gynaecologists. At present, such treatments have a recognised place in the management of abnormal menstrual loss.

Transcervical resection of the endometrium (TCRE)

In TCRE, the diathermy resectoscope, which is a modification of the prostatic resectoscope is used. This is comprised of a 26 French gauge unmodified continuous flow resectoscope fitted with a 4 mm forward-oblique telescope. Most surgeons prefer an 8 mm cutting loop which, when inserted in its full radius, cuts out tissue of 4 mm depth and destroys the endometrium to a further depth of 2–3 mm.[23] The use of a 4 mm loop avoids the repeat pass with the increased risks of perforation and/or thermal damage. The 4 mm loop may be preferred, especially by beginners, for areas of restricted access such as the tubal ostial areas and, if passed through once, is less likely to perforate the uterus. The recently introduced 6 mm loops are preferred by some as a compromise.

Currently, the loop is a monopolar device in which the electric current passes through the loop electrode attached to the operating hysteroscope. A non-electrolyte medium such as glycine 1.5% is used via the inner inflow sheath for distension of the uterine cavity.

An intrauterine pressure of 80–120 mmHg is usually required. The aim is to maintain adequate uterine cavity distension providing a better view and greater safety whilst avoiding excessively high pressures which increase the risk of fluid overload. Appropriate intrauterine pressure can be achieved by simple gravity alone or with the additional help of a sphygmomanometer cuff inflated around the bag. Alternatively, a commercially available irrigation pump may be used. Flux of irrigant is achieved by continuous suction through the outer sheath of the hysteroscope with a negative pressure of -50 mmHg.

Constant monitoring of fluid balance by a dedicated member of the theatre staff is mandatory. Fluid absorption during TCRE depends on a number of factors such as: the use of thinning agents for endometrial preparation, the size of the loop used, the state of the tubes (patent or occluded), and also the duration of surgery and intrauterine pressure. Fluid absorption is increased further if hysteroscopic myomectomy is performed exposing wider areas of the endometrial vascular bed. Glycine is a non-physiological solution and therefore in the event of increased absorption electrolyte disturbance such as hyponatraemia occurs (**Table 10.1**).

The endometrium is excised in a systematic manner starting at the cornua followed by the fundus, postero-laterally and finally the anterior uterine wall. The diathermy current used is a mixture of cutting (100 W) and coagulation (50 W) electrical energy. The depth of excision is extended down until the fibres of the superficial myometrium are visible. The depth of destruction depends mainly on the size of the loop, the electrical current used and the time that the tissues are exposed to the

Table 10.1 Effect of fluid absorption and necessary action during hysteroscopic surgery

Volume absorbed	Effect	Action
<1 L	Well tolerated by healthy patients	Continue surgery
1–2 L	Mild hyponatraemia	Complete surgery quickly
<2 L	Severe hyponatraemia	Stop surgery

diathermy energy. Slower movement of the loop and higher power produce greater tissue damage.

Great care needs to be exercised particularly on resecting the tubal ostia where the myometrium may be only 4 mm thick, increasing the risk of perforation. The entire endometrium is treated terminating at the level of the internal cervical os; this requires clear anatomical demarcation or may be marked on the sheath of the hysteroscope at 4 cm from the external cervical os. The depth of cut of the loop is 3–4 mm; thus timing of the TCRE in the immediate post-menstrual phase is ideal, as the endometrial thickness is 3 mm during that time. However, this timing may be difficult from the administrative and logistical point of view. Consequently, endometrial suppression (thinning) agents, such as Danazol or gonadotrophin releasing hormone agonists (GnRH-agonist) may be used pre-operatively to ensure the presence of an atrophic endometrium. This results in easier surgery, homogeneity of endometrial destruction and enhanced effectiveness of the procedure. Recent evidence[24] suggests that following endometrial preparation with GnRH-agonists, TCRE is significantly shorter in duration, easier to perform and results in significantly more patients with amenorrhoea compared to controls.

Due to the autonomic nerve supply of the uterus, TCRE may be performed without general anaesthesia.[25] This may be achieved by giving preoperative sedation and analgesia, intraoperative anxiolytics and analgesia, and para- or/and intra-cervical local anaesthesia. However, the majority of TCREs in the UK are performed under general anaesthesia. Regional anaesthesia (spinal) may be used as an alternative.

When TCRE is performed under local anaesthesia, two major hazards of hysterectomy are avoided, major abdominal surgery and general anaesthesia. This is particularly important for patients in whom hysterectomy has been thought to be undesirable, dangerous or impossible.[26] Postoperative recovery is usually swift and patients may be discharged from hospital within 3–4 h. Therefore, TCRE is an ideal procedure for day-case surgery, whatever type of anaesthesia is used.[27]

Rollerball electrical ablation

A variety of electrodes in variable shapes and sizes are available on the market. A small, 2 mm diameter electrode is more effective than the 4 mm electrode as it has a higher density for a given power. This allows rapid movement and the use of a lower power, which reduces the risk of perforation. Additionally, the smaller electrode allows a wider field of view for the endoscopist. The electrodes vary in shape; a ball-shape has the advantage of being adaptable to endometrial irregularities. Low-wattage coagulation current is used and this balances the need for adequate depth of destruction and surgical speed. Coagulation should be pursued in a systematic fashion maintaining a steady slow pace. Great care should be exercised in coagulating the tubal ostia where complications are more likely to arise.

Nd:YAG laser ablation of the endometrium (ELA)

The Nd:YAG laser has the ability to transmit high power through optical fibres which penetrate the endometrium to a depth of 5 mm ensuring adequate tissue destruction. Other laser modalities such as CO_2, potassium-titanyl-phosphate (KTP) and argon lasers are considered less suitable.

The procedure is performed under general or regional anaesthesia. Physiological saline or Ringer's lactate may be used for uterine distension. Laser energy at a power of at least 50 W of continuous wave is transmitted down quartz fibres of 600–1200 μm diameter passed through a channel of an operating hysteroscope. Power density depends on the diameter of the fibre, with wider fibres having lower power densities. A bare fibre is used with no artificial tip and no coolant channel. It is imperative that laser safety standards should be followed at all times and the operating team are appropriately trained in the use of lasers.

Laser ablation is performed using the dragging technique; the fibre is placed on the surface of the endometrium and parallel furrows are created by firing the laser while the fibre is being withdrawn towards the surgeon. The procedure takes around 30 min in a normal-sized uterus.

Radiofrequency endometrial ablation

The use of tissue hyperthermia (heating tissue above 43°C) has been used for many years in the treatment of malignant disease. Phipps,[21] in 1990, reported on the use of hyperthermia in the treatment of dysfunctional uterine bleeding. The aim of the procedure is to induce cell death. The endometrium is heated for approximately 20 min by a probe releasing radiofrequency electromagnetic energy.

The main difference between this method and TCRE, rollerball ablation or ELA, is that it is not performed under direct hysteroscopic vision. There is no need for a uterine distension medium and therefore no risk of fluid overload.

A conductive angulated probe is placed within the endometrial cavity. An insulated belt electrode placed around the patient's waist ensures a closed circuit by way of a return cable to the radiofrequency source. A 27.12 MHz signal is applied to the thermal probe and the endometrial surface is heated to around 62–65°C for approximately 20 min. The power applied varies, usually between 150–400 W, during the procedure in order to maintain therapeutic temperatures. The radiofrequency generator is combined with the temperature monitoring apparatus and is now available commercially in an all-in-one machine (MENOSTAT, Rocket Medical, Watford, UK).

The patient may be treated under general or regional anaesthesia and the procedure is suited for day case surgery. With the patient in lithotomy, the uterine cavity is sounded, the cervix dilated to 10 mm and the length of the cervical canal estimated using a special angulated probe for the detection of the internal os. The estimated length of the cervical canal is subtracted from the total uterine length. This determines the size of the probe used which should spare the cervical canal from heating. A thermal guard is inserted in the vagina sitting in the fornices; this is held in place with the use of two stay sutures. A safety check is performed before the generator is switched on to ensure there is no contact between the patient and metal. During treatment the probe is rotated slowly by 360°. Severe uterine cramping lasts approximately 6 h and patients are discharged between 8–24 h after the operation. A watery, blood-stained vaginal discharge occurs for a period of 4–6 weeks. A number of non-operator related complications had led to discontinuation of this treatment in some countries[28] until safety issues were addressed.

Complications of hysteroscopic surgery

(1) Operative complications

Uterine perforation and trauma. During cervical dilatation and hysteroscopy the cervix may be traumatised and the uterus perforated with the dilators or the hysteroscope. In the event of perforation the procedure should be immediately abandoned as the perforated uterus cannot hold the distension medium. This is not a serious complication and observation and conservative management is usually all that is needed. Perforation during operative-hysteroscopy however, carries the additional risk of mechanical and/or thermal injury to adjacent structures such as bladder, ureter, bowel and blood vessels. In this case, intra-abdominal damage needs to be excluded and this should be performed by laparoscopy with an early resort to laparotomy if necessary. Uterine perforation should be suspected when there is sudden decrease of intra-uterine pressure, sudden rise in the fluid deficit or when there is abdominal distension.

Incomplete and unrecognised perforations remain the main pitfalls. In the event of incomplete perforation the resultant rapid intravasation should alert the surgeon. In the case of an unrecognised perforation, thermal energy may be conducted to surrounding vessels and viscera. Particularly thin areas such as tubal ostia and uterine scars should be treated with great care. Postoperatively, any undue symptoms such as pain not settling with simple analgesia, fever, diarrhoea or haematuria should be treated with great suspicion.

Uterine perforation has been documented in all the series of hysteroscopic surgery for the treatment of menorrhagia. In the early years the rates of uterine perforation following TCRE were reported to range between 1–3.7%.[27,29–31] In contrast, the roller-ball technique appeared safer with a 1.5% uterine perforation rate.[32] The consensus was that the rate of uterine perforation was greatly related to operator's experience. Indeed, in Magos *et al's*[27] series of 250 resections, uterine perforations occurred in the first 57 cases. In a postal survey of 3000 uterine ablations,[32] 33% of the perforations occurred in the first ever procedure performed and 57% during the first five procedures. Recent evidence however has refuted this and demonstrated that, apart from uterine perforation, operative complications did not depend on a surgeon's experience.[10,33]

Garry *et al*[34] reported an even lower incidence of uterine perforation following ELA (0.4%) and a 1% total complication rate. All perforations occurred during the insertion of the rigid hysteroscope, none involved damage of adjacent organs and all were managed by simple observation and postponement of the procedure to a later date.

However, cases of bowel injury associated with ELA have been reported.[35] Until 1994 there was a growing feeling that TCRE was a more dangerous procedure than ELA. This was summarised by the statement that "laser ablation using the drag technique has a lower risk of complications than resection or electrocoagulation."[36] However, in the Aberdeen randomised study,[37] uterine perforation and overall complication rates were comparable in both procedures. One laparotomy was performed for small bowel obstruction following a full thickness cornual burn in an ELA patient. There was one perforation in TCRE and that was made with the dilator and none with the resectoscope. In the Scottish audit,[10] 978 patients were recruited between 1991 and 1993; 65% of them were treated by TCRE and 32% by ELA. Uterine perforation occurred in 1% of patients with no significant difference between the two procedures.

In the Mistletoe study,[33] significantly less perforations occurred with the use of the laser (0.65%) and roller ball alone (0.64%) than with loop alone (2.47%) or the loop and ball in combination (1.27%). The rate of perforation was 2.14% with radiofrequency and no perforations were reported after 36 cases of cryoablation.

Haemorrhage: Primary intraoperative bleeding is relatively uncommon and may be due to perforation, or cervical trauma and may necessitate hysterectomy. It may also arise from deep endometrial vessels and can be managed by coagulating the bleeding areas. If it persists, a size 12–14 Foley's catheter may be inserted and inflated with 30 ml saline/water and kept in the uterus for 6–8 h. If these measures fail then a hysterectomy may become necessary. In the Scottish hysteroscopic surgery audit,[10] excessive haemorrhage occurred in 3.5% of cases and was managed conservatively in all but 2 patients who required hysterectomy. In the Mistletoe study,[33] the overall rate of haemorrhage was 2.38% (0.97% associated with rollerball alone, 1.17% with laser, 2.57% with loop and ball and 3.53% with loop alone). There were no cases of haemorrhage associated with radiofrequency and cryoablation techniques. These differences were only statistically significant at the 5% level.

Fluid overload: Fluid absorption and its consequences are much greater during operative hysteroscopy than during a diagnostic one. This is due to the longer time it requires, the presence of open blood vessels and the nature of the distension medium used. In particular this applies to non-ionic solutions such as glycine 1.5% which are used for electrosurgical resection/ablation. Excess fluid absorption may cause hyponatraemia, hypotension, haemolysis and bradycardia, and in severe cases congestive heart failure, pulmonary and/or cerebral oedema leading to confusion, coma or even death.

It is therefore vital that fluid deficit absorbed is monitored carefully during the procedure by frequently measuring the volume of fluid used and collected. Detectable falls in the haemoglobin and serum albumin concentrations occur but of greater significance is the resultant hyponatraemia which, in the case of glycine, is directly proportional to the volume (> 2 L) of fluid absorbed.[38]

Symptomatic fluid overload is probably the commonest potentially serious complication of ELA. This was recognised in the first series of ELA[16] and was found to be associated with the duration of the procedure. In the Aberdeen study,[37] the only significant finding was that of a higher volume of fluid absorbed in the laser group (766 ml) than in the TCRE group (414 ml) but this did not have any clinical significance. However, the numbers were too small (50 patients in each group) to exclude differences in rare complications. In the Scottish hysteroscopic surgery audit,[10] there were significantly more cases of fluid overload with ELA ($p < 0.001$) than with resection. In none of these cases however, was there clinical pulmonary oedema. Apart from one death from toxic shock syndrome following an uncomplicated TCRE, and significantly more cases of fluid overload with ELA, there were no other difference in complication rates. Similarly, the Mistletoe study[33] reported significantly more fluid absorption with the use of laser. Fluid absorption of more than 2 L was noted in 5.1% of ELA as compared with 1.5% of loop, 1.2% of roller ball and 1.0% of loop and ball combined procedures.

It must be noted, however, that due to the usage of normal saline in ELA, fluid absorption leads to fluid volume effects rather than hyponatraemia. In contrast, absorption greater than 2 L of glycine leads to both volume overload and hyponatraemia.[39]

It is not clear why ELA has a higher rate of fluid absorption than TCRE. It may be due to the shorter duration of TCRE compared to ELA, although fluid absorption during TCRE is not strictly related to its duration.[39] It could also be due to the differences between the techniques in the form of blood vessel destruction. Furthermore, during ELA there is a constantly high intrauterine pressure whereas in TCRE this is relieved periodically with the removal of the resectoscope.

In view of the above, there are now strict guidelines regarding fluid balance estimation and management (**Table 10.1**). Furthermore, the surgeon should be able to identify pre-operatively the group of patients at increased risk of excessive fluid absorption: those with patent fallopian tubes, those where no endometrial preparation has been used and those with large fibroids.[27]

Staff risks: These should not be underestimated. A burn may result if the surgeon touches the activated loop during TCRE. The Nd:YAG laser can potentially cause skin burns and irreversible blindness if the eye is exposed to the beam. Adequate training of staff and adherence to safety precautions are therefore vital. These include never activating the laser beam outside the uterine cavity, wearing protective goggles (including the anaesthetist and patient), laser proof barriers on all glass windows with adequate warning signs, and an interlocking system which switches off the laser if the theatre door is opened inadvertently during the operation.

Gas embolism: This is a rare, but potentially fatal complication. It had been reported with ELA[40] and endometrial resection.[41]

Death: It had also been reported following ELA and TCRE.[40,41] In the Scottish hysteroscopy audit[10] one death occurred due to toxic shock syndrome following an uncomplicated TCRE. In the Mistletoe study,[33] ten deaths were reported but only two appeared to be directly related to hysteroscopic surgery. One was due to brain stem coning associated with a malignant glioma, and occurred during a combined procedure and the other was due to streptococcal septicaemia

3 weeks following a loop resection. Direct mortality rates were 2 in 10,000 for the loop/ball combined procedure and 3 in 10,000 for the loop alone.

Burns: This serious complication has been associated with radiofrequency endometrial ablation. Skin burns or thermal damage in the uterus deeper than the expected few millimetres have been reported. The latter are more difficult to control and appear to be dependent on uterine blood flow and circulatory changes after pelvic surgery. Thermal damage has resulted in extensive transmural necrosis and vesicovaginal fistula formation.[28,42]

(2) Postoperative complications
Infection: Inflammatory reaction invariably follows endometrial destruction and therefore women experience a profuse serosanguinous vaginal discharge for several weeks afterwards. Prophylactic antibiotics may be used, although there is no clear proof of their effectiveness. Severe fatal septicaemia though rare, has been reported.[10,33]

Secondary haemorrhage: This should be managed by antibiotics, curettage or, rarely, hysterectomy.

Cyclical pain: Patients may present with amenorrhoea and cyclical lower abdominal pain in the absence of haematometra as described by Asherman.[22] It may be due to the presence of intrauterine synechiae and/or iatrogenic adenomyosis. This complication may be difficult to treat and ultimately hysterectomy may be required. If haematometra is suspected, the diagnosis is readily made by ultrasound examination and pain may be relieved by cervical dilatation. At present, there is no proof that postoperative uterine probing, as practised by some, reduces the incidence of haematometra.

Pregnancy: Whenever applicable, a form of contraception should be practised by all women who undergo endometrial ablative techniques. Pregnancies (intrauterine or tubal) have been reported after both TCRE and ELA.[43] Two main problems may be encountered; (i) Impaired uterine vasculature with its consequences on placentation and the possibility of foetal growth retardation and, (ii) Morbid placental adherence.[44] Although many pregnancies are terminated or spontaneously miscarry, uneventful pregnancies have been reported with no obvious complications.[30]

Uterine malignancy: Although there should be no increased risk of endometrial cancer following hysteroscopic surgery, the main concern is the theoretical possibility of endometrial cancer arising from buried islands of residual endometrium presenting late. When hormone replacement therapy is indicated, a form of combined hormone should be used, either cyclically or, perhaps preferable, continuously. Endometrial glands and tissue are present even in amenorrheoic women. Cases of endometrial carcinoma after resection have been reported. However, a review of the literature[45] suggested that pre-existing endometrial hyperplasia was a common denominator and hence should be considered as a contraindication to ablation.

Treatment failure: This occurs with all methods of hysteroscopic surgery and should be part of the preoperative counselling.

Summary of complications

In the early 1990s, it was felt that ELA was probably safer than TCRE. Recent evidence however, suggests there was little, if any, difference in the safety of the two techniques.[37] The overall complications rate, uterine perforation and significant fluid overload were similar and additionally, no statistical difference in the occurrence of complications between experienced and less experienced operators was noted.[10]

In the Mistletoe study,[33] 686 women were registered prospectively between April 1993 and October 1994. Laser and rollerball ablations had consistently fewer immediate operative complications (haemorrhage, perforation,visceral burns, cardiovascular and respiratory complications) than loop alone or loop and ball combined together. Additionally, there were fewer occasions where additional surgery was needed following ELA or rollerball. Laser ablation was significantly less likely to result in an emergency hysterectomy than the loop alone.

There were extremely small numbers of immediate post-operative complications (within 24 h) between the four main techniques (complication rates between 0.77% and 2.86% with the exception of cryoablation group 8.33%). The combined diathermy group produced significantly fewer total immediate postoperative complications than the loop alone approach. Similarly, long term (up to 6 weeks) post-operative complications were uncommon, ranging between 1.25% and 4.58%.

There was no significant difference in the complication rates between doctors who had attended a training course and those who did not. Interestingly, increasing operator's experience was associated with fewer uterine perforations in the loop group alone and there was no overall level of experience above which women were less likely to have complications.

Effectiveness of conventional endometrial ablation techniques

Initial reports were based on personal series of small numbers of patients and limited periods of follow-up. There are now both randomised trials and large audit data which compare hysteroscopic surgery results with hysterectomy. The results can be divided into effect on menses (amenorrhoea, hypomenorrhoea, persistent menorrhagia), return to normal activity, patient satisfaction and additional benefits (premenstrual tension, dysmennorhoea). **Table 10.2** outlines the advantages and disadvantages of hysteroscopic surgery and hysterectomy to the patients and the health service.

In the Aberdeen study,[37] the results were identical on the effectiveness of TCRE and ELA. At 12 months, 22% of patients were amenorrhoeic and 62% hypomenorrhoeic. Similarly, 43% reported less and 42% no dysmenorrhoea, with no change in 5% of patients and worsened symptoms in 10% of women. Non-menstrual benefits included reduction of premenstrual symptoms and breast discomfort. Overall, 78% of patients were very satisfied and 18% moderately satisfied with the outcome of their treatment. Longer-term follow up, however, is not available.

The Scottish Audit[10] reported no significant difference in patient outcome between TCRE and ELA at 6, 12 and 24 months of follow-up. Overall, there was amenorrhoea in 25%, brown discharge in 18%, significant hypomenorrhoea in 42%, slight hypomenorrhoea in 11% and unchanged or heavier menstruation in 5%. Dysmenorrhoea was absent in 51%, reduced in 31%, unchanged in 11% and worse in 7% of women. At 24 months post-surgery, 53% of women were very satisfied and 31% satisfied with the results. Although the satisfaction rate at 12 months was significantly worse in the group under 40 years compared to the older group of patients (79% vs 88% respectively), the audit suggests that results from both methods are still acceptable in the younger group.

A randomised study comparing TCRE with abdominal hysterectomy[6] with an average follow-up of 2.8 years, reported that women randomised to hysterectomy experienced more of an improvement in menstrual symptoms and higher satisfaction rates with some evidence of superior health-related quality of life. Although the cost of TCRE was lower, further study was required to determine the relative cost effectiveness of the 2 procedures.

A large randomised controlled study comparing TCRE with hysterectomy (abdominal or vaginal)[46] showed that following TCRE there were less operative and post-operative complications, less analgesic requirement and hospital stay as well as quicker return to normal activity and

Table 10.2 Advantages and disadvantages of hysteroscopic surgery.

Advantages	
For the patient	**For the National Health Service**
Day case procedure	No need for inpatient admission
Shorter duration of procedure	Shorter theatre time
Rapid recovery and convalescence	Short hospital stay (2–4 hours)
Possibility of local anaesthetic/conscious sedation	Probably more cost-effective
No surgical scar	
Less minor complications than hysterectomy	
Majority (around 80%) of patients satisfied	
Avoidance and alternative to hysterectomy	
Disadvantages	
For the patient	**For the National Health Service**
Complications (operative and postoperative)	High initial set-up cost
Treatment failure in 20%	Training costs
A proportion will need further treatment	Possible need for further surgery
Majority will continue to menstruate	Need for long-term follow-up
Some will continue to have dysmenorrhoea	Cost effectiveness remains debatable
Contraception required	Possible increase in litigation due to operative complications
Cervical screening required	
Need for combined hormone replacement therapy	
Very long-term (over 5 years) success and complications unknown	
Possible late presentation of endometrial cancer	

work. On follow-up for up to 3 years (mean 2 years), women treated hysteroscopically had a higher chance of requiring further surgery but 1 in 8 women in the hysterectomy group also underwent additional surgery. Patient satisfaction at 3 years was higher, though not significantly, with hysterectomy (96%) than TCRE (85%). This translates into significant savings to the health service and at 3-year follow-up, the mean costs for the two procedures were reported as £554 for TCRE and £1,225 for hysterectomy. Life table analysis showed that over a 5-year period, women treated with TCRE had a 91% chance of avoiding hysterectomy and 80% chance of avoiding any further surgery. Results were best in older women and in those with dysfunctional uterine bleeding, but even women with fibroids and uterine size greater than 12 weeks had greater than 50% chance of being satisfied.[47]

Both TCRE and ELA suffer from the same problem, that menstrual results are better than patient satisfaction. In all the above-mentioned large studies, some women were not satisfied with the technique despite having good menstrual results. Lack of satisfaction may be due to pain, or to patient's perception of inappropriate menstrual loss. This highlights the need for adequate counselling and appropriate selection preoperatively.

In a cost-utility analysis of abdominal hysterectomy versus TCRE,[48] it was reported that by 2 years, TCRE costs only 71% that of abdominal hysterectomy. However, the author concluded that under the most plausible parameter values, and on the basis of health state values elicited from the sample of women with menorrhagia, abdominal hysterectomy was likely to be considered more cost-effective. This would be valid only if purchasers were willing to pay an additional cost of at least £6,500 per extra quality-adjusted life-year generated by hysterectomy!

New techniques

Several clinicians continue to have reservations concerning existing conventional hysteroscopic techniques and systems. Additionally, the constant drive to simplify and expedite endometrial ablation procedures has led in recent years to the development of new technology. In this section, we will describe these innovative techniques and provide, whenever possible, an up-to-date analysis of their effectiveness. They include, microwave endometrial ablation, balloon ablation systems, hydrothermal ablation, cryoablation and photo-dynamic ablative techniques.

With all these therapies it is essential that appropriate criteria for patient selection are implemented. These normally include appropriate assessment of patient expectations and desire to conserve their uteri, absence of anatomical abnormalities in the uterus including polyps and fibroids, uterine cavity depth not greater than 100–120 mm, exclusion of cervical and uterine malignancy, and absence of previous uterine surgery. Choice of anaesthesia should be determined by individual patient's choice, pain tolerance, need for cervical dilatation and presence or absence of medical indications.

Microwave ablation

The use of microwave to destroy the endometrium was first reported by Sharp.[49] The microwave applicator (8.5 mm in diameter) consists of a circular metal pipe dielectric-filled waveguide and dielectric radiating tip to propagate microwave energy at 9.2 GHz into the uterine cavity. The tip produces a hemispherical field of heating in tissues and allows the endometrium to be destroyed to a depth of 5–6 mm. The power level used is 30 W and is controlled via a foot-switch operated by the surgeon. The temperature achieved inside the uterus is monitored continuously by thermocouples on the exterior surface of the waveguide. A computer displays the temperature fluctuations graphically in real time, thus enabling the surgeon to control the movement of the applicator within the endometrial cavity to produce a uniform layer of tissue destruction, while gradually withdrawing the probe. The duration of treatment varies according to the depth of the uterine cavity. A normal size uterus (75–85 mm) typically requires 2–3 min while a large uterus (100–110 mm) will require 6–7 min.

The technique is simple and easy to learn, with a number of safety measures being incorporated into the system. No intraoperative complications have been reported and early results are encouraging. Over 1500 patients have been treated to date with a reported 90% satisfaction rate.[50]

Cooper *et al* published their results from a randomised controlled trial comparing MEA™ to rollerball/resection in 1999.[51] Two hundred and sixty-three women were initially randomised within their study centre to treatment with either MEA™ (n = 129) or rollerball/ resection (n = 134) ablation. This size of study had an 80% chance of detecting a minimum of 15% difference in satisfaction between the two methods, assuming that 78% of patients would be satisfied by the rollerball/ resection treatment (0.05 level of significance, 80% power).

The study was performed on a pragmatic basis to enable results to be as generalisable as possible. Therefore, trial exclusion criteria were minimal and pre-operative assessment using ultrasound or hysteroscopy was discouraged unless indicated by clinical examination, or an endometrial biopsy could not be obtained. Notably, whilst the two lead surgeons were experienced hysteroscopic surgeons (having performed at least 50 endometrial resections), they had only performed five MEA™ procedures when the trial was started.

All of the 263 women prospectively randomised received 3.6 mg goserelin 5 weeks pre-operatively in order to promote endometrial thinning. A general anaesthetic was used for all procedures (MEA™ or rollerball/resection), this was the practice of the surgeons at that time, and, as one of the primary endpoints of the study was patient satisfaction, it eliminated any potential bias from using different methods of analgesia.

Intra-operatively, submucous fibroids of greater than 2 cm were found in 32 women, in these cases, the treatment proceeded as originally intended, with the exception of one woman in the rollerball/resection group who required a two-stage procedure, and one woman in the MEA™ group who underwent an endometrial resection. Four other women originally randomised to MEA™ underwent rollerball/resection as a result of the MEA™ equipment failing (this study used an earlier model to the device currently available, personal communication, I. Feldberg, Microsulis plc.) In those women randomised to rollerball/resection, one woman underwent MEA.

Blunt perforation with an inactive hysteroscope or MEA™ probe occurred to one patient in each group, the MEA™ patient with perforation declined an attempt at a repeat procedure, and later requested a hysterectomy. The perforation in the rollerball/resection patient caused bleeding into the broad ligament, which was managed intra-operatively by converting to a hysterectomy. A hysterectomy was also required in another of the rollerball/resection treated patients, who presented 2 weeks after the original procedure with abdominal/pelvic pain.

Primary haemorrhage occurred in 5 patients treated by rollerball/resection, this was managed by inserting a 14 gauge Foley catheter into the uterus for 6 h; there were no cases of primary haemorrhage in the MEA™ group. Readmission after discharge occurred in 6 women treated by rollerball/resection; 3 complained of pelvic pain, 2 required repeat procedures, and one patient had chest pain. Four women treated by MEA™ were subsequently readmitted; three with minor secondary haemorrhage treated by antibiotic therapy.

Rates of satisfaction with, and acceptability of treatment were high for both techniques at 12-month follow-up, and the results were similar to previous trials of endometrial ablation. Of the eight health-related quality of life dimensions in the Short Form-36, all were improved after MEA™ (six significantly) and seven were improved after TCRE (all significantly). Although amenorrhea was not used as an outcome to define success, this was achieved in 40% of treated patients for both techniques. Dysmenorrhea and peri-menstrual symptoms also improved in most treated women, with only 4% and 8% of MEA™ and rollerball/resection treated women respectively complaining of "new" pelvic pain after treatment. Cooper's study validated MEA™ as an endometrial ablation technique with good safety, and comparable safety to rollerball/resection.

Balloon endometrial ablation techniques

A number of balloon endometrial ablative techniques have been described recently. They include devices utilising heated fluid within a balloon (ThermaChoice™, Gynecare, Ethicon Ltd., USA and Cavaterm™, Wallsten Medical SA, Switzerland) or electrodes mounted on the surface of the balloon (Vesta™, Valleylab, Colorado, USA).

(1) ThermaChoice™ ablation system

The ThermaChoice™ uterine balloon ablation system was first described by Neuwirth.[51] It consists of a 16 cm long by 4.5 mm wide catheter with a latex balloon at its distal end, which houses the heater element. The catheter is connected to a control unit that monitors, displays and controls pre-set intrauterine balloon pressure, temperature and duration of treatment (**Figure 10.1**). After the balloon catheter insertion, sterile 5% dextrose water is injected into the balloon until the intrauterine pressure stabilises between 160 and 180 mmHg. The fluid within the balloon is heated to approximately 87°C and the treatment automatically

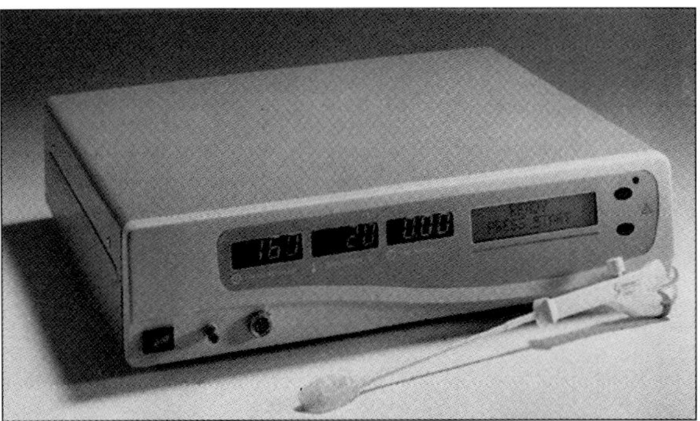

Figure 10.1 The ThermaChoice™ uterine balloon therapy controller.

continues at that temperature for 8 min. For safety, the device automatically deactivates if the pressure or the temperature fluctuate below or above preset values.

Measurement of serosal temperatures and depth of thermal injury generated by the ThermaChoice™ system were studied both in *ex vivo* and *in vivo* uteri.[52,53] *In vivo* serosal temperatures from 12 anatomic locations did not exceed 39.9°C with a mean of 36.1°C. Histological examination revealed deep endometrial and superficial myometrial damage to all areas. The greatest depth of myometrial injury occurred in the midfundus (3.4 mm).[52] By electron microscopy, no thermal effect could be demonstrated in the myometrium beyond 15 mm from the endometrial surface following up to 16 min of therapy.[53]

A number of studies have reported on the outcome following this treatment.[54,55] In a large observational multi-centre study,[55] no intra-operative complications were reported. There was minimal postoperative morbidity and treatment led to a significant reduction in the severity and duration of menstrual flow and dysmenorrhoea by 15% in 88% of women who reverted to eumenorrhoea or less. Increasing age, higher balloon pressure, smaller uterine cavity and a lesser degree of pre-procedure menorrhagia were associated with significantly improved results.

In a randomised study comparing ThermaChoice™ endometrial ablation with rollerball ablation[56] no operative complications occurred with balloon therapy while two cases of fluid overload, one uterine perforation and one case of cervical laceration occurred in the rollerball group (3.2% of cases). One year follow-up data did not show any significant difference between the two groups in:

- percentage of women whose diary score decreased by 90% or less;
- patients highly satisfied (balloon 85.6% vs. rollerball 86.7%);
- impact of treatment on quality of life;
- dysmenorrhoea scores.

However, a greater percentage of women in the rollerball were amenorrhoeic at 12 months (27% vs 15%, $p<0.05$). In the balloon group, more procedures were carried out under sedation or local anaesthesia (47% vs 16%) and the mean operating time was significantly shorter in the balloon group (27.4 vs 39.6 minutes). In 71% of cases, the procedure was completed in 30 min or less, compared with 28.6% in the rollerball group ($p<0.05$).

Increasingly, the procedure is being carried out under local anaesthesia or conscious sedation.[55–59] Careful pre-operative assessment to determine the patient's tolerance of pain is essential. Pre-medication with non-steroidal anti-inflammatory drugs given either orally or rectally to alleviate uterine pain is obligatory. Intra-operative medication may include local injection of 1% lidocaine or bupivicane with or without epinephrine 1:100,000 and/or a combination of a rapid, short acting opioid such as fentanyl and a benzodiazepine such as midazolam. The combination is given intravenously shortly before the operation to provide the required sedation and amnesiac effects of the former and the analgesic effects of the latter. A dedicated nurse should be available at the patient's bedside throughout the operation to reduce their anxiety and provide the necessary feedback to the clinician. The operation is usually well tolerated by the majority of patients and with a high satisfaction rate after 24 h.[57,59]

(2) Cavaterm™ ablation system

The technique was first described by Friberg in 1996.[60] The system consists of a silastic balloon catheter connected to a central unit. The procedure begins with dilation of the cervix to 9 mm, then the depth of the uterine cavity is measured in order to adjust the balloon length of the catheter before insertion. The balloon is then filled with glycine 1.5% until a pressure of about 180 mmHg is achieved. The internal heating pump circulates the fluid and maintains the fluid temperature around 75°C. The treatment cycle begins when the fluid temperature reaches 66°C and lasts for 15 min.

To date, the reported success rates following therapy are limited to small series. Follow-up periods have also been variable. In one series of 60 patients followed for between 12–37 months, 70% had amenorrhoea or minimal bleeding and 94% of patients reported excellent satisfaction with the outcome. Seven patients had a hysterectomy during the 3-year follow-up period.[61] Fifty-one patients were examined with hysteroscopy and saline infusion sonography 11–28 months after therapy. It was reported that those with minimal or no bleeding had more uterine fibrosis than patients bleeding more.[62] To date, only one small comparative study between the Cavaterm™ ablation system with rollerball has been reported. Romer's[64] study assessed the outcomes of Cavaterm™ versus rollerball in 20 women, (10 patients in each arm of the study). Again, women were excluded if they had any intrauterine abnormalities (submucous myomas, uterine septae, suspicion of uterine wall weakness, or uterine cavity length <4 cm or >10 cm) or histological pathology, however Romer pre-treated both groups with 2 injections of gonadotrophin-releasing hormone analogues (GnRHa). Follow-up at 15 months found almost identical results in the two treatment arms of the study, with all 20 women expressing satisfaction with their treatment.

This study has gross methodological weaknesses: there is no power study to calculate the number of women needed to demonstrate if a statistically significant difference exists between the 2 treatments, and, as such, its results must be treated with caution until larger studies are performed.

(3) Vesta™ DUB treatment system

Endometrial ablation using an inflatable multi-electrode balloon was first reported by Soderstorm in 1996.[63] In its current format, the Vesta™ DUB Treatment System (Valleylab, Boulder, Colorado, USA) consists of a handset for the introduction of an electrode carrier, a controller to monitor and distribute the electrical energy, and a Valleylab Force 2™ electrosurgical generator. The generator is set to supply 'pure cut' mode current at 45–50 W. The silicone inflatable electrode carrier has a triangular shape that unfurls when its insertion sheath is withdrawn. There are six ventral and six dorsal flexible electrode plates covering the surface of the carrier, each with its own thermistor. The cornual plates have a set temperature of 72°C while that of the remaining plates is set at 75°C. Distension of the carrier lumen ensures that the electrodes are kept in intimate contact with the endometrium. The control unit monitors generator output as well as the temperature and impedance of the 12 electrodes throughout the warm-up and treatment phases (**Figures 10.2, 10.3 and 10.4**).

The cervix is dilated to 9–10 mm followed by introduction of the handset. Once appropriately positioned, the sheath is withdrawn and the silicone carrier is inflated with 8–12 ml of air. The therapy cycle begins with a warm-up phase, programmed to occur within 3 min, and during which all electrodes should reach their pre-set temperatures, following which the controller automatically shifts to a 4 min treatment phase. This produces a uniform thermal destruction to a depth of 4–5 mm into the myometrium in the presence of early proliferative endometrium.

Early studies in extirpated uteri showed that in 88% of sections the necrosis depth into the

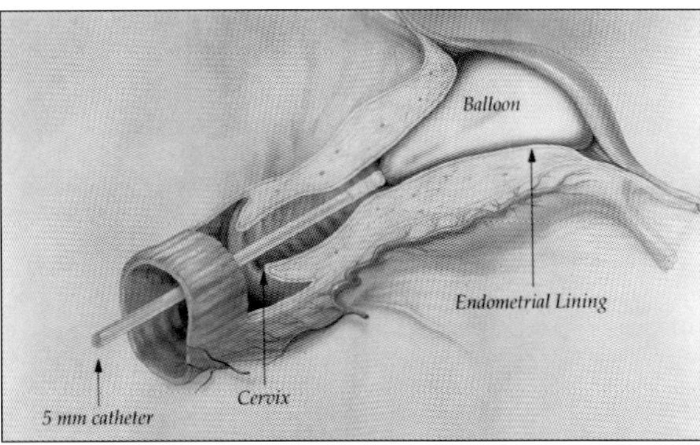

Figure 10.2 The ThermaChoice™ uterine balloon catheter with a diameter under 5 mm often allows a endometrial ablation to be performed without cervical dilation.

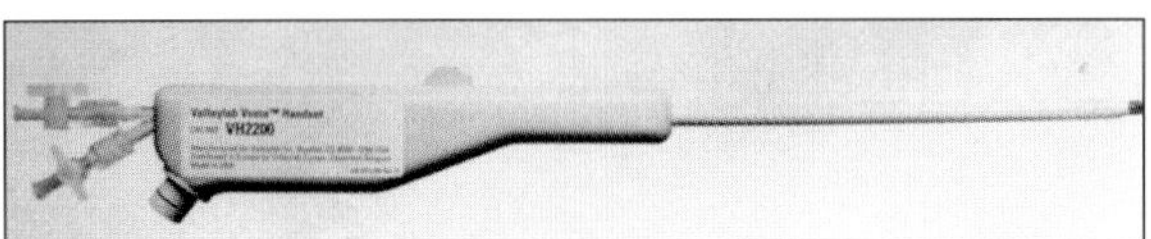

Figure 10.3 The Vesta™ DUB treatment system.

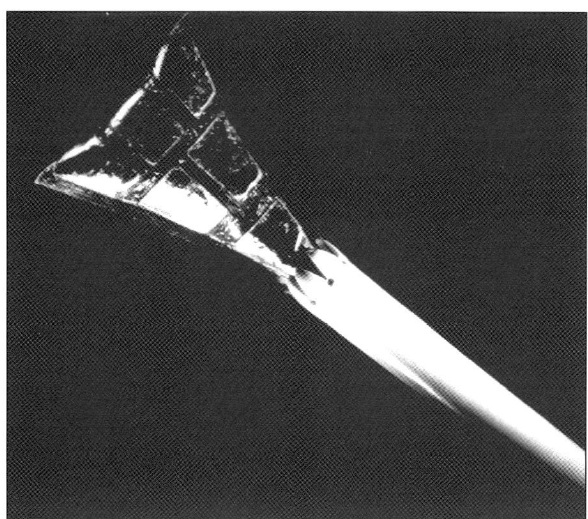

Figure 10.4 Enlarged view of the Vesta™ catheter tip showing the electrode plates with their thermistors.

myometrium was between 2–4 mm depending on the treatment variables and the degree to which the electrode balloon conformed to the uterine cavity. Early clinical experience indicated amenorrhoea and hypomenorrhoea rates of 40% and 49% respectively.[63] A subsequent study[64] reported an amenorrhoea rate of up to 38% after 6 months. It was also reported that 88% of patients should expect to be free of menorrhagia, dissatisfaction or need for a second operation after 24 months. Preliminary results from a randomised study evaluating the Vestablate system with rollerball/TCRE suggest comparable outcomes at 6 months (amenorrhoea rate: 34% vs 37%; decrease in menstrual score to 75 or less 86% vs 83% respectively).[65]

Hydrothermal ablation techniques

The Hydro ThermAblator™ – HTA (BEI Medical Systems Company, Inc., USA), unlike traditional ablation technology, utilises circulation of heated saline that is in direct contact with the entire endometrial lining under direct hysteroscopic vision.[66] It is far less experience dependant than traditional endometrial ablation techniques. Additionally, anatomical variations such as a partial septate uterus or a small submucous fibroid do not prevent effective treatment.

The system includes a control unit which prompts the operator to follow the steps involved in the preparation for treatment. After positioning of the patient in the dorsolithotomy position, the cervix is dilated to 8–9 mm and the HTA sheath (7.8 mm in diameter including the hysteroscope) is introduced into the uterine cavity. Room temperature saline flows under gravity (maximum fluid pressure less than 55 mmHg) to flush the uterine cavity then the warming process starts allowing a gradual increase of the circulating saline temperature. The 10-min treatment cycle starts when the saline temperature reaches the ablating level (90°C). At its conclusion, room temperature saline automatically flushes hot saline from the sheath and cools the uterine cavity and the control unit, when appropriate, it prompts the operator to remove the sheath from the patient. It is presumed that the heating temperature applied for the treatment cycle would result in uniform and adequate depth of endometrial destruction, but not involving the cervix.

A number of safety controls are incorporated in the operating system. The fluid level reservoir provides gravity flow control and continuous monitoring of circulating fluid volume. Thus, loss of 10 ml of fluid automatically interrupts treatment. The low pressure presumably avoids escape of fluid through the fallopian tubes or cervical canal.[67] The insulated continuous flow sheath protects the cervical canal from thermal effect and the externally heated saline rather than internal focused energy source presumably reduces potential risks associated with intrauterine sources of energy, such as laser tips, electrodes or internal heaters.

The technique is in its early days and large numbers of treated women followed for a reasonable period of time (one year or more) are not yet available. Further, it is essential that improvement on current new techniques should enable this treatment to be conducted in an office environment and under conscious sedation. The need for cervical dilation may hinder its widespread application. It remains to be shown that the technique has added benefits over other minimally invasive techniques and whether there is a need to undertake the procedure under hysteroscopic control at all.

Another system (EnAbl™, InnerDyne Inc, Sunnyvale, Ca, USA) is currently being developed. It works on the principle of in-situ heating (80°C) of the endometrium with small volumes of circulating saline solution for 15 min.[68]

There are numerous other techniques aalso being developed and are still in case study or small cohort published series. Safety studies and early clinical results have been published for photosensitisation,[69,70] cryoablation,[71] and interstitial laser heating.[72,73]

Summary

It is beyond doubt that this multitude of techniques provided patients with suitable alternatives to hysterectomy and conventional ablation procedures. However, it is imperative that these techniques are thoroughly evaluated in properly conducted randomised controlled studies to establish safety, long-term outcome, cost-effectiveness, patient acceptability and satisfaction, as well as suitability for sedation in the office or outpatient environment.

The notion of a simple, safe, cost-effective, office-based technique with high patient satisfaction offers millions of women world-wide the choice to treat their menorrhagia without the need for hysterectomy and with minimal interruption to their family or social life. Cost implications to health care systems will be equally significant.

New developments are taking place in this field very rapidly. The reader is advised to seek up to date information on the second generation endometrial ablation devices from published journals.

REFERENCES

1. Consumers' Association Ltd. Drugs for menorrhagia: Often disappointing. *Drug Ther Bull* 1990; **28**: 17–20.
2. Gath D, Osborn M, Bungay G *et al.* Psychiatric disorder and gynaecological symptoms in middle aged women: a community survey. *BMJ* 1987; **294**: 213–218.
3. Garry R. Endometrial ablation and resection: validation of a new surgical concept. *Br J Obstet Gynaecol* 1997; **104**: 1329–1331.
4. Coulter A, Bradlow J, Agass M, Martin-Bares C, Tulloch A. Outcomes of referrals to gynaecology outpatient clinics for menstrual problems: an audit of general practice records. *Br J Obstet Gynaecol* 1991; **98**: 789–796.
5. Vessey MP, Villard-Mackintosh L, McPherson K, Coulter A, Yates D. The epidemiology of hysterectomy: findings in a large cohort study. *Br J Obstet Gynaecol* 1992; **99:** 402–407.

6. Sculpher M, Dwyer N, Byford S, Stirrat G. Randomised trial comparing hysterectomy and transcervical endometrial resection: effect on health related quality of life and costs two years after surgery. *Br J Obstet Gynaecol* 1996; **103**: 142–149.

7. Wingo PA, Huezo CM, Rubin GL, Ory HW, Peterson HB. The mortality risk associated with hysterectomy. *Am J Obstet Gynecol* 1985; **803:** 8–13.

8. Dicker RC, Greenspan JR, Strauss LT. Complications of abdominal and vaginal hysterectomy among women of reproductive age in the United States. *Am J Obstet Gynecol* 1982; **144**: 842–848.

9. Thakar R, Manyonda I, Satanton SL, Clarkson P, Robinson G. Bladder, bowel and sexual function after hysterectomy for benign conditions. *Br Obstet Gynaecol* 1997; **104**: 983–987.

10. A Scottish audit of hysteroscopic surgery for menorrhagia: complications and follow up. Scottish Hysteroscopy Audit Group. *Br J Obstet Gynaecol* 1995; **102**: 249–254.

11. Cooper KG, Parkin DE, Garratt AM, Grant AM. A randomised comparison of medical and hysteroscopic management in women consulting a gynaecologist for the treatment of heavy menstrual loss. *Br J Obstet Gynaecol* 1997; **104**: 1360–1366.

12. Pantaleoni DC. On endoscopic examination of the cavity of the womb. *Medical Press Circular* 1869; **8**: 26–27.

13. Baumann A. Electrocoagulation of endometrium and cervical mucosa for uterine hemorrhage and leukorrhea (in German) *Geburtshilfe Frauenheilkd* 1948; **8**: 221–226.

14. Droegemueller W, Greer B and Makowski E. Cryosurgery in patients with dysfunctional uterine bleeding. *Am J Obstet Gynecol* 1971a; **38**: 256–258.

15. Droegemueller W, Makowski E, Mascalka R. Destruction of the endometrium by cryosurgery. *Am J Obstet Gynecol* 1971b; **110**: 467–469.

16. Goldrath MH, Fuller TA, Segal S. Laser photovaporization of the endometrium for the treatment of menorrhagia. *Am J Obstet Gynecol* 1981; **140**: 14–19.

17. DeCherney AH, Polan ML. Hysteroscopic management of intrauterine lesions and intractable uterine bleeding. *Obstet Gynecol* 1983; **61**: 392–397.

18. DeCherney AH, Cholst I, Naftolin F. The management of intractable uterine bleeding utilizing the cystoscopic resectoscope. In Siegler AM and Lindeman HJ (eds) *Hysteroscopy: Principles and Practice* 1984; pp 140–142.

19. Lin BL, Miyamoto N, Tonomatu M *et al.* The development of a new hysteroscopic resectoscope and its clinical applications on transcervical resection and endometrial ablation. *Japan J Gynecol Obstet Endosc* 1988; **4**: 56–59.

20. Vaincaillie TG. Electrocoagulation of the endometrium with the ball ended resectoscope. *Obstet Gynecol* 1989; **74**: 425–427.

21. Phipps JH, Lewis BV, Roberts T *et al.* Treatment of functional menorrhagia with radiofrequency endometrial ablation. *Lancet* 1990; **335**: 374–376.

22. Asherman JG. Traumatic intra-uterine adhesions. *J Obstet and Gynaecol Br Empire.* 1950; **57**: 892–896.

23. Hill OJ, Maher PPJ. Intrauterine surgery using electrocautery. *Aust N Zeal J Obstet Gynec* 1990; **30**: 145–146.

24. Donnez J, Vilos G, Gannon MJ, Stampe-Sorenson S, Klinte I, Miller RM. Goserelin acetate (Zoladex) plus endometrial ablation for dysfunctional uterine bleeding: a large randomized, double-blind study. *Fertil Steril* 1997; **68**: 29–36.

25. Magos AL, Baumann R, Cheung K and Turnbull AC. Intra-uterine surgery under intravenous sedation: an outpatient alternative to hysterectomy. *Lancet* 1989a; **ii**: 925–926.

26. Lockwood M, Magos AL, Baumann R, Turnbull AC. Endometrial resection when hysterectomy is undesirable, dangerous or impossible. *Br J Obstet Gynaecol* 1990; **97**: 656–658.

27. Magos AL, Baumann R, Lockwood GM, Turnbull AC. Experience with the first 250 endometrial resections for menorrhagia. *Lancet* 1991; **337**: 1074–1078.

28. Thijssen RFA. Radiofrequency induced endometrial ablation: an update. *Br J Obstet Gynaecol* 1997; **104**: 608–613.

29. Sturdee D and Hogart B. Problems with endometrial resection. *Lancet* 1989; **337**: 1474.

30. Maher PJ and Hill DJ. Transcervical endometrial resection for abnormal uterine bleeding – report of 100 cases and review of the literature. *Aust N Zeal Obstet Gynec* 1990; 30 **4**: 357–360.

31. Pyper RJD and Haeri AD. A review of 80 endometrial resections for menorrhagia. *Br J Obstet Gynaecol* 1991; **98**: 1049–1054.

32. Macdonald R and Phipps J. Endometrial ablation: a safe procedure. *Gynaecol Endos* 1992; **1**: 7–9.

33. Overton C, Hargreaves J, Maresh M. A national survey of the complications of endometrial destruction for menstrual disorders: the MISTLETOE study. *Br J Obstet Gynaecol* 1997; **104**: 1351–1359.

34. Garry R, Erian J, Grochmal S. A multicentre study into the treatment of menorrhagia by Nd-YAG laser ablation of the endometrium. *Br J Obstet Gynaecol* 1991; **98**: 357–362.

35. Perry CP, Daniell JF, Gimpelson RJ. Bowel injury from Nd-YAG endometrial ablation. *J Gynaecol Surg* 1990; **6**: 199–203.

36. Royal College of Obstetricians and Gynaecologists. Report of the RCOG Working Party on Training in Gynaecological Endoscopic Surgery. London: *RCOG Press*, 1994.

37. Pinion SB, Parkin DE, Abramovich DR, Naji A, Alexander DA, Russell T, Kitchener HC. Randomised trial of hysterectomy, endometrial laser ablation, and transcervical endometrial resection for dysfunctional uterine bleeding. *Br Med J* 1994; **309**: 979–983.

38. Baumann R, Magos AL, Kay JDS, Turnbull AC. Absorption of glycine irrigating solution during transcervical resection of the endometrium. *Br Med J* 1990; **300**: 304–305.

39. Byers GF, Pinion S, Parkin DE, Chambers WA. Fluid absorption during transcervical resection of the endometrium. *Gynaecol Endosc* 1993; **2**: 21–23.

40. Baggish MS, Daniell JF. Catastrophic injury secondary to the use of coaxial gas-cooled fibres and artificial sapphire tips for intra-uterine surgery. *Lasers in Surgery and Medicine* 1989; **9**: 581–584.

41. Wood SM, Roberts FL. Air embolism during transcervical resection of the endometrium. *Br Med J* 1990; **300**: 945.

42. Phipps JH, Lewis BV, Prior MV, Roberts T. Experimental and clinical studies with radio frequency induced thermal endometrial ablation for functional menorrhagia. *Obstet Gynecol* 1990; **76**: 876–881.

43. Whitelaw NL, Garry R, Sutton CJG. Pregnancy following endometrial ablation: two case reports. *Gynaecol Endosc* 1992; **1**: 129–132

44. Whitelaw N, Sutton C. Nine years experience of endoscopic surgery in a District General Hospital. In Sutton CJG (ed.) *New Surgical techniques in Gynaecology* 1993; Carnforth, Lancs: Parthenon Publishing.

45. Gimpelson RJ. Not so benign endometrial hyperplasia: endometrial cancer after endometrial ablation. *J Am Assoc Gynecol Laparosc* 1997; **4**: 507–511.

46. O'Connor H, Broadbent J, Magos A, McPherson K. Medical Research Council randomised trial of endometrial resection versus hysterectomy in management of menorrhagia. *Lancet* 1997; **349**: 897–899.

47. O'Connor H, Magos A. Endometrial resection for the treatment of menorrhagia. *NEJM* 1996; **335**: 151–156.

48. Sculpher M. A cost-utility analysis of abdominal hysterectomy versus transcervical endometrial resection for the surgical treatment of menorrhagia. *International Journal of technology assessment in health care* 1998: **14**(2): 302–319.

49. Sharp NC, Cronin N, Feldberg I, Evans M, Hodgson D, Ellis S. Microwaves for menorrhagia: a new fast technique for endometrial ablation. *Lancet* 1995; **346**: 1003–1004.

50. Feldberg IB, Cronin NJ. A 9.2 GHz microwave applicator for the treatment of menorrhagia. *IEEE MTT-S Digest* 1998; WE3E-1: 755–758.

51. Cooper KG, Bain C, Parkin DE. Comparison of microwave endometrial ablation and trans-cervical resection of the endometrium for treatment of heavy menstrual loss: a randomised trial. *Lancet* **354**: 27 Nov 1999, 1859–1863.

52. Neuwirth RS, Duran AA, Singer A, Macdonald R, Buldoc L. The endometrial ablator: A new instrument. Obstet Gynecol 1994; **83**: 792–796.

53. Shah AA, Stabinsky SA, Klusak T, Bradley KR, Steege JF, Grainger DA. Measurement of serosal temperatures and depth of thermal injury generated by thermal balloon endometrial ablation in ex vivo and in vivo models. *Fertil Steril* 1998; **70**: 692–697.

54. Anderson LF, Meinert L, Rygaard C, Junge J, Prento P, Ottesen BS. Thermal balloon endometrial ablation: safety aspects evaluated by serosal temperature, light microscopy and electron microscopy. *Eur J Obstet Gynecol Reprod Biol* 1998; **79**: 63–68.

55. Vilos GA, Fortin CA, Sanders BA, Pendley L, Stabinsky SA. Clinical trial of the uterine thermal balloon for the treatment of menorrhagia. *J Am Assoc Gynecol Laparosc* 1997; **3**: 383–387.

56. Amso NN, Stabinsky SA, McFaul P, Blanc B, Pendley L, Neuwirth R. Uterine thermal balloon therapy for the treatment of menorrhagia: the first

300 patients from a multi-centre study. International collaborative uterine thermal balloon working group. *Br J Obstet Gynaecol* 1998; **105**: 517–523.

57. Meyer WR, Walsh BW, Grainger DA, Peacock LM, Loffer FD, Steege JF. Thermal balloon and rollerball ablation to treat menorrhagia: a multicentre comparison. *Obstet Gynecol* 1998; **92**(1): 98–103.

58. Fortin C, McColl MB. Gynecare UBT system under local anaesthesia. *J Am Assoc Gynecol Laparosc* 1996; **3**(4, Supplement): S13.

59. Fernandez H, Capella S, Audibert F. Uterine Thermal balloon therapy under local anaesthesia for the treatment of menorrhagia: a pilot study. *Hum Reprod* 1997; (**12**) (11): 2511–2514.

60. Amso NN, Abramovich, Cullimore J, Parker M, Stabinsky S. Uterine balloon therapy under local analgesia: A feasibility study. Presented at 7th annual meeting of the International Society of Gynaecologic Endoscopy, Sun City, South Africa, 15–18 March 1998.

61. Friberg B, Persson BR, Willen R, Ahlgren M. Endometrial destruction by hyperthermia – a possible treatment of menorrhagia. An experimental study. *Acta Obstet Gynecol Scand* 1996; (**75**): 330–335.

62. Friberg B. Balloon endometrial destruction by hyperthermia for the treatment of menorrha. Three years follow-up on the Cavaterm™. Presented at the 6th annual meeting of the International Society of Gynaecologic Endoscopy, Singapore, 16–19 April 1997.

63. Friberg B, Joergensen C, Ahlgren M. Endometrial thermal coagulation – degree of uterine fibrosis predicts treatment outcome. *Gynecol Obstet Invest* 1998; (**45**): 54–7.

64. Romer T, Die therapie rezidivierender menorrhagien – Cavaterm™-balloon Kaogulation versus roller-ball endometrium Koagulation – eine prospektive randomiserte vergleichstudie. *Zentralblatt fur Gynakologie* 1998; **120**(10): 511–514.

65. Soderstorm RM, Brooks PG, Corson SL *et al.* Endometrial ablation using a distensible multielectrode balloon. *J Am Assoc Gynecol Laparosc* 1996; **3**: 403–407.

66. Dequesne J, Gallinat A, Garza-Leal JG, Sutton CJG, van der Pas HFM, Wamsteker K, Chandler JG. Thermoregulated radiofrequency endometrial ablation. *Int J Fertil* 1997; **42**(5): 311–318.

67. Corson SL, Brill AI, Brooks PG, Cooper JM, Indman PD, Liu JH, Soderstrom RM, Vaiscaille TG. Interim Results of the American Vesta™ trial of endometrial ablation. *J Am Ass Gynecol Laparosc* 1999; **6**(1): 41–49.

68. Goldrath MH, Barrionuevo M, Husain M. Endometrial ablation by hysteroscopic instillation of hot saline solution. *J Am Assoc Gynecol Laparosc* 1997; **4**: 235–240.

69. Bustos-Lopez HH, Baggish M, Valle RF, Vadilla-Ortega F, Ibarra V, Nava G. Assessment of the safety of intrauterine instillation of heated saline for endometrial ablation. Fertil Steril. 1998; **69**(1): 155–160.

70. Fehr MK, Madsen SJ, Svaasand LO *et al.* Intrauterine light delivery for photodynamic therapy of the human endometrium. *Hum Reprod* 1995; **10**: 3067–3072.

71. Pitroff R, Majid S, Murray A. Transcervical endometrial cryoablation (ECA) for menorrhagia. *Int J Gynecol Obstet* 1994; **47**: 135–140.

72. Rutherford TJ, Zreik TG, Troiano RN, Palter SF, Olive DL. Endometrial cryoablation, a minimaly invasive procedure for abnormal uterine bleeding. *J Am Assoc Gynecol Laparosc* 1998; **5** (1): 23–28.

73. Donnez J, Polet R, Mathieu PE, Konwitz E, Nisolle M, Casanas-Roux F. Endometrial laser interstitial hyperthermy: A potential modality for endometrial ablation. *Obstet Gynecol* 1996; **87**(3): 459–464.

11

Laparoscopic Myomectomy

Techniques and results

J. B. Dubuisson
C. Chapron
A. Fauconnier

Introduction

Although uterine myomas are common (between 20–25% of sexually-active women have fibroids[1]), the diagnosis of a myoma should not be taken as the sole indication for surgery. Asymptomatic myomas discovered incidentally during clinical examination or ultrasound should be observed. Myomas causing symptoms (menorrhagia, pain or dragging feeling in the pelvis, urinary symptoms, constipation) warrant treatment.

Recently in the field of gynaecological surgery, there has been a marked interest in endoscopic surgery. The possibilities offered by these new surgical approaches (hysteroscopy, laparoscopy) have now brought the management of uterine myomas back into the limelight. There is now sufficient surgical skill and adequate instrumentation to enables myomectomies to be carried out via laparoscopy. This novel technique has only been reported by a few centres.[2–6] Initially, the objectives of these published studies were to evaluate the possibility of performing such operations by laparoscopy. The authors have been able to confirm that laparoscopic myomectomy is feasible, but it is now important to evaluate what the indications, results and risks are of such procedures. These points will be discussed later in this chapter after a description of the operative techniques for laparoscopic myomectomy.

Laparoscopic myomectomy

(1) Operative procedure

Anaesthesia and positioning of the patient

Laparoscopic myomectomy is performed under general anaesthesia. The patient is placed in lithotomy stirrups at the beginning of the procedure. This enables a uterine cannula to be introduced and a dilute methylene blue dye solution to be injected.[6] The methylene blue dye stains the endometrium, which facilitates the cleavage of myomas which are close to the uterine cavity, and closure of the myometrium after an accidental or voluntary opening of the cavity. After the methylene blue has been injected, we replace the cannula with a uterine mobiliser (we use the same instrument when performing a laparoscopic hysterectomy).[7] The uterus is positioned to give optimal access to the myomas: an anteverted position for a posterior myoma, a retroverted position for an anterior myoma. To facilitate manipulation of the ancillary instruments, low lithotomy stirrups are used.

Positioning of the suprapubic trocars

Three suprapubic trocars (two lateral 5 mm, and one midline 10 mm) are positioned carefully to optimise the safety and ergonomics of the operation. Their relative positions depend on:

- the uterine/ myoma size;
- the number of myomas;
- the location of the myoma.

The trocars should be introduced 3 cm above the uterine fundus, with the two iliac trocars inserted lateral to the epigastric vessels.

Instrumentation

Five mm monopolar scissors or hook is used for coagulation and electro-section of the uterus. The electrosurgical unit is usually set to deliver 50–80 W of power. Two 5 mm atraumatic forceps, a 10 mm grip forceps, curved scissors and a pelvicleaner (Storz-Endoscopy, Paris, France) are used to enucleate the myoma. A 5 mm bipolar forceps enables haemostasis to be performed during the hysterotomy and enucleation procedures. A 5 mm needle holder is used to close the uterus, with either 2–0, 3–0 or 4–0 Vicryl (Polyglactine 910, Ethicon, Neuilly, France) intraperitoneal sutures. Extra-abdominal sutures may also be required. The myoma is then removed by either morcellation,[8] or through a minilaparotomy or colpotomy incision.

Principles of the technique

It is necessary to accurately determine the anatomical relationship of the myoma to the round ligaments and fallopian tubes. The ureters should be visualised if the myoma is located within the broad ligament. As myomectomy is a conservative and minimally invasive procedure performed in relatively young women, it is important to bear in mind the principles of atraumatic infertility surgery at every stage of the technique. Magnification, meticulous haemostasis and impeccable closure of the myometrium are required. A 'microsurgical' technique prevents bleeding, adhesions and postoperative complications. The technique varies according to the location of the myomas.

1. For pedunculated myomas, the technique is easy and consists of coagulation and electrosection of the implantation surface. We occassionally use a loop suture, but when the implantation surface is small, no sutures may be required.

2. For sessile subserous and/or interstitial myomas, a hysterotomy is performed at the site of the myoma. A direct incision limits the bleeding. A vertical incision is most commonly used, although in some cases, a horizontal incision may be performed.

The authors use monopolar scissors or a hook for the incision. Complementary coagulation of the myometrial vessels is often performed using a bipolar forceps. Vasoconstrictive agents may also be used. Atraumatic enucleation is performed using a 10 mm grasping forceps, monopolar curved scissors and a pelvicleaner. The uterine cavity is not intentionally opened. The hysterotomy is closed if the incision is deep, long (>2 cm) or bleeding. Sutures are used to prevent haemorrhage, rupture of the myometrium in a subsequent pregnancy and to reduce the risk of adhesion formation. The uterus is usually closed in one layer (sometimes two layers) with interrupted 2–0 or 3–0 Vicryl.[9] The sutures are normally placed every 5 mm along the hysterotomy incision. After suturing, there should be complete haemostasis; if bleeding occurs, another suture should be placed.

Removal of the myoma

Myomas must always be extracted to avoid peritoneal reimplantation, and to allow histological examination. The myoma can be extirpated by a variety of techniques. Abdominally this can be achieved by using one of the suprapubic puncture sites after enlarging the incision (to 20 mm). This was traditionally performed by removing one of the trocars and bringing the resected myoma to the port site incision where it is held by a single tooth tenaculum. The myoma is then pressed against the peritoneum to prevent loss of the CO_2 pneumoperitoneum, and then fragmented under laparoscopic control using a small blade passed through the incision. This technique is long and difficult in overweight patients and with large myomas. Recently, electrosurgical morcellators have been developed for use, these can be inserted through a trocar, and are a significant improvement on the previous technique.[8] The myoma may also be removed through a posterior colpotomy. This is an easy and elegant technique. After removal of the myoma, the peritoneal cavity is irrigated with saline solution and a further check is made for complete haemostasis. No drainage is used.

A laparoscopically assisted myomectomy (LAM) is performed in specific cases where uterine suturing and/ or removal of the myoma is difficult.[10]

Results of our experience

From January 1989 to November 1997, we performed 328 laparoscopic myomectomies according to the techniques described above. The mean age of our patients was 37.5 ± 6.7 years (range 18–64).[11]

The indications for surgery were:

1. persistent bleeding despite medical treatment (n = 87; 26.5%)

2. pelvic pain (n = 105; 32%)
3. pressure symptoms (n = 33; 10.1%)
4. large myomas (n = 42; 12.8%)
5. infertility (n = 111; 33.8%)
6. recurrent abortion (n = 3; 0.9%)

The average duration of the operation was 129 +/– 59 min (range 30–320). Six hundred and ten myomas were removed, the mean number per patient was 1.9 +/– 1.6 (range 1–14). Only one myoma was removed in 205 patients (62.5%). Two myomas were removed in 53 patients (16.6%), three in 31 patients (9.5%) and four or more in 39 women (1.8%). The mean diameter of the largest myoma was 54.6 +/– 23 mm and the range was between 50 and 70 mm in 34.5% (113 cases), between 70 and 90 mm in 18% (59 cases) and 90 mm or more in 10.6% (35 cases). The type of the largest myoma removed was intramural in 43% of the cases (n = 141), subserous in 41.8% (n = 137) and pedunculated in 15.2% (n = 50).

Two hundred and eighty-seven women (87.5%) were treated using a laparoscopic myomectomy. In 31 women, a laparoscopic assisted myomectomy was required (LAM) (9.4%). In these cases, the uterine suture and extirpation were performed through a transverse minilaparotomy incision (4 cm long) using the 'long' instruments from a laparotomy instrument set. In 10 cases (3%) conversion to laparotomy was necessary. The two main reasons for conversion were difficulties in suturing or significant bleeding. However, no woman in our series had a blood transfusion. In one case a conversion to laparotomy was performed because of sudden hypercapnia. In another case conversion to laparotomy was performed because of difficulty in dissecting an 8 cm diameter myoma from the myometrium. The histology subsequently confirmed the presence of adenomyosis.

The complication rate for LM was 7.6% (25 cases). Apart from the 10 patients who required conversion to a laparotomy, 15 other patients had complications. These operative complications were haemorrhage (11 cases, 3%) hypercapnia (1 case, 0.3%), subcutaneous emphysema (2 cases, 0.6%), uterine perforation (1 case, 0.3%). One major late post-operative complication was observed; a uterine rupture during pregnancy.[12] This patient had undergone a bilateral salpingostomy and LM for infertility secondary to bilateral tubal disease and an intramural posterior wall myoma measuring 3 cm. The uterus was repaired with 3–0 vicryl stitches. The patient later presented as an emergency with pelvic pain at 34 weeks gestation. The diagnosis of uterine rupture was made immediately and an emergency laparotomy performed. A large uterine rupture at the location of the hysterotomy scar was noted. It was apparent that the placenta and the body of the fetus had delivered into the abdominal cavity through a large postero-fundal uterine rupture. The rupture was enlarged with a scalpel and the baby was delivered. The post-operative course was uneventful for the mother and baby.

Discussion

Diagnosing a uterine myoma does not necessarily imply surgery. Only myomas which are complicated or large, those which increase rapidly in size and those whose symptoms persist in spite of correct medical treatment should be operated upon. When surgery is indicated, the problem arises as to which technique should be used. The development of endoscopic surgical techniques permits, in certain cases, the operation to be carried out by either hysteroscopic or laparoscopic means. The indications for these two surgical techniques are completely different. Hysteroscopic surgery is indicated for treating some sub-mucous myomas.[13,14,16] This technique is only suitable if both of the following conditions are fulfilled:

- The intracavity portion of the myoma must represent at least half of the volume of the myoma
- The myoma must not be larger than 4–5 cm

Hysteroscopic treatment may consist of either resection with a diathermy loop 13–16 or Nd-Yag laser myolysis.[15,17] For intramural myomas (subserous and/or interstitial) as well as pedunculated myomas, myomectomy, which previously always required a laparotomy, may in certain situations now be performed using laparoscopic surgery.

LM is a difficult technique; in our experience the rate of conversion to laparotomy was 3% and a laparoscopic-assisted myomectomy was needed in 9.4%. The overall complication rate was 7.6%.[11]

LM as an operation involves four specific difficulties. (**Figures 11.1–11.8**)

1. The location of the hysterotomy.
2. The type of hysterotomy.
3. The uterine suture.
4. The removal of the myoma.

The correct location for the hysterotomy incision is paramount. For an intramural myoma, the larger the subserous component, the easier it is to identify where to place the incision. For deeply embedded interstitial myomas, it is essential to use pre-operative ultrasonography. This guides the optimum location for the hysterotomy incision and can also measure the relative distances between the myoma, the serosa and the endometrium.

The second difficulty lies in the choice of direction for the uterine incision. The standard option is a vertical hysterotomy.[18] However, as most of the uterine vasculature runs almost transversely,[19,20] it may seem more logical to make a transverse incision. Theoretically, this type of incision would enable blood loss to be reduced, especially where an intramural myoma is deeply embedded and well vascularised. The authors cannot confirm this and still prefer vertical hysterotomy incisions. From a practical viewpoint, vertical incisions are easier to suture laparoscopically.

Difficulty in suturing the uterus is in our experience the main indication for converting to a laparotomy or LAM. The uterine suture may be performed in different ways, with either continuous suturing or separate stitches. The knots may be tied either intra- or extra-corporeally (in which case they are taken into the pelvis with a knot pusher). The choice of technique depends mainly on the surgeon's experience, and he/she should use the technique that they are most adept at. There is no gold standard for this, and we use separate stitches, as we do for laparotomy. If the myomas are deeply embedded in the myometrium, the suture can be made along two planes. The quality of the scar after LM has yet to be assessed.

Whereas the risk of uterine rupture after myomectomy via laparotomy is low,[21,22] there have, to the authors' knowledge, been three cases of uterine rupture after LM.[12,23,24] Rupture is related to defective healing of the hysterotomy. To obtain a 'healthy' scar and limit the risk of dehiscence during pregnancy, we propose some general recommendations:

- atraumatic technique;
- limited use of electro-coagulation to minimise tissue necrosis;
- no opening of the uterine cavity[24];
- meticulous suture technique;
- conversion to a LAM or laparotomy if any problem occurs.

Extirpating the myoma is the last main difficulty with this operation. Different techniques are available:[1]

- extraction via one of the suprapubic trocar ports following fragmentation using a scalpel;
- using an electric morcelator;
- via posterior colpotomy;
- extraction via LAM.

The authors prefer to use an electric morcelator or perform a posterior colpotomy. If a colpotomy is chosen, in cases of limited vaginal access and/or voluminous myomas, the myoma may need to be morcellated via the vagina in order to remove it.

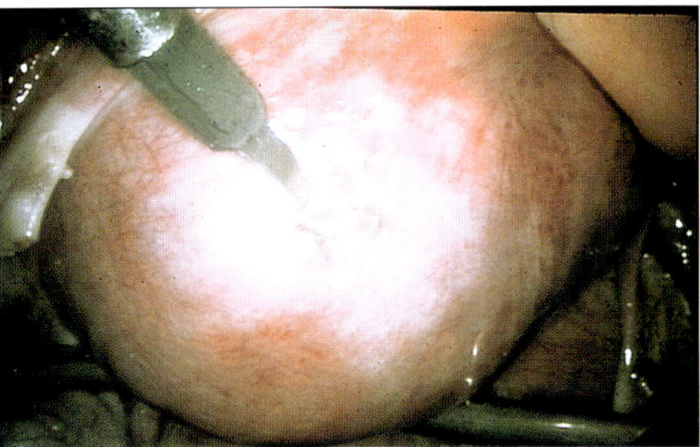

Figure 11.1 Posterior intramural myoma.

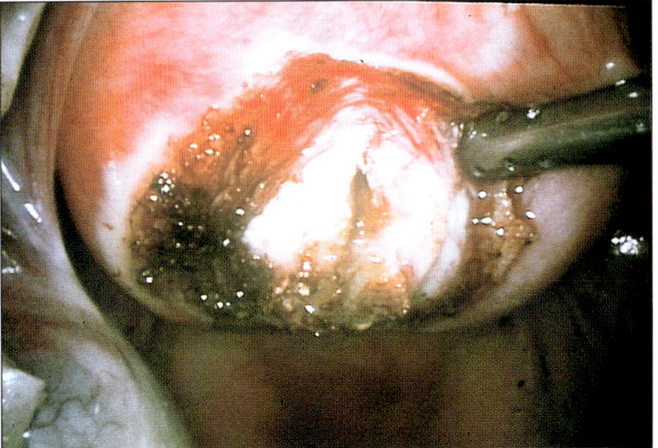

Figure 11.2 Vertical hysterotomy until the capsule of the myoma.

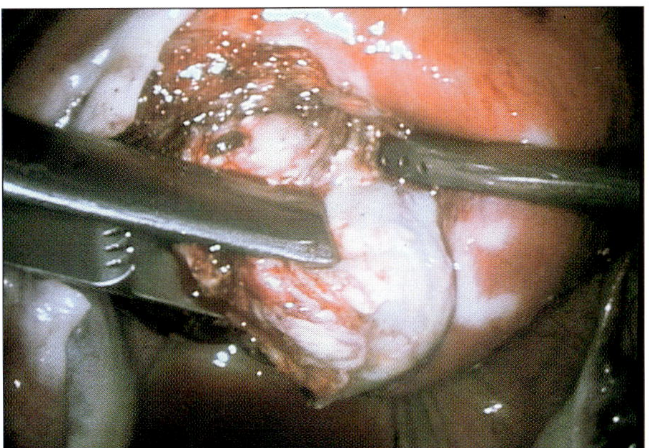

Figure 11.3 Enucleation of the myoma.

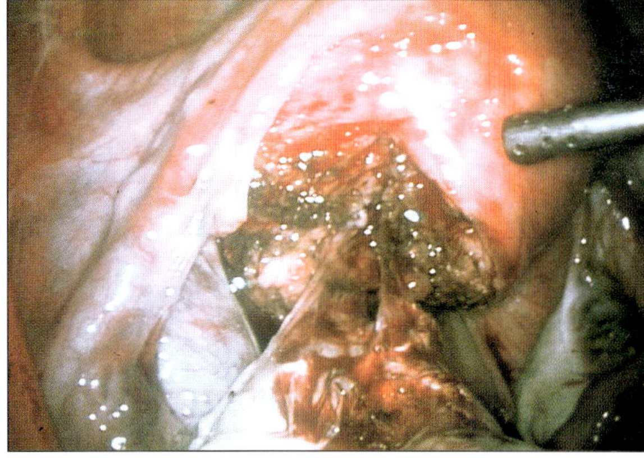

Figure 11.4 The enucleation is achieved.

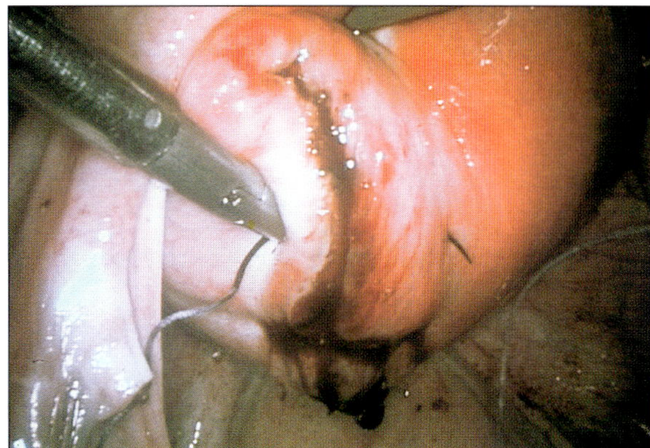

Figure 11.5 Suture of the hysterotomy.

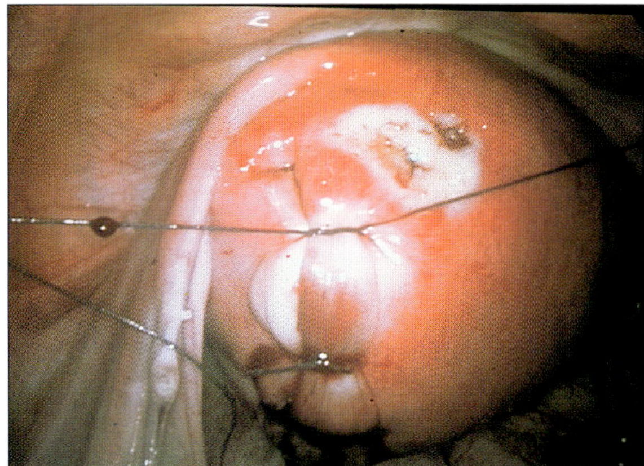

Figure 11.6 Suture using intracorporeal knots.

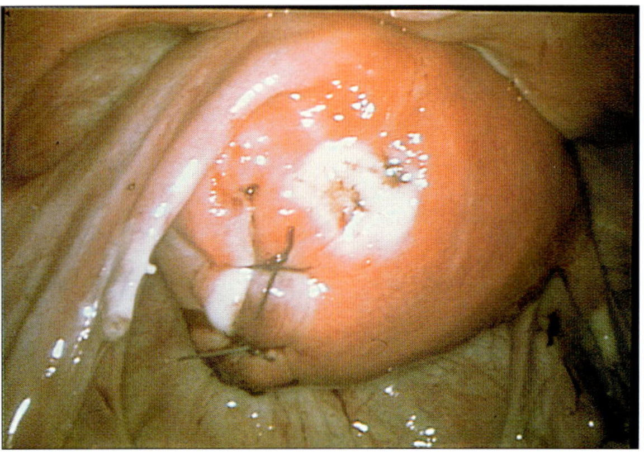

Figure 11.7 The suture is achieved.

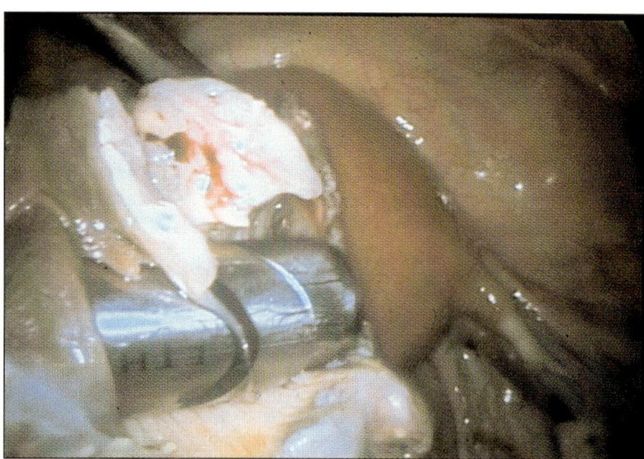

Figure 11.8 Extraction of the myoma using electric morcelation.

Although our results underline that LM is a difficult technique, the feasibility of the operation has been definitively proven. Moreover, it is a reproducible technique, as other centres have also reported encouraging results.[3,4,5] The factors which appear to limit its use are the size and number of the myomas. The authors consider that the operation should ideally only be performed when the size of the myoma is less than 8–10 cm and there are less than 3 myomas (of more than 4 cm diameter) to be resected.[9]

The operative technique for LM is now well defined and the indications for this operation are ever more specific. Further studies must be done to evaluate the risk of adhesions for this operation and the results of this technique for infertile patients.

Conclusion

Laparoscopic myomectomy is feasible. The technique requires an experienced laparoscopic surgeon with considerable endoscopic suturing skills. Laparoscopic myomectomy appears to be a safe and reproducible technique, with several teams already reporting their experience. The contra-indications are myomas of over 8–10 cm and/or multiple myomas. If these contra-indications are observed, laparoscopic myomectomy may usually be safely carried out. Preliminary results are encouraging with respect to the post-operative course and the quality of the uterine scar, but large scale series or randomised trials will have to confirm these initial results.

REFERENCES

1. Novak ER, Jones GS and Jones HW. Myomes utérins. In: Novak ER, Jones GS, Jones HW (eds). *Gynécologie Pratique*, Editions Maloine, Paris, 1970, pp 309–322.
2. Dubuisson JB, Lecuru F, Foulot H, Mandelbrot L, Aubriot FX and Mouly M. Myomectomy by laparoscopy – a preliminary report of 43 cases. Fertil and Steril 1991; **1**(56): 827.
3. Daniell JF, Gurley LD. Laparoscopic treatment of clinically significant symptomatic uterine fibroids. J Gynecol Surg 1991; **7**: 37–40.
4. Hasson HM, Rotman C, Rana N, Sistos F, Dmowski WP. Laparoscopic myomectomy. Obstet Gynecol 1992; **80**: 884–888.
5. Nezhat C, Nezhat F, Silfen SL, Schaffer N, Evans D. Laparoscopic myomectomy. Int J Fertil 1991; **36**: 275–280.
6. Dubuisson JB, Chapron C, Mouly M, Foulot H, Aubriot FX. Laparoscopic myomectomy. Gynaecol Endosc 1993; **2**: 171–173.
7. Chapron C, Dubuisson JB, Aubert V, Morice P, Garnier P, Aubriot FX, Foulot H. Total laparo-

scopic hysterectomy: preliminary results. Human Repro 1994; **9**: 2084–2089.

8. Steiner RA, Wight E, Tadir Y, Haller U. Electrical device for laparoscopic removal of tissue from the abdominal cavity. Obstet and Gynecol 1993; **81**: 471–474.
9. Dubuisson JB, Chapron C, Chavet X, Morice P, Aubriot FX. Laparoscopic myomectomy: Where do we stand? Gynaecol Endosc 1995; **4**: 83–86.
10. Nezhat C, Nezhat F, Bess 0, Nezhat CH, Mashiach R. Laparoscopically assisted myomectomy: a report of a new technique in 57 cases. Int J Fertil Menopausal Stud 1994; **39**: 39–44.
11. Dubuisson JB, Chapron C, Fauconnier A. Laparoscopic myomectomy. Operative technique and results. Ann N Y Acad Sci. 1997 Sep; **26**: (828) 326–31.
12. Dubuisson JB, Chavet X, Chapron C, Morice P. Uterine rupture during pregnancy after laparoscopic myomectomy. Human Repro 1995; **10**: 1475–1477.
13. Corson SL & Brooks PG. Resectoscopic myomectomy. Fertil Steril 1991; **55**: 1041–1044.
14. Neuwirth RS. A new technique for an additional experience with hysteroscopic resection of submucous fibroids. Am J Obst Gynecol 1978; **131**: 91–95.
15. Parent B, Barbot J, Guedj H, Nodarian P (Eds). Hystéroscopie chirurgicale Lasers et techniques classiques; Editions Masson, Paris, 1994, pp 48–60.
16. Siegler Am,Valle RF. Therapeutic hysteroscopic procedures. Fertil Steril 1988; **50**: 685–701.
17. Baggish MS, Sze EHM, Morgan G. Hysteroscopic treatment of symptomatic subraucous myomata uteri with the ND-YAG laser. J Gynecol Surg 1989, **5**: 27–31.
18. Verkauf B.S. Myomectomy for fertility enhancement and preservation. Fertil Steril 1992; **58**: 1–15.
19. Farrer-Brown G, Beilby JOW, Tarbit MH. The vascular patterns in myomatous uteri. J Obst Gynaecol Br Commonwealth 1970; **77**: 967–970.
20. Igarashi M. Value of myomectomy in the treatment of infertility. Fertil Steril 1993; **59**: 1331–1332.
21. Brown AB, Chamberlain R, Te Linde RW. Myomectomy. Am J Obstet and Gynecol 1956; **71**: 759–763.
22. Davids A. Myomectomy – Surgical technique and results in a series of 1150 cases. Am Obstet Gynecol 1952; **63**: 592–604.
23. Harris WJ. Uterine dehiscence following laparoscopic myomectomy. Obstet and Gynecol 1992, **80**: 545–546.
24. Friedmann W, Maier RF, Luttkus A, Schafer APA and Dudenhausen JW. Uterine rupture after laparoscopic myomectomy. Acta Obstet Gynecol Scand 1995, **75**: 683–684.

12

Management of Vaginal Prolapse after Hysterectomy

P. Hogston

Introduction

Prolapse is a common gynaecological condition; the true incidence of which is unknown. Not all patients are symptomatic, whilst others accept their symptoms and do not wish to have treatment. Women with prolapse may also suffer urinary incontinence. Prolapse after hysterectomy may affect any part of the vagina but when the vaginal vault is involved, treatment is more complex, carries a greater risk and is more prone to failure.

Epidemiology and aetiology

The epidemiology of vaginal prolapse, particularly after hysterectomy is poorly documented for many reasons (**Table 12.1**). Not all patients have symptoms nor present to a doctor. A specialist is required to differentiate the types of prolapse and it can affect women of a wide age range.

Uterovaginal prolapse accounts for between 5–29% of hysterectomies in reported series.[1] Denervation of the pelvic floor due to childbirth is the main risk factor[2] but it is suggested that collagen changes are also important.[3] Age, heavy lifting at work, bowel dysfunction and joint hypermobility have also been reported to increase the risk of prolapse.

The importance of prior hysterectomy as an aetiological factor is difficult to ascertain as long-term follow up of large numbers of women is required. Mant from Oxford reported a cohort study of 17,032 women between the ages of 25 and 39 over 17 years, where he examined the epidemiology of genital prolapse.[1] His data showed that a woman undergoing hysterectomy for prolapse had a risk of a subsequent pelvic floor repair at 15 years, 5.5 times higher than a woman who had a hysterectomy for other reasons. This increased risk is linear and there is every reason to believe that this risk will continue to increase as prolapse can present more than 15 years after hysterectomy.

Table 12.1

Aetiological factors in prolapse
- Childbirth
- Hysterectomy
- Age
- Menopausal status
- Heavy lifting at work
- Joint hypermobility
- Bowel dysfunction
- Incontinence surgery

Despite the argument that uterovaginal prolapse will be prevented by better obstetric care and more caesarean section, the rate of surgery for prolapse is increasing.[4] However with improved anaesthesia and more ready access to a specialist the threshold for surgery has undoubtedly fallen. The widespread use of colposuspension for stress incontinence also predisposes to vaginal vault prolapse and enterocoele in up to 17% of cases.[5]

With an increase in life expectancy, the number of women requiring treatment for prolapse is likely to increase for the foreseeable future (**Figure 12.1**).

Comprehensive assessment of the patient with prolapse and documentation

The diagnosis is usually obvious, although vaginal cysts, urethral mucosal prolapse or uterine

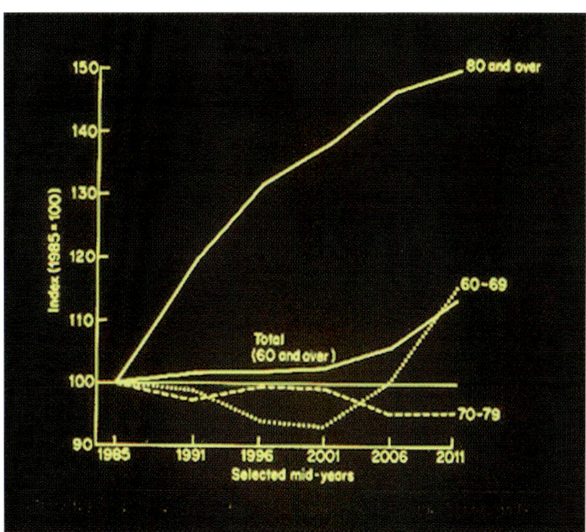

Figure 12.1 Predicted number of women requiring prolapse treatment

inversion may confuse the inexperienced. The supine position may underestimate the degree of prolapse, as may examination first thing in the morning or if a pessary has been in use.

There is no universally accepted system for describing the position of the pelvic organs and experienced gynaecologists do not always agree in their assessment of the same patient. Vaginal vault prolapse is invariably associated with other vaginal support defects (**Table 12.2**).

British textbooks tend only to refer to the three degrees of cervical/uterine descent although this can also be used for any anterior or posterior wall prolapse[6]. The term procidentia is often used for third degree uterine prolapse but it is simply another word for prolapse. When the uterus is outside the introitus (total vaginal eversion) all vaginal supports have failed. Many such cases of total vaginal eversion are in fact severe second degree prolapse and the cervix has undergone elongation and hypertrophy.

In the USA, American gynaecologists commonly use Baden's half-way system which refers to each part of the vaginal prolapse with reference to the hymen (**Figure 12.2**).[7] In order to standardise the terminology the International Continence Society has recently introduced the Pelvic Organ Prolapse Quantitation (POP-system), which allows accurate description of physical findings as well as meaningful comparisons between published data.[8] Once instructed thoroughly, it is an accurate and reproducible method of documentation.[9]

Table 12.2

Vaginal vault prolapse is associated with:

Anterior compartment prolapse
- Central defect
- Paravaginal defect

Posterior compartment prolapse
- Enterocoele
- Rectocoele
- Perineal body disruption

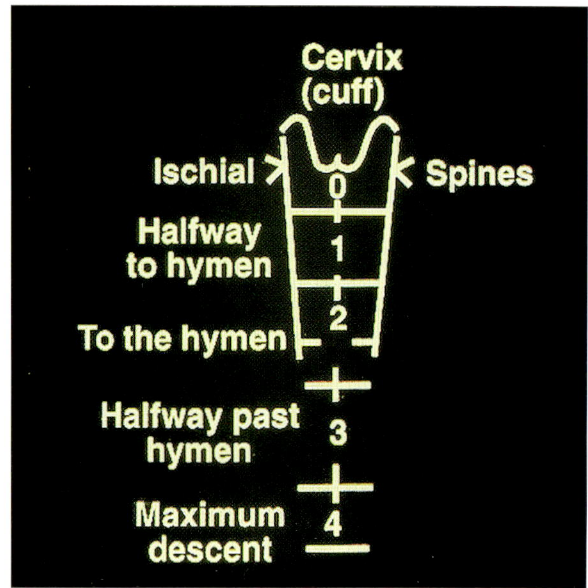

Figure 12.2 Baden's half way system.

Investigations

Although unusual, upper tract problems such as hydronephrosis and even renal failure have been described with complete prolapse and hence renal assessment by biochemistry and ultrasound need to be considered in such patients.[6]

Post-micturition residual urine measurement by catheterisation or ultrasound will identify patients in chronic retention who may also have voiding difficulty after any surgery.

Additional investigations such as cystometry will be required if incontinence is present but occult stress incontinence is increasingly recognised as a potential problem.

Veronikis reported that 83% of patients with massive pelvic organ prolapse have occult stress incontinence by using urethrocystometry and urethral pressure profiles after prolapse reduction,[10] whereas Versi only reported occult stress incontinence occurring in 28% of patients by using video-urodynamics.[11] Occult detrusor instability can also occur.[12] The availability of these investigations will determine their use but if surgery is contemplated in women with severe prolapse some assessment for occult stress incontinence is essential.

Investigations such as dynamic fluoroscopy or ultrasound can demonstrate the presence or absence of an enterocoele which can save tedious dissection in the operating theatre.[13] Several authors have now described MRI of the pelvic floor in patients with prolapse but it may also help our anatomical knowledge and allow study of normal women.[14] However, the test is performed supine, normal controls are limited and presumed abnormalities are not defined with objective measurements. Therefore its use should remain confined to research protocols.

Treatment

Conservative measures such as pelvic floor exercises, electrical stimulation or weighted cones are particularly useful for young women without a completed family and where urinary incontinence is also a problem. Vaginal pessaries are useful in the frail or infirm but no treatment may be an option in this group also.

For most women requiring treatment, surgery will usually provide the best option and approximately 10% of women undergo an operation for incontinence or prolapse in their lifetime. Particular care is required for patients with medical problems, but age *per se* is not a major risk factor under 80 years.[15] A study of 66,478 patients over 65 undergoing surgery for stress incontinence showed a mortality of 3.3 per 1,000.[16] Only 2.6% of patients were over 85 and the mortality for this group was 1.6%. However, the over 80 years population is growing and will place increasing demands on medical and surgical services (**Figure 12.1**).The rate and quality of healing depends on oestrogen[17] and the use of hormone replacement therapy before surgery in post- menopausal women is recommended.[18]

Prevention of vault prolapse at hysterectomy

The uterosacral-cardinal ligament complex is required to support the vaginal vault after hysterectomy and maintenance of vaginal length is important.[20] At surgery the ligament is severed, shortened and then reattached to the vaginal skin. The distance between the cervix and ureters increases with the severity of the prolapse allowing up to 15 cm of shortening in severe cases.[19] Many techniques of vault support are described, most using the pedicle sutures themselves to resuspend the vault.

McCall described his technique of cul-de-plasty (culdoplasty) in 1957, later modified by Nicholls[20] (**Figure 12.3**).

After excising any enterocoele sac, a separate suture is placed through the full thickness of the vaginal vault at a point selected to become the highest point of the reconstructed vault. The suture then

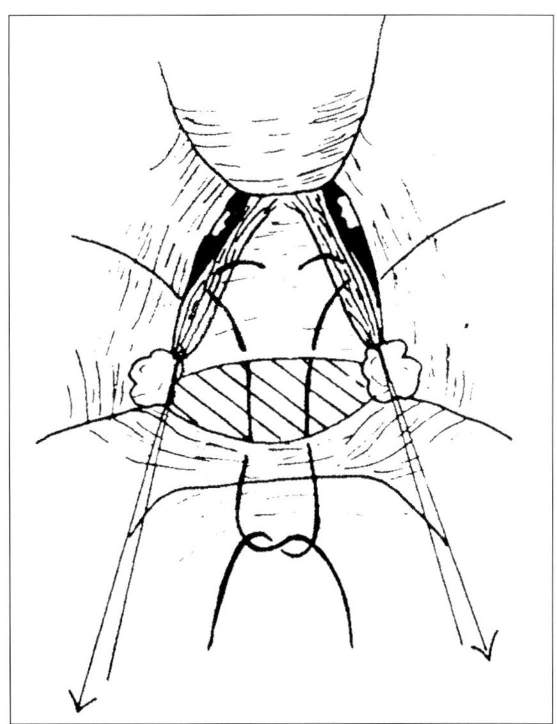

Figure 12.3 McCall's cul-de-plasty using a separate delayed absorbable suture to support the vaginal vault.

also picks up peritoneum and the uterosacral ligament at the level to which the vault will be fixed. The suture then takes the same tissue on the other side and returns through the vaginal skin to be tied. McCall originally used silk but a delayed absorbable material such as Polyglactin or Polyglycolic Acid will cause less problems with suture erosion and granulation tissue. Scientific evaluation of this method suggests an 85% success rate at 9 years.[21] Information from the Mayo Clinic in a series of 693 patients with post-hysterectomy vault prolapse identified only 47 (6.8%) patients with a previous vaginal hysterectomy and McCall's culdoplasty by this technique.[22]

Treatment of concurrent genuine stress incontinence (GSI)

Vaginal surgery consistently shows lower success rates than suprapubic operations, and needle suspensions are no better than anterior repairs.[23] To successfully repair a woman's prolapse only to leave her incontinent is every surgeon's nightmare. The reported success rate from anterior colporrhaphy for prolapse is 92% with up to 8-year follow-up.[24] In the presence of stress incontinence, however success rates are closer to 70%.[23]

By attention to technique and suture material, individual surgeons have produced good results from vaginal surgery. Beck reports a 94% success rate but only operated on 20 patients a year.[25] Grody reports a technique of paraurethral fascial sling urethropexy and vaginal paravaginal repair in 75 patients using Polytetrafluoroethylene (PTFE® Gore, Inc., Flagstaff, Az).[26] At 2 years, 92% of women were dry but larger series using these techniques are required. Furthermore, work from Austria has shown evidence of denervation of the urethra after vaginal surgery leading to a decrease in maximum closure pressure, which requires further study.[27] The surgeon is thus left with the dilemma of a combined vaginal and abdominal operation with increased operating time and morbidity.

Treatment of occult genuine stress incontinence (GSI)

The late David Nichols addressed the issue of occult stress incontinence and advocated pubourethral ligament plication in massive prolapse in order to elevate the urethra and urethrovesical junction.[20] Kelly's plication of the bladder neck is also necessary to eliminate funnelling but urethral plication is avoided as it narrows the lumen.

Despite the logic of his argument, data to support his thesis is not presented. Columbo and colleagues from Milan have addressed this issue in a randomised controlled trial of cystopexy alone versus cystopexy and pubourethral ligament plication in 102 continent patients undergoing surgery for prolapse.[28] At 1 year, 4 patients in each arm (8%) had post-operative stress incontinence at one year. They then investigated surgery in women undergoing surgery for prolapse and either stress incontinence or potential stress incontinence, defined as "a positive stress test with repositioning" by randomising 109 patients to either concomitant pubourethral ligament plication or Pereyra suspension.[29] With a minimum five-years follow up, Pereyra suspension provided significantly better results for potential incontinence (100% vs 76% objective). However for incontinent patients the cure rate was only 57% and not significantly different in either arm.

Complications were higher for the Pereyra group, particularly the risk of reoperation. Veronikis reported however a 56% incidence of low-pressure urethra as a cause of occult GSI and proposed a sling urethropexy using Mersilene mesh or fascia lata with a 100% success at one year. The optimum therapy for patients with GU prolapse and occult GSI remains to be determined.

Suture material

The ideal suture for vaginal surgery does not exist. If one regards prolapse in the same way as a hernia i.e.

a breakdown in connective tissue support then the surgeon would use nonabsorbable sutures of great strength. This is largely impractical in the vagina because of the substantial risk of fistula and the problems of dyspareunia. However nothing less than delayed absorbable suture is logical as connective tissue will only have 25% of its strength at 3 weeks, by which time rapidly absorbable sutures will have disappeared.[4] This should therefore be used for culdoplasty (see above) and rectocoele repair. In the anterior compartment, Polytetrafluoroethylene (PTFE®) has many attractive features, being a permanent monofilament suture that handles well and is incorporated into adjacent structures during healing.[26] Some practice with knot tying is required as they tend to slip.

The use of permanent 2-0 Ethibond® (Ethicon Ltd), and polyester and polypropylene for posterior compartment repair is described. However suture erosion is a problem and follow-up data is still required.[30]

Repair of post-hysterectomy vault prolapse

Pelvic floor repair for post-hysterectomy prolapse can be technically challenging and may involve repair of all vaginal supports (**Figure 12.4**).

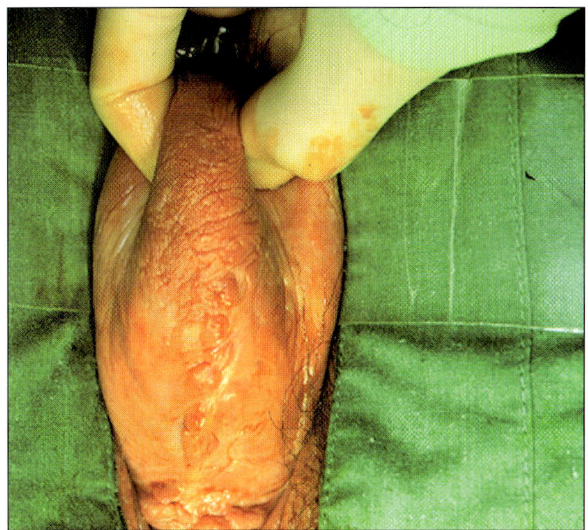

Figure 12.4 Complete vaginal vault eversion.

Anaesthetic considerations are paramount and regional anaesthesia may be appropriate to reduce opiate use if nothing else. Adequate time must be allowed for pelvic reconstructive surgery and the aim is to restore structure and function, particularly for sexually active women. Post-operative care is also important, particularly for the elderly and strategies to avoid post-operative confusion and hypothermia need to be considered.[4]

Vaginal approach

Traditional techniques include closure of the enterocoele sac and plication of the uterosacral ligaments (culdoplasty) or closure of the vagina by colpocleisis. Because these operations are often said to fail and prevent intercourse, other techniques[31] have been described (**Table 12.3**). The Mayo Clinic, however report the use of culdoplasty in 693 patients with post-hysterectomy prolapse.[22]

Complications such as infection and bladder or rectal damage were low at 3% and there were no long term sequelae. A postal survey of 660 patients operated on between 1976 and 1987 produced an 80% response. Only 36 (5.2%) patients had a definite second operation and 493 (71%) patients, after a mean of 8.8 years, had not had a further operation. Data on 164 (23.7%) were incomplete. Therefore, culdoplasty is a very successful low morbidity operation and should still be considered the operation of first choice.

Patients with total vaginal eversion are unlikely to have sufficient cardinal-uterosacral ligament

Table 12.3

Techniques for posthysterectomy vault prolapse

- Endopelvic fascia vault fixation
- McCall's culdoplasty
- Sacrospinous ligament fixation
- Iliococcygeal fixation
- Colpocleisis
- Sacrocolpopexy

strength and Nichols popularised sacrospinous ligament fixation for this indication.[20] After opening the posterior vaginal wall and incising the right rectal pillar, the sacrospinous ligament is identified. Two permanent sutures are placed through the ligament, two finger-breadths medial to the ischial spine. The sutures are attached to the vaginal mucosa and held until the vagina is two-thirds closed. The vaginal apex is thus firmly attached to the surface of the sacrospinous ligament without a suture bridge. Unilateral fixation is usually sufficient but bilateral fixation can be considered in severe cases.[32] Over 1,200 cases are reported in the literature but follow-up times are often not specified or less than 1 year. The number of procedures performed in the UK is estimated between 2,000 and 3,500 per year (Cory Bros, personal communication) but the success rate and complications have been reported in the literature for less than 100 patients.[33] The overall success rate in published series is between 77% and 92% but early reports use absorbable sutures which are not recommended.[31]

The advantages of the vaginal route include a high success rate, fewer complications, less pain and a shorter hospital stay. There is the ability to repair other defects and maintain vaginal length and thus coital function. Specific complications include buttock pain due to damage of a small nerve running through the sacrospinous ligament in 3%, which settles spontaneously by six weeks.[31] Gluteal pain and lumbar plexus neuropathy require immediate removal of sutures that have been incorrectly placed. Cystocoele is frequently reported as a long-term problem but only Smilen *et al* have compared long-term results of similar patients undergoing pelvic floor repair with and without sacrospinous fixation.[34] They found recurrent cystocoele in similar numbers suggesting other factors than the sacrospinous fixation determine subsequent cystocoele. Stress incontinence is rare. Although infrequent, serious complications have been reported, and with the more widespread use of the technique many are likely to go unreported. Life-threatening haemorrhage from laceration of the hypogastric venous plexus or inferior gluteal artery (resulting in death) has occurred.[35] The anatomic variations mean the inferior gluteal artery may arise from the posterior division of the internal iliac artery and hence ligation of the hypogastric artery may increase pulse pressure and worsen rather than help (**Figure 12.5**). Vascular clips, packing or embolization are suggested in these difficult situations and involvement of other colleagues is vital.

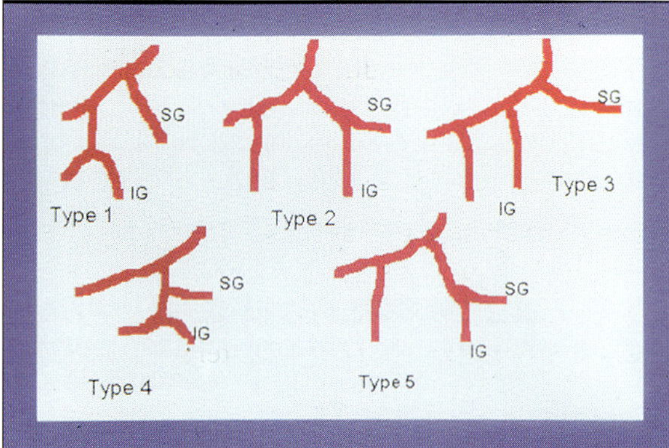

Figure 12.5 Vascular anatomical variations.

Other vaginal operations include endopelvic fascia fixation and iliococcygeal fixation of the vagina.[31] Partial vaginectomy seems to have been performed concomitantly, which is itself a treatment, but will also result in a short vagina.

Abdominal approach

Several authors have described the use of sacrocolpopexy interposing mesh between the vagina and sacrum.[4] The disadvantage of laparotomy is particularly clear in the elderly with more complications and a longer recovery time. Positioning the mesh retroperitonealy involves careful dissection to avoid the ureter, middle sacral vessels, common iliac vein and mesocolon. Nonabsorbable sutures are used to attach the mesh to the vagina and sacrum with careful assessment of the length to avoid overcorrection, Synthetic mesh is commonly Marlex, Mersilene or GoreTex® and success rates in excess of 90% at 5 years are reported.[36] A concomitant colposuspension can be performed if stress incontinence is present and it is often necessary to repair vaginally any rectocoele and deficient perineum. Serious operative complications occur in low numbers in the literature but are under-reported by occasional operators. Severe haemorrhage and death can occur from presacral veins and the surgeon needs to be aware of the options including thumbtacks and magnetic applicators. Post-operative intestinal obstruction can occur if the mesh is not buried and graft extrusion and vaginal rupture can occur due to poor vascularity of the cuff itself.

The abdominal procedures have also been performed via laparoscopy as opposed to laparotomy.[37] Operating time is longer but the risks of surgery seem similar in experienced hands. Initial success seems acceptable but longer-term results are awaited.

Post-hysterectomy vault prolapse – which operation?

Experienced operators report high success rates with both procedures, with vaginal operations having less morbidity. In younger women with concomitant urinary stress incontinence, the abdominal approach is likely to be more appropriate since colposuspension would be the operation of choice for the stress incontinence. In the absence of incontinence or cystocoele, however success rates are similar for both operations and the major difference is in complications. For elderly patients it is clear that vaginal surgery carries less risk, lower morbidity, shorter hospital stay and faster return to normal activities.[31]

A comparative study from Canada reports a large personal series of 130 vaginal sacrospinous fixations and 80 abdominal sacrocolpopexies over 6 years.[38] It is not clear why one operation was chosen over the other, although 59 of the abdominal group (74%) had a colposuspension as well. The failure rate over a mean of 3 years was 2% in both groups perhaps highlighting good case selection for the procedures. Benson has reported the only randomised study of vaginal versus abdominal surgery for recurrent prolapse.[39] Of 101 patients randomised, 88 completed the study and half the patients had complete pelvic organ prolapse. Abdominal sacrocolpopexy showed a higher success rate and the need for fewer subsequent operations.

Conclusion

Vaginal vault prolapse is a difficult condition to manage and is not suitable for the occasional operator. From published series both approaches appear equally effective and individual patient assessment by a surgeon regularly performing such procedures would appear to be the key to success rather than the procedure *per se*.

REFERENCES

1. Mant J, Painter R, Vessey M. Epidemiology of genital prolapse: observations from the Oxford Family Planning Association study. *Br J Obstet Gynaecol* 1997; **104**: 579–585.
2. Smith ARB, Hosker GL, Warrell DW. The role of partial denervation of the pelvic floor in the aetiology of genitourinary prolapse and stress incontinence of urine. A neurophysiological study. *Br J Obstet Gynaecol* 1989; **96**: 24–28.
3. Versi E, Cardozo L, Brincat M, Cooper D, Montgomery J, Studd J. Correlation of urethral physiology and skin collagen in postmenopausal women. *Br J Obstet Gynaecol* 1988; **95**:147–152.
4. Grody MHT. *Benign Postreproductive Gynaecologic Surgery*. New York. McGraw Hill. 1995.
5. Wiskind AK, Creighton SM, Stanton SL. The incidence of genital prolapse after the Burch colposuspension. *Am J Obstet Gynaecol* 1992; **167**: 399–405.
6. Cardozo L. Urogynaecology. Churchill Livingstone 1997.
7. Baden WF, Walker T. *Surgical repair of vaginal defects* Lippincott, Philadelphia. 1992.
8. Bump RC, Bo K, Brubaker L, DeLancey J, Karskov P, Schull B *et al.* The standardisation of terminology of female pelvic organ prolapse and pelvic floor dysfunction. *Am J Obstet Gynaecol* 1996; **175**: 10–17.

9. Steele A, Mallipeddi P, Welgoss J, Soled S, Kohli N, Karram M. Teaching the pelvic organ prolapse quantitation system *Am J Obstet Gynaecol* 1998; **179**: 1458–1464.

10. Veronikis DK, Nichols DH, Wakamatsu MM. The incidence of low-pressure urethra as a function of prolapse-reducing technique in patients with massive pelvic organ prolapse (maximum descent at all vaginal sites). *Am J Obstet Gynaecol* 1997; **177**: 1305–1314.

11. Versi E, Griffiths DJ, Giovanini D. Video-urodynamic diagnosis of occult GSI in patients with pelvic organ prolapse (abstract). *Int Urogynecol J* 1997; **8**(1): S079.

12. Rosenzweig BA, Pushkin S, Blumenfield D, Bhatia NN. Prevalence of abnormal urodynamic test results in continent women with severe genitourinary prolapse. *Obstet Gynaecol* 1992; **79**: 539–542.

13. Smith C, Brubaker LT, Saclarides TJ. *The Female Pelvic Floor: Disorders of Function and Support.* Philadelphia: Davis 1996.

14. Aronson MP, Bates SM, Jacoby AF, Chelmow D, Sant GR. Periurethral and paravaginal anatomy: an endovaginal magnetic resonance imaging study. *Am J Obstet Gynaecol* 1995; **173**: 1702–1710.

15. Muller K. Operating on the elderly woman. *Curr Opinion Obstet Gynaecol* 1997; **3**: 300–305.

16. Sultana CJ, Campbell JW, Pisanelli WS, Sivinski L, Rimm AA. Morbidity and mortality of incontinence surgery in elderly women: An analysis of Medicare data. *Am J Obstet Gynaecol* 1997; **176**: 34–48.

17. Ashcroft GA, Dodsworth J, Van Boxtel E, Tarnuzzer RW, Horan MA, Schultz GS, Ferguson MW. Estrogen accelerates cutaneous wound healing associated with an increase in TGF-B1 levels. *Nature Medicine* 1997; **3**: 1209–1215.

18. Obanye R, Hogston P. The pre-operative use of oestrogen for vaginal surgery *J Br Menopause Soc* 1996; **3**: 23–26.

19. DeLancey JO, Strohbehn K, Aronson MP. Comparison of ureteral and cervical descents during vaginal hysterectomy for vaginal prolapse. *Am J Obstet Gynaecol* 1998; **179**: 1405–1410.

20. Nichols DH, Randall CL. *Vaginal Surgery* 4th edn. Baltimore: Williams & Wilkins 1996.

21. Colombo M, Milani R. Sacrospinous ligament fixation and modified McCall culdoplasty during vaginal hysterectomy for advanced vaginal prolapse. *Am J Obstet Gynaecol* 1998; **179**: 13–20.

22. Webb MJ, Aronson MP, Ferguson LK, Lee RA. Posthysterectomy vaginal vault prolapse: primary repair in 693 patients. *Obstet Gynaecol* 1998: **92**: 281–285.

23. Jarvis GJ. Surgery for genuine stress incontinence. *Br J Obstet Gynaecol* 1996; **101**: 371–374.

24. Weber AM, Walters MD. Anterior vaginal prolapse: review of anatomy and techniques of surgical repair. *Obstet Gynaecol* 1997; **89**: 311–318.

25. Beck RP, McCormick S, Nordstrom L. 25 year experience with 519 anterior colporrhaphy procedures. *Obstet Gynaecol* 1991; **78**: 1011–1018.

26. Grody MHT, Nyirjesy P, Kelley LM, Millar ML. Paraurethral fascial sling urethropexy and vaginal paravaginal defects cystopexy in the correction of urethrovesical prolapse. *Int Urogynecol J* 1995; **6**: 80–85.

27. Zivkovic F, Tamussino K, Ralph G, Schied G, Auer-Grumbach M. Effect of vaginal surgery on the lower urinary tract. *Curr Opinion Obstet Gynaecol* 1997; **9**: 329–331.

28. Columbo M, Maggioni A, Zanetta G, Vignalli M, Milani R. Prevention of postoperative stress urinary incontinence after surgery for genitourinary prolapse. *Obstet Gynaecol* 1996; **87**: 266–271.

29. Columbo M, Maggioni A, Scalambrino S, Vitobello D, Milani R. Surgery for genitourinary prolapse and stress incontinence. A randomised trial of posterior pubourethral ligament plication and Pereyra suspension. *Am J Obstet Gynaecol* 1997; **176**: 337–343.

30. Cundiff GW, Weidneer AC, Visco AG, Addison WA, Bump RC. An anatomic and functional assessment of the discrete defect rectocoele repair. *Am J Obstet Gynaecol* 1998; **179**: 1451–1457.

31. Sze EH, Karram MM. Transvaginal repair of vault prolapse: a review. *Obstet Gynaecol* 1997; **89**: 466–475.

32. Pohl JF, Frattarelli JL. Bilateral transvaginal sacrospinous colpopexy: preliminary experience. *Am J Obstet Gynaecol* 1997; **177**: 1356–1362.

33. Carey MO, Slack MC. Transvaginal sacrospinous colpopexy for vault and marked uterovaginal prolapse. *Br J Obstet Gynaecol* 1994; **101**: 536–540.

34. Smilen SW, Saini J, Wallach SJ, Porges RF. The risk of cystocoele after sacrospinous ligament fixation *Am J Obstet Gynaecol* 1998; **179**: 1465–1472.

35. Barksdale PA, Elkins TE, Sanders CK, Jaramillo FE, Gasser RF. An anatomic approach to pelvic haemorrhage during sacrospinous ligament fixation of the vaginal vault. *Obstet Gynecol* 1998; **91**: 715–718.

36. Snyder TE, Krantz KE. Abdominal retroperitoneal sacral colpopexy for the correction of vaginal prolapse *Obstet Gynaecol* 1991; **77**: 944–949.

37. Mahendran D, Prashar S, Smith AR, Murphy D. Laparoscopic sacrocolpopexy in the management of vaginal vault prolapse *Gynecol Endosc* 1996; **5**: 217–222.

38. Hardiman PJ, Drutz HP. Sacrospinous vault suspension and abdominal colposacropexy: success rates and complications. *Am J Obstet Gynaecol* 1996; **175**: 612–616.

39. Benson JT, Lucente V, McClellan E. Vaginal versus abdominal reconstructive surgery for the treatment of pelvic support defects: A prospective randomised study with long term outcome evaluation. *Am J Obstet Gynaecol* 1996; **175**: 1418–1422.

13

Recent Advances in Gynaecological Oncology Surgery

R. A. F. Crawford

Patterns of gynaecological cancer

The patterns of gynaecological cancer seen in the UK are changing with an increase in ovarian cancer and less cervical cancer. Gynaecological cancer, in the most part associated with the post-menopausal woman, will become more important as the aged proportion of the population increases. It accounted for approximately 6,400 deaths in England and Wales in 1997 with a rate of 24 per 100,000 women. This death rate is largely due to ovarian cancer which continues to be one of the leading causes of cancer death in women. Due to the success of the cervical screening programme in which 85% of women between 25 and 64 years have had a cervical smear in the previous five years, overall incidence and mortality from cervical cancer is falling. There were 2740 new cases of cervical cancer in England and Wales in 1997 which represents a 26% fall in incidence over the last five years (NHS Cervical Screening Programme). Since 1991, mortality from cervical cancer has fallen by 7% per year with only 1222 deaths from cervical cancer in 1997. In the UK, care of gestational trophoblastic disease (GTD) has been centralised since 1973. Surgery has little role to play in the management of GTD other than at the initial diagnosis. No further comment will be made about GTD other than to mention that it is more common than vulval cancer and yet its centralisation of care has not been detrimental to the gynaecological service in the UK. Gynaecological cancer accounts for less than 10% of the total gynaecological budget in the district general hospital and, therefore, the transfer of women with cancer for specialist surgery and further management is unlikely to affect the unit significantly. The benefits for the woman are likely to be an improved survival and better quality of life.

In this chapter, the following topics will be discussed:

1. the changing approach to ovarian cancer;
2. the exciting surgical concepts being used in cervical cancer;
3. the changes in the surgical management of women with endometrial cancer and vulval cancer.

Operative laparoscopy for lymphadenectomy

Operative laparoscopy has progressed dramatically in the last 10 years with most operative procedures now having an endoscopic equivalent. Gynaecological cancer has attracted the attention of the skilled laparoscopist because the laparoscopic equivalent to the open radical surgery approach could potentially be performed without the apparent morbidity. In using the laparoscopic approach, there is improved exposure in the true pelvis due to the significant magnification. There is a reduced incidence of ileus due to less bowel handling and post-operative analgesia requirement is less. This, in turn, reduces hospital stay and also the cosmetic outcome is better. The disadvantage of the laparoscopic approach is that it is technically more difficult and required theatre time is longer. Complications have been reported, and the relative high incidence of these may be related to lack of appropriate training and expertise. It may also be related to honest reporting of complications as well as difficulties encountered in developing a new procedure.

The laparoscopic transperitoneal pelvic lymphadenectomy has become a standard operation since it was first described by Professor Querleu.[1] Two monitors are placed just beyond the patient's feet, allowing a comfortable operating position for the two surgeons. The bladder is kept empty with a Foley catheter. The technique which the author uses is similar to most and involves a 10 mm laparoscope through a subumbilical incision. Three further ports are used for manipulation, dissection, haemostasis and specimen retrieval. Two 5 mm ports are used in the iliac fossae and a 10–12 mm port is used in the midline suprapubic area. The 5 mm ports are placed laterally to allow a good angle for operating on the contralateral pelvic sidewall. The larger midline port allows for specimen retrieval and the use of a Ligaclip applicator or linear stapler/cutter. The use of a clear port with a flap valve allows easy tissue retrieval as the lymph nodes can be observed as they are withdrawn from the abdomen. As usual for operative laparoscopy, a thorough inspection of the abdomen is performed. A steep Trendelenburg position allows the small bowel to fall out of the pelvis. The round ligament is divided with diathermy allowing access to the pelvic sidewall. If the lymphadenectomy is diagnostic and the uterus is being left in situ, the round ligament can be left intact. There are virtues in using either monopolar or bipolar diathermy for this manoeuvre. The author has now changed to bipolar and does not find this causes undue difficulty. Using scissors and dissectors, the external iliac vessels are visualised. The temptation is to begin the dissection too laterally which leads to damage of the genito-femoral nerve and the psoas muscle. The paravesical and pararectal spaces are developed as in the open procedure. The author usually strips the external iliac vessels first but some operators clear the obturator fossa early as bleeding will stain the tissues reducing the clarity of the picture. The obturator fossa is easily entered by slipping medially over the external iliac vein. Alternatively, access to this area can be obtained by dissecting behind the external iliac vessels and retracting them medially. Attention is paid to preserving the obturator nerve by identifying it before any sharp dissection or diathermy is performed. At present, the author uses a laparoscopic 10 mm Babcock forcep to retrieve the nodal tissue. Alternatively, the three pronged Ceolio-extractor (Lépine, Lyon, France) can be used. The contamination of the port site with malignant tissue is a potential problem of more significance with ovarian cancer rather than cervical carcinoma.[2]

Laparoscopic para-aortic lymphadenectomy, described in 1992 by Childers[3] and then in 1993 by Querleu,[4] has a role in endometrial, ovarian and some cases of cervical cancer. The monitors are placed adjacent to the head of the patient. It is convenient to have the surgeon operating between the legs of the patient and the camera operator standing to the left of the patient. Identification of the landmarks is important and steep Trendelenberg aids with displacement of the small bowel into the upper abdomen. On occasion, a further port can be useful for a fan retractor. An incision is made at the level of the bifurcation of the aorta over the common iliac artery. This allows the development of the retroperitoneal space and at the same time uses the peritoneum to keep the small bowel from obscuring the field. As in the open lymphadenectomy, the nodal tissue is identified by finding the adventitia of the aorta with sharp dissection and diathermy. The fat pad containing the lymph nodes is then removed. Ligaclips can be useful for the perforating vessels. Bipolar diathermy is used in preference to monopolar diathermy as it is more precise. Care must be taken in identifying the inferior mesenteric pedicle and the ureters. The Harmonic scalpel (Ultracision – Ethicon Endosurgery – an ultrasound cutting coagulating device) may be useful in performing the lymphadenectomy as it will reduce the changing of instruments during the procedure.

Fowler[5] compared the yield from laparoscopic and open lymphadenectomies. In this study, between 62% and 97% of the total lymph nodes were sampled laparoscopically. It was noted that there was a significant learning curve with laparoscopic lymphadenectomy. Interestingly, no patient with negative nodes at laparoscopy had positive pelvic nodes at laparotomy.

Ovarian cancer

In advanced epithelial ovarian cancer, which accounts for about 75% of cases, management of the woman in a multidisciplinary setting with the surgery provided by an appropriately trained gynaecological oncologist gives the best outcome (a 25% increased survival at 3 years in women with stage 3 disease compared to a general gynaecologist, Junor, in press). The gynaecological oncologist achieves a greater rate of cytoreduction than the general gynaecologist.[6] Although never proven in a prospective randomised trial, it appears that reduction of the tumour burden in advanced disease is associated with an improvement in the patient's symptoms as well as survival. However, even in experienced hands, not all women have disease that can be resected to less than 0.5 cm. The EORTC (European Organisation for Research and Treatment of Cancer) gynaecological cancer collaborative group have established a trial to examine the role of primary surgery versus primary chemotherapy. Both arms allow for the use of interval debulking surgery. Interval debulking surgery is performed part way through the scheduled chemotherapy, typically after three courses, and this has been shown to have a survival benefit of 6 months.[7] The MRC is running a trial looking at the value of interval debulking surgery in the UK (OVO6 started in 1998 and is recruiting patients).

Van Dam[8] used laparoscopy to assess the operability of women with advanced ovarian cancer in a pilot study of 83 cases. This was an attempt to define a group of patients who would benefit from immediate primary surgery (with the intent to leave no macroscopic residual disease). Forty eight per cent of the cases underwent primary surgery and 89% of these women had no residual disease remaining after surgery. A further 40% underwent interval debulking surgery after platinum chemotherapy but only 42% of this group had complete cytoreduction. The remaining 12% of patients had progressive disease despite first and second-line chemotherapy. In this last group, it is unlikely that aggressive surgery would have been beneficial. The result of further trials in this area are awaited to see whether this will be an advance in the surgical management of ovarian cancer.

In the group of patients who have their early ovarian carcinoma diagnosed unexpectedly on pathology, the original staging may be less than optimal. It is well documented that restaging of early ovarian cancer will lead to an upstaging in over 30% of cases.[9] The result of this upstaging leads to chemotherapy for those upstaged and a better survival for those who are true early stage. This restaging may be done laparoscopically.[4] Problems associated with laparoscopic intervention in women with suspect adnexal masses and ovarian cancer[10] will not be discussed in this chapter.

Cervical cancer

Laparoscopic surgical staging of cervical cancer by evaluating the status of the lymph nodes in the pelvic and para-aortic areas has been used. The Gynecological Oncology Group (GOG – the research arm of the Society of Gynecologic Oncologists in the USA) has always used surgical staging of the lymph nodes in protocols for advanced cervical cancer. Open para-aortic lymphadenectomy, whether transperitoneally or extraperitoneally, is associated with about 4% serious morbidity.[11] Enteric late complications from radiation after surgical staging are over 10%. Laparoscopic staging has been used in an attempt to reduce this problem. In a prospective series from Monash Medical Centre, Melbourne Australia, 4/14 cases had positive para-aortic nodes and their radiation fields were extended (Jobling T – *personal communication*). This led to changes in radiation fields in 25% of the cases with advanced disease. Posover[12] reviewed the Jena experience of laparoscopic staging. All patients with cervical cancer underwent laparoscopic para-aortic and bilateral pelvic lymphadenectomy and then a radical vaginal procedure if appropriate. Positive para-aortic nodes were found in 14% of cases, all of which were advanced. The radiation treatment was changed in 10 cases (either to include extended field therapy or to restrict the fields). No survival or long-term morbidity was included in these studies. In the UK, it is not the standard approach to perform para-aortic node dissection for cervical cancer as the positivity in operable cases is very low (3.1%).[13] Petereit[14] reviewed the role of para-aortic node evaluation and its impact upon treatment decisions. The absolute yield for surgically evaluating all stages of cervical cancer is low since those patients most likely to have involved para-aortic nodes have the lowest probability of cure due to high pelvic and metastatic failures, while those patients with the highest probability of cure are least likely to harbour occult para-aortic disease. They recommended the use of surgical staging for those patients who have positive and/or bulky lymph nodes on imaging (and with a reasonable chance of pelvic control). A second group was recommended for laparoscopic surgical staging where the patient had advanced disease (for which there was a reasonable chance of pelvic control) and negative imaging in relation to the para-aortic area. In this group, if the para-aortic region was clear of metastases, the radiation would then be limited to the pelvis and so reduce the overall morbidity.

The Schauta radical vaginal hysterectomy has been largely ignored as a method of treatment of early cervix cancer in the developed world as it was felt to require two operations – the vaginal operation and separate incisions for the lymphadenectomy. Proponents through this century have included Amreich in Berlin in the 1930s and Navratil in Graz Austria in the 1950s. Dargent[15] reintroduced this operation in the late 1980s. He used the laparoscopic pelvic lymph node dissection for staging and then went on to perform a radical vaginal hysterectomy if the lymph nodes were negative. This work demonstrated that it was possible to perform radical vaginal surgery with a minimum of morbidity and with good outcomes. Various published[16,17,18] and unpublished series have addressed the use of radical vaginal surgery in cervical cancer. It appears that radical vaginal surgery is possible and easier than total laparoscopic approaches. The morbidity is less than the abdominal approach even though the extent of the radicality can be greater than at the abdominal procedure. It will remain to be seen whether a laparoscopic vaginal approach will overtake the use of the abdominal approach. We are seeing a reduction in the incidence of cervical cancer and it is unlikely that in the UK we shall be able to provide randomised study data which will confirm the superiority of one approach over the other. The advantage of a two stage procedure (laparoscopic pelvic lymphadenectomy and then when the nodes are confirmed negative to proceed to a central radical hysterectomy either vaginal or abdominally) is that it reduces the use of adjuvant radiotherapy. The avoidance of dual radical treatments reduces the complication rate greatly.[19] The other advantage of learning the techniques of radical vaginal surgery is that it allows the surgeon to perform the radical trachelectomy.

In recent years, there has been an increase of 77% in the incidence of invasive carcinoma of the cervix in young women, aged between 25–34 years.[20] This mostly represents screen detected cases and, therefore, these women present with early stage small volume disease.[21] Whilst there is general acceptance in the UK that conisation of the cervix is acceptable treatment for superficial invasive cervical cancer (stage 1Ai) for those women wanting to preserve their fertility,[22] invasive cancer beyond this has traditionally been treated with either radical surgery or radiotherapy. These radical treatments have produced excellent survival results, but both modalities are associated with subsequent sterility and often significant morbidity.

Following changes in the FIGO staging rules in 1985, Burghardt[23] described 16 women with small volume stage 1B cancers managed conservatively with cone biopsy or simple hysterectomy alone and there was no case of recurrence after 5-years follow-up. In line with this and the view that radical management represented over-treatment for a proportion of the very early tumours led to the investigation of the use of less radical techniques particularly in women with an overwhelming desire to preserve their fertility. In a landmark paper, Dargent[24] reported a modification of the radical vaginal hysterectomy to provide adequate local resection of the tumour along with the sampling of the draining pelvic lymph nodes, thus dealing with the invasive cancer in an acceptable oncological manner. Dargent has performed more than 60 cases over the last 14 years (*personal communication*). Two women have had recurrent disease which has been distant from the pelvis and 16 women have given birth to healthy infants. Schneider[25] has reported two cases using a similar technique in 1995. We have reported our experience of this procedure.[26] The experience in London (St. Bartholomew's/ Royal Marsden and St. Thomas' Hospitals) has now increased to more than 20 cases since 1994 with seven live births. Roy[27] has reported a larger series (50 cases with 4 live births) from Canada.

All patients consented to the radical trachelectomy procedure as described below knowing that further treatment might be necessary and that the overall survival results are both unknown and might be worse than achieved with conventional therapy. The patients and their partners also received counselling and support from a clinical nurse specialist. The women selected for this technique had:

1. a strong desire to preserve their potential fertility;
2. a cancer which located on the ectocervix with little or no extension in the endocervical canal;
3. a small volume invasive cancer of the cervix as defined on excisional biopsy (either large loop excision of the transformation zone [LLETZ] or cold knife cone biopsy).

For the radical trachelectomy, the patient was placed in the lithotomy position as for a vaginal hysterectomy. No Schuhardt incision was used for additional vaginal access. Infiltration of the vaginal epithelium using bupivicaine and adrenaline facilitated the formation of the vaginal cuff. A sleeve was formed by incising the vagina circumferentially approximately 2 cm distal to the cervix. Sharp dissection was used to separate the vagina from adjacent structures and this cylinder of tissue was sewn over the cervix to protect it during the subsequent operation.

The vesicovaginal space was further developed in the preparation of the anterior part of the specimen. The bladder pillars were defined by the formation of the uterovesical space in the midline and the paravesical spaces laterally. The ureter was then palpated in the bladder pillar and further mobilised cranially with blunt dissection. The descending vaginal and cervical branches of the uterine artery were ligated and divided. The posterior part of the specimen was prepared by mobilising the Pouch of Douglas in the midline and sweeping the peritoneum in a cranial direction. The uterosacral ligaments were identified, ligated and divided approximately 1–2 cm from the cervix. The cardinal ligaments were identified between the paravesical space anteriorly and the pararectal space posteriorly. Again 1–2 cm of tissue was obtained lateral to the cervix to ensure an adequate margin of resection. Care was taken to ensure that the ureter and uterine artery were not included in the ligatures.

The endocervical canal was identified using a Hegar dilator (size 6) and the cervical isthmus was transected using diathermy. The anterior and posterior aspects of the uterus were secured with tissue holding forceps to facilitate the later anastomosis. The specimen was sent to pathology and a frozen section was taken from the endocervical margin to ensure there was no tumour present. A single monofilament non-absorbable suture (1 nylon) was inserted in the remains of the isthmus as a cervical cerclage. This was tied tight around the Hegar 6 dilator. Using polyglycolic sutures, the vaginal epithelium was reanastomised to the isthmic endocervical epithelium at the uterine margin ensuring that the canal was open. The remaining vaginal epithelium was closed transversely. The bilateral pelvic lymphadenectomy was performed either transperitoneally laparoscopically or extraperitoneally at open operation. All women were advised to use contraception for 6 months following surgery.

The radicality of cancer surgery is being questioned in all aspects of oncology and nowhere is this more relevant than in the management of the young woman with invasive cervical cancer. It is now common practice in the UK to treat superficially invasive lesions (FIGO stage 1A) with a cone biopsy to preserve potential fertility. The use of this approach is based on the observation that in these lesions, the likelihood of parametrial extension and distant metastases to lymph nodes is very small (less than 1%) in early stromal invasion. In 1977, Burghardt[28] stated that 'there was no therapeutic necessity for the removal of the uterine fundus and the adnexa in the management of small volume tumours. As the tumour volume enlarges, the likelihood of parametrial invasion and distant metastasis increases. The radical trachelectomy technique represents a midway point between the conservative (cone biopsy or simple hysterectomy) and radical (radical hysterectomy) treatments for cervical cancer. It is an attempt to provide satisfactory locoregional treatment for selected women with small volume invasive cervical cancers which according to the textbook should be treated in a radical fashion. The novelty of the approach is that these women are given a further chance to have a family and, at the same time have their cancer dealt with adequately. In the London group, we have had no cases to date with recurrent disease. The presence of positive nodes in three cases demonstrates the need to perform a pelvic lymphadenectomy in women with invasive carcinoma of the cervix other than early stromal invasion. In view of the excellent survival rate for women with small volume cervical tumours, we will never be able to guarantee that there is no increased mortality using this technique as the sample size for statistical significance would preclude a randomised study.

This new management may potentially risk suboptimal treatment for the woman if the size of tumour is wrongly assessed. It is also not possible to extrapolate from the successful cure of cervical cancer by radical hysterectomy and necessarily anticipate good results with a lesser procedure. However, the limited radicality may be analogous to the changes in practice seen in the last decade in vulval cancer where the same survival results have been achieved with the reduced morbidity of lesser surgery. The trachelectomy cannot be offered as standard treatment replacing the radical hysterectomy until further work and time have shown the efficacy of the procedure. In the UK, there is limited expertise with respect to radical vaginal surgery and this type of surgery should not be undertaken lightly, without appropriate training.

Smith *et al*[29] devised another approach to the treatment of early cervical cancer with a view to preserving fertility. The abdominal radical trachelectomy is a version of the radical total hysterectomy but the cervix is transected and the uterine corpus is anastomosed to the vaginal resection margin. The blood supply is maintained by the ovarian pedicle. There have been no live births yet following this procedure, which has only been performed in a few hospitals. It has been reported that there have been significant pelvic adhesions following this open abdominal approach to the cervix. It appears to be more sensible to learn the appropriate techniques for radical vaginal and laparoscopic surgery than use this hybrid operation.

Endometrial carcinoma

Endometrial carcinoma has typically been treated with a simple abdominal hysterectomy and bilateral salpingo-oophorectomy. The use of laparoscopy allows good assessment of the peritoneal cavity, the removal of the adnexae, the preparation for a vaginal hysterectomy as well as obtaining peritoneal fluid for cytology. Pelvic and para-aortic lymphadenectomy may also be performed if required. The MRC ASTEC study is looking at the value of pelvic lymphadenectomy and also at the effect of external beam radiotherapy. It is now actively recruiting. It allows the use of laparoscopy if the operator has sufficient expertise. The laparoscopic/vaginal approach is ideal for endometrial carcinoma as the patients have a minimum of morbidity and a short hospital stay. However, even in the most capable hands, the very obese patient may preclude a laparoscopic approach and the woman with a significant vaginal stenosis may stop a vaginal approach.

Vulval cancer

Vulval cancer is rare in the UK with less than 900 new cases a year. This means that each obstetric and gynaecology consultant will see less than one case a year. The management of this disease is being increasingly centralised. Whilst surgical advances led to a greatly increased survival rate with the advent of the butterfly incision, there was a significant morbidity associated with this surgery. A more conservative approach has now been taken with the wide local excision of the tumour and then separate incisions for the inguino-femoral lymphadenectomy. The radical local excision of the primary lesion spares the patient the psychosexual consequences of radical vulvectomy. Local recurrence occurs in up to 10% of cases regardless of whether a radical vulvectomy was performed or not. This recurrence can usually be treated with further surgery. By contrast, recurrence in the groin is usually fatal, so any patient with a lesion more than 1 mm stromal invasion should have at least an ipsilateral inguinal-femoral lymphadenectomy performed. Postoperative groin and pelvic radiation should be given for patients with 3 or more micrometastases, one macrometastasis (>10 mm) or any evidence of extra-capsular nodal spread. The future role of lymphatic mapping to decrease the morbidity associated with complete inguinal-femoral lymphadenectomy awaits further investigation. Trials evaluating the role of the sentinel node are underway.[30]

Conclusion

Laparoscopy has had a major impact on the operative repertoire of the surgical gynaecological oncologist. New operations with a slant towards conservative management are being seen in all forms of oncology. The review of practice has lead to improvements in the accepted gold standard operations as well as developments which given time may prove very beneficial. The appropriate use of multi-centred research will allow the changes to be evidence based.

REFERENCES

1. Querleu D, Leblanc E, Castelain B. Laparoscopic pelvic lymphadenectomy in the staging of early carcinoma of the cervix. *Am J Obstet Gynecol* 1991; **164**: 579–581.
2. Fidalgo de Matos CJ, Querleu D, Leblanc E. Pelvic endoscopic lymphadenectomy in the assessment of early cancer of the uterine neck: survey of 25 French hospital centers. *Rev Med Brux* 1993; **14**:163–168.
3. Childers JM, Hatch KD, Tran AN & Surwitt EA. Laparoscopic para-aortic lymphadenectomy in gynecologic malignancies. *Obstet Gynecol* 1993; **82**:741–747.
4. Querleu D & Leblanc E. Laparoscopic infrarenal para-aortic lymph node dissection for restaging of carcinoma of the ovary or fallopian tube. *Cancer* 1994; **73**: 1467–1461.
5. Fowler JM, Carter JR, Carlson JW, Maslonkowski R, Byers LJ, Carson LF, Twiggs LB. Lymph node yield from laparoscopic lymphadenectomy in cervical cancer: a comparative study. *Gynecol Oncol* 1993; **51**: 187–192.
6. Junor EJ, Hole DJ, McNulty L, Mason M, Young J. Specialist gynaecologists and survival outcome in ovarian cancer: a Scottish national study of 1866 patients. *Br J Obstet Gynaecol* 1999; **106**: 11: 1130–1136.
7. Eisenkop SM, Spirtos NM, Montag TW, Nalick RH & Wang H. The impact of sub-specialty training on the management of advanced ovarian cancer. *Gynecol Oncol* 1992; **47**: 203–209.
8. van der Burg MEL, Lent M van, Buyse M, Kobierska A, Colombo N, Favalli G, Lacave AJ, Nardi M, Renard J & Pecorelli S. The effect of debulking surgery after induction chemotherapy on the prognosis in advanced epithelial ovarian cancer. *NEJM* 1995; **332**: 629–634.
9. van Dam P, Decloedt J, Tjalma W and Vergote I. Is there a role for diagnostic laparoscopy to assess operability of advanced ovarian cancer? *Int J Gynecol Cancer* 1997; **7**: S28.
10. Young RC, Decker DG, Wharton JT, Piver S, Sindelar WF, Edwards BK & Smith JP. Staging laparotomy in early ovarian cancer. *JAMA* 1983; **250**: 3072–3076.
11. Crawford RAF, Gore ME & Shepherd JH. Ovarian cancers related to minimal access surgery. *Br J Obstet Gynaecol* 1995; **102**: 726–730.

12. Heller PB, Malfetano JH, Bundy BN, Barnhill DR, Okagaki T. Clinical-pathologic study of stage IIB, III and IVA carcinoma of the cervix: extended diagnostic evaluation for para-aortic node metastases – a gynecologic oncology group study. *Gynecol Oncol* 1990; **38**: 425–430.

13. Posover M, Krause N, Khne-Heid R, Schneider A Value of laparoscopic evaluation of para-aortic and pelvic lymph nodes for treatment of cervical cancer. *Am J Obstet Gynecol* 1998; **178**: 806–810.

14. Monaghan JM, Ireland D, Mor-Yosef S, Pearson SE, Lopes A, Sinha DP. Role of centralization of surgery in stage 1b carcinoma of the cervix: a review of 498 cases. *Gynecol Oncol* 1990; **37**: 206–209.

15. Petereit DG, Hartenbach EM & Thomas GM. Para-aortic node evaluation in cervical cancer: the impact of staging upon treatment decisions and outcome. *Int J Gynecol Cancer* 1998; **8**: 353–364.

16. Dargent D. A new future for Schauta's operation through pre-surgical retroperitoneal pelviscopy. *Eur J Gyn Oncol* 1987; **8**: 292–296.

17. Querleu D. Laparoscopically assisted radical vaginal hysterectomy. *Gynecol Oncol* 1993; **51**: 248–254.

18. Roy M, Plante M, Renaud M-C & Tétu B. Vaginal radical hysterectomy versus abdominal radical hysterectomy in the treatment of early-stage cervical cancer. *Gynecol Oncol* 1996; **62**: 336–339.

19. Posover M, Krause N, Schneider A. Identification of the ureter and dissection of the bladder pillar in laparoscopic assisted radical vaginal hysterectomy. *Obstet Gynecol* 1998; **91**: 139–143.

20. Landoni F, Maneo A, Colombo A et al Randomised study of radical surgery versus radiotherapy for stage 1b-11a cervical cancer. *Lancet* August 23 1997, **350**: (9077) 535–40.

21. CRC (1994) Cervical cancer screening. Factsheet 13.1.

22. Herbert A, Breen C, Bryant TN, Hitchcock A, MacDonald H, Millward-Sadler GH, Smith J. Invasive cervical cancer in Southampton and South-West Hampshire: effect of introducing a comprehensive screening programme. *J Med Screen* 1996; **3**: 23–28.

23. Morgan PR, Anderson MC, Buckley CH, Murdoch JB, Lopes A, Duncan ID, Monaghan JM. The RCOG microinvasive carcinoma of the cervix study: preliminary results. *BJOG* 1993; **100**: 664–668.

24. Burghardt E, Girardi F, Lahousen M, Pickel H, Tamussino K. Microinvasive carcinoma of the uterine cervix (International Federation of Gynecology and Obstetrics stage 1A). *Cancer* 1991; **67**: 1037–1045

25. Dargent D, Brun JL, Roy M, Mathevet P, Remy I. La Trachélectomie Élargie (TE) Une alternative a l'hystérectomie radicale dans le traitement des cancers infiltrants développés sur la face externe du col utérin. *J Ob Gyn* 1994 **2**: 285–292.

26. Schneider A, Krause N, Kühne-Heid R, Noschel H. Erhaltung der Fertilität bei frühem Zervixkarzinom: Trachelektomie mit laparoskopischer Lympho-nodektomie. *Zentralbl Gynakol* 1995; **118**: 6–8.

27. Shepherd JH, Crawford RA, Oram DH. Radical trachelectomy: a way to preserve fertility in the treatment of early cervical cancer. *Br J Obstet Gynaecol* 1998; **105**: 912–916.

28. Roy M, Plante M. Pregnancies after radical vaginal trachelectomy for early-stage cervical cancer. *Am J Obstet Gynecol* 1998; **179**:1491–1496.

29. Burghardt E & Holzer E. Diagnosis and treatment of microinvasive carcinoma of the cervix uteri. *Obstet Gynecol* 1977; **49**: 641–653.

30. RCOG working Party Report. Clinical recommendations for the management of vulval cancer. RCOG Press, July 1999.

14

What is the Current Role of Endometrial Ablation and Resection

D. E. Parkin

Introduction

"Endometrial ablation and resection is one of the most carefully evaluated of surgical procedures." wrote Garry in an editorial in 1997.[1] This statement is even more valid as more scientifically reliable studies are published. In this article the role of ablative methods is assessed, concentrating on the most robust studies and comparing them to less sound evidence. For ease, all methods are referred to as endometrial ablation, including resection and the non-hysteroscopic methods.

The story of endometrial ablation to date has had five phases. The first phase was characterised by extreme enthusiasm promoted by the pioneers. They were claiming that hysterectomy for menorrhagia was a thing of the past with the development of these procedures, which gave excellent results with few risks. The second phase was a reactionary backlash by those who had tried hysteroscopic ablative methods and found that either they were difficult to perform, gave unexpected major complications or discovered that the results were not as good as claimed by the proponents. This was partly because training courses were not yet available and not all gynaecologists were able to self teach themselves to the same level as achieved by the pioneers. As long-term results were not yet available, patient expectation was perhaps too high, especially if amenorrhoea was the expected and desired outcome leading to a degree of disillusionment. The third phase was the publication of the first randomised trials (especially those comparing transcervical resection of the endometrium (TCRE) to hysterectomy) along with the first large uncontrolled series. This gave credibility to these procedures and substantiated their continued use, evaluation and development. The fourth phase was (and still is) the further randomised trial results including their long-term follow up, the long-term follow up of the uncontrolled series and the national audit carried out in England and Wales. This wealth of data has ensured the place of endometrial ablation in the gynaecologist's repertoire. It has also lead to production of the first evidence-based guidelines on endometrial ablation. The fifth phase is the search for new techniques of endometrial ablation (second generation methods) which may be easier to perform with less skill and training, possible to perform under local anaesthetic and as effective as the classical hysteroscopic methods.

The history of endometrial ablation

Endometrial ablation began with Goldrath pioneering endometrial laser ablation (ELA) in 1981. Though in the UK Magos is thought of as the originator by introducing TCRE into Britain in 1989, ELA had already been in use in Glasgow by Davis since 1985.[2] Despite this early start in the UK, the rapid expansion of these techniques did not occur until the early 1990s. This is probably because the equipment for TCRE was far more readily available and affordable than that for ELA. This rapid expansion pre-dated both the evidence base to support its widespread use and the training courses for the techniques. The equipment manufacturers must take their share of the blame for this, as there was an active sales drive at this time. In the USA, rollerball ablation (RBA) was the leading method though has not been widely used in the UK.

Uncontrolled studies of a reasonable size then began to appear of both TCRE and ELA which gave support to their continued use.[3,4] When Nicholson *et al* independently followed up the patients treated with TCRE by Magos they found less convincing results suggesting that follow up may be biased by the patient's desire to please their surgeon.[5] It is conflicting evidence such as this which made results of randomised controlled trials (RCT) so vital.

Why do we need randomised controlled trials?

The main reason is to remove bias. This was perhaps less important in the very early days of endometrial ablation as we were unsure as to even the very basic safety and efficacy of endometrial ablative methods. As soon as these were available it was vital to compare them with hysterectomy. A randomised comparison was vital, if for no other reason than the satisfaction after hysterectomy is less than the perceived 100% and any comparison assuming that to be so is immediately flawed. Now that prognostic factors for a successful outcome after endometrial ablation are well recognised,[6] it is possible to produce an uncontrolled series achieving apparently good results. An example of this would be to include patients aged over 40, with proven excess menstrual loss and who wished the procedure. Some studies presented at conferences have even included postmenopausal women and used the amenorrhoea rate as an outcome measure. This rather cynical manipulation of data in small studies can only reflect poorly on the standing of gynaecological endoscopy.

The use of a RCT removes this bias as both arms are from the same population. Better still is an RCT using a clinically relevant and not overly exclusive population. In this case the results are both believable and applicable to every day practice.

In this new climate, where many second generation methods of ablation are being promoted by manufacturers, there is an increased need for unbiased evidence-based medicine in this field. At the 1999 meeting of the European Society of Gynaecological Endoscopy there were 13 second generation methods demonstrated in the trade exhibition and available for purchase.

Of these, only Vesta™ and MEA™ have been rigorously compared to the acknowledged "gold standards"- trans-cervical resection or laser ablation. Two other devices (ThermaChoice™ and Cavaterm™) have been compared to rollerball ablation - a technique which itself has never been directly compared in a RCT setting to hysterectomy. The remaining instruments' results are all based on case series, and cohorts (**Table 14.1**), with the limitations that are inherent in these studies.

Table 14.1 Published studies on second generation methods of ablation

Instrument	Type of study
Enabl™	Cohort
BEI™	Cohort
ThermaChoice™	Cohort, RCT
Cavaterm™	Cohort, RCT
Menotreat™	Cohort
MEA™	Cohort, RCT
Novasure™	Cohort
Vesta™	Cohort, RCT
ELITT™	Cohort
Menostat™	Cohort
First Option™	Cohort
Cryogen™	Cohort
Photodynamic therapy	Case reports

There is considerable market competition in this area, and the author feels that some manufacturers may be reticent about participating in RCTs lest their instrument proves inferior, with consequent waste of the investment put into development.

The final reason for promoting RCTs is the expansion of both evidence-based guidelines and systematic reviews.[7] Both of these approaches rely on the grading of evidence. This means that level I evidence (evidence produced from a RCT or meta-analysis of RCTs) will have a much greater impact than observational data (level 3) and may lead to changes in practice. Grade A recommendations can only be made from class I evidence.[7]

The evidence-based role of endometrial ablation

Structured reviews and guidelines stratify on the basis of the quality and therefore the grade of the evidence.[7] Therefore my discussion will be based around the evidence from RCTs, though using the best available evidence from other studies where a RCT has not been performed. The Cochrane Collaboration[8] have recently published on the use of endometrial destruction techniques compared to hysterectomy, and I will discuss their findings also.

Is endometrial ablation an alternative to hysterectomy?

There have been four RCTs comparing TCRE or TCRE and ELA to hysterectomy for the treatment of menorrhagia. Two of these were methodologically sound with 1:1 randomisation at the time that surgery was decided upon, the Bristol study from Dwyer *et al* and the Aberdeen study of Pinion *et al.*[9,10] A very important point is that both studies had an upper limit of uterine size of 10 weeks of pregnancy and allowed fibroids. Pre-operative hysteroscopy was not used to select out patients so making these patients a clinical entity which is generally understood by practising gynaecologists.

The follow up of these two studies varied, with only 4 months follow up in the Dwyer study compared to 6 and 12 months in the Pinion study. The other two RCTs either had recruitment when already on the waiting list for hysterectomy as in the study by Gannon *et al* or a 3:1 randomisation to TCRE with a high rate of patients declining to be randomised and a prolonged recruitment time as in the MRC multi-centre study headed by Magos.[11,12] The Cochrane Collaboration also includes Crosignani's paper[13] on the effect on long-term quality of life and clinical outcomes between patients undergoing endometrial resection or vaginal hysterectomy.

Despite these methodological differences the short-term results of the Dwyer, Pinion and MRC studies are remarkably similar. Dwyer found a satisfaction rate of 84% after TCRE compared to 93% for hysterectomy and Pinion at 12 months found a 78% satisfaction with TCRE/ELA and 89% with hysterectomy. Both studies showed the now well-established benefits of reduced risks and greatly shortened recovery time for endometrial ablation.[9,10] The other feature is that hysterectomy does not lead to 100% patient satisfaction when carried out for excessive menstrual loss despite giving complete amenorrhoea (except if a subtotal has been performed when a small amount of bleeding sometimes occurs). The role of ablation as a genuine alternative to hysterectomy, at least in the short-term was therefore firmly established. These short term results, though giving an evidence base to continue the development, still left the procedure open to the accusation that ultimately most or all women will end up needing a hysterectomy.

Long-term results of large uncontrolled series are now becoming available. The two that give the best estimate as to the long-term outcome are the long-term follow up of TCRE from the Magos team and ELA from Garry's team. Magos followed up 525 women for up to five years. Despite the apparent long-term nature of this study, the mean follow up was only 31 months and only 43 women were followed up for the full 5 years. Despite these limitations, the hysterectomy rate was only 9% and 80% avoided further surgery.[14] This is a robust response to those who usually feel that ultimately all women will end up with a hysterectomy following endometrial ablation. Garry and his team have reported long-term follow up of 1000 ELA procedures, but in fact only involving 746 women followed up for up to 6 years. The rate of repeat surgery was 15% during the period of follow up, but by using life table analysis they predicted a hysterectomy rate of 21% at 6.5 years.[15] Despite the size of these studies, they are flawed by the fact that follow up is not complete for the entire cohort over the whole time period and therefore they rely on statistical assessment to estimate the final hysterectomy rate. The other drawback is the fact that in an uncontrolled series the degree of symptomatology of these women at the start of treatment is unknown.

A genuine long-term review has been prepared by Pinion of the Aberdeen RCT for TCRE/ELA against hysterectomy.[16] These women were followed up by questionnaire and case note review between 4 and 6 years post-operatively with a mean of 61 months. Hysterectomy was avoided in

76%, with no overall difference in satisfaction between the hysterectomy and resection and ablation groups. Life table analysis showed that hysterectomy was unusual once women were 36 months after their hysteroscopic surgery. This result is reassuring as it shows that in this group of women hysterectomy was avoided in three quarters of them. This is despite the fact that they were expecting a hysterectomy and its associated amenorrhoea and were operated on early on in our learning curve. Based upon this and the short-term follow up of the RCTs against hysterectomy we can be assured that ablative surgery, especially with TCRE, is a genuine alternative to hysterectomy.

What is the role of endometrial ablation and medical treatment?

When ablative methods were introduced the general feeling was that as these were proposed alternatives to performing a hysterectomy, the same criteria as for selection for hysterectomy should apply. To try and stop a great increase in the total number of surgical procedures and because of the then unquantified risks of ablative surgery, it was thought by many, including myself, that patients had to earn their ablation (as for hysterectomy) by trying and then failing to be satisfied with the results of medical treatment. We then carried out a pragmatic RCT comparing TCRE as an initial treatment with medical treatment in women attending the gynaecology clinic for the first time. The results of patients randomised to initial TCRE were not surprising with the 78% of women being very satisfied with the result of their surgery at 4 months and an amenorrhoea rate of 38%. In the TCRE arm there was an increase in haemoglobin levels, especially in those who were mildly anaemic preoperatively. In the medical group however, only 20% of women were happy to continue with their prescribed treatment and there was no change in haemoglobin levels. Perhaps more importantly, the use of a health-related quality of life score; the Short Form 36 (SF36)[16,17] demonstrated that these women were significantly disabled by their symptoms at the start of the trial. At four months, the women in the TCRE group returned to normal values for their age, whilst the women in the medical group did not.[17] When Cooper *et al* followed these women up at 2 years, the same differences were still present. By this time, 49% of the women randomised to medical treatment had undergone TCRE and 15% hysterectomy. Only 20% of the TCRE group required any further treatment and only 10% underwent hysterectomy. There were fewer hysterectomies among those randomised to immediate TCRE which is reassuring. Of interest and concern was the fact that those women randomised to medical treatment who subsequently had a TCRE never achieved the same normal SF36 score of those randomised to an initial TCRE. This may be due to dissatisfaction if an acceptable improvement in symptoms is delayed by first using an ineffective medical treatment, despite the fact that there is no reason to believe that there would be any difference in the efficacy of TCRE between the two groups.[18] The conclusion from these papers is that patient choice must be taken into account when deciding on the management of menorrhagia. If a woman is keen or willing to be treated medically in the first instance then immediate endometrial ablation would not be appropriate. However, if a woman does not wish medical management then it would be unreasonable to withhold surgical treatment with endometrial ablation as if she is not satisfied with the outcome of the chosen medical management she may not ultimately achieve the same level of satisfaction.

The Mirena Intra Uterine System may be an option in this situation. Preliminary studies have shown promising rates of satisfaction and amenorrhoea when used for dysfunctional bleeding. Large RCTs comparing Mirena to ablative methods need to be performed to validate their roles, however individual patient preferences are making recruitment for randomised trials in this area increasingly difficult.[19] One possible role of Mirena may be in the woman aged less than 40 years complaining of DUB. We know that these women do not have as high a success rate as in older women. If this is successful, then an ablation once she reaches the age of 40 may be indicated.

Which patients are best suited for endometrial ablation?

Prognostic factors are now well recognised for success of endometrial ablation based on randomised trials and the large audit studies. These have been recently summarised.[6] Women who genuinely have excessively heavy periods have a better outcome after TCRE than those with normal menstrual blood loss. Gannon showed that in women whose menstrual blood loss was above 80 ml per cycle the subjective failure rate was 9% compared to 18% in women who perceived their periods to be heavy but who had normal menstrual loss.[20] Patient age appears to be important, with younger women having a lower satisfaction than older women. The Scottish Audit of Hysteroscopic Surgery showed a lower satisfaction in women under 40 years of age. In this study the satisfaction rate 1 year after treatment was 88% in women aged over 40, but only 79% in women below this age.[21]

The amenorrhoea rate in the early studies was closely matched to the proportion of women claiming to be very satisfied with the procedure.[9,10] This finding was especially found in the studies comparing ablation to hysterectomy where one arm virtually guarantees amenorrhoea. This factor may be less important now that the results are well known and patients can be counselled more appropriately. The presence of irregular periods or menstrual dysmenorrhoea has been thought to predict a poor outcome. However, our RCT comparing TCRE and ELA in 372 patients failed to find any difference in satisfaction using either of these criteria.[22]

Success or failure of resection or ablation of the endometrium is certainly multifactorial, with genuine and perceived severity of symptoms, patient expectation and uterine pathology all playing their part. There may also be subtle psychological factors needing more formal evaluation using tools such as the Short Form-36.[17,18] In addition, there is the efficacy and performance of the procedure as well as the pathological healing processes in the uterus.

The histopathological status of the removed uterus following failure of electrothermal endometrial ablation (rollerball) has recently been studied by Davis *et al.*[23] Though this study was on patients following rollerball ablation, the method has not been compared to other methods or hysterectomy in any published randomised trials. The results of rollerball in uncontrolled studies seem similar to the other ablation methods and a hysterectomy rate of 15% is not dissimilar to other series in the literature.[24] Davis found that failure is related to three pathological groupings. These are:

1. continued dysfunctional bleeding due to either regrowth or persistence of endometrium and adenomyosis;

2. complications of healing especially cervical stenosis;

3. unrelated lesions - in women still complaining of excessive bleeding they found endometrium to be present focally but not diffusely in the uterine cavity. They also found that hysterectomy for failure of ablation was associated with the finding of fibroids in 30% and adenomyosis in 27%.[23]

A study such as this does not tell us what "pathology" would be found women after successful endometrial ablation. In Pinion's study, women with a clinical diagnosis of dysfunctional uterine bleeding and randomised to either hysterectomy or ablation have been shown to have fibroids in 20%, endometriosis in 8% and adenomyosis in 17%, yet even after 4-6 years the hysterectomy rate was only 22%.[10] The conclusion must therefore be that many women undergoing endometrial ablation will be satisfied with the result despite having such pathology. The finding of such pathology at hysterectomy in those who fail may overestimate the importance of that abnormality and shows the value of a randomised trial. We still cannot reliably inform an individual woman of the outcome of endometrial ablation, though we now know some of the prognostic factors.

Which method of endometrial ablation?

The three-hysteroscopic methods, TCRE, ELA and rollerball all have their disciples. The major problem with comparing one uncontrolled series against another is that not only are you comparing the technique, but also the surgeon and the patient selection. There has been an unpublished trial of TCRE compared to ELA in the UK, otherwise there is only one RCT in the literature. In this study, TCRE was compared to ELA in 372 patients. This showed that TCRE was faster and caused less fluid absorption both as a mean value and in terms of large volume absorption. There were no differences in complications between the two methods, indeed the only major complication was a case of small bowel damage after ELA. There was no difference in outcome as measured by satisfaction (90%), amenorrhoea rate (45%), or hysterectomy rate (20%) between the two methods.[20]

The Scottish Audit of Hysteroscopic Surgery was a prospective study of both complications and efficacy in nearly 1000 women with an estimated 95% reporting rate. Approximately a quarter of the patients were treated by ELA and nearly all of the remainder by TCRE. No difference could be found between either of the methods in terms of complications (apart from fluid absorption) or efficacy.[21] The only dissenting voice is the UK audit (MISTLETOE) of 10,000 women. In this study, there was a higher rate of uterine perforation and emergency hysterectomy with TCRE than ELA.[25] This is concerning, but may relate to training and the fact that there are few occasional users of ELA because of the cost and scarcity of the equipment. The conclusion has to be that there is little or no difference between TCRE and ELA in any regard.

Second generation endometrial ablation methods

Because of the training and eye/hand co-ordination needed to safely perform the hysteroscopic methods, the search has been on to develop easier methods of ablating the endometrium. A further advantage of non-hysteroscopic methods is removal of any risk of excessive irrigation fluid absorption. As stated earlier at the time of writing there are 13 new methods available and these were displayed and presented at the 8th Congress of the European Congress of Gynaecological Endoscopy in December 1999. The two methods with the most apparent promise are discussed below.

Balloon methods
These methods rely on a combination of heating and pressure within the uterine cavity to achieve destruction of the endometrium and the superficial myometrium. The distensibility of the balloons should allow them to take up the shape of the endometrial cavity. There seems to be a reluctance to use these methods in anything other than a regular 8 cm cavity in the absence of fibroids. Singer, in 1994, published a series of 18 women treated with balloon endometrial ablation (BEA) under general anaesthetic. In this small series, 83% had a degree of improvement.[26]

The Thermachoice™ system was used in a RCT of 275 patients comparing it to rollerball ablation.[27] In this method the balloon is inflated in the uterine cavity to a pressure of 160–180 mmHg and then heated to 87°C for 8 min. In this series, only women with a normal cavity were included. Myer's study was a landmark in the validation of the new second-generation endometrial ablation techniques, and the results were generally reassuring.[27] The study showed that the operation time for Thermachoice was less than for rollerball with fewer complications. After 24 months follow up that there was no difference in the ability of each method to reduce the bleeding score to a normal value, but there was a greater reduction in menstrual blood loss scores for the rollerball group.[27]

The Cavaterm™ system uses a balloon inflated to 180–200 mmHg and a temperature of 75°C for 15 min. There is circulation of the fluid inside the balloon to maintain an even temperature. A series of 200 patients has been presented giving a 94% success rate, but only after patients with fibroids or any 'cavity change' have been excluded.[28]

The Cavaterm™ system has also been compared in a randomised controlled trial to rollerball endometrial ablation. Romer's study[29] assessed the outcomes of Cavaterm versus rollerball in 20 women, (10 patients in each arm of the study). Again, women were excluded if they had any intrauterine abnormalities (submucous myomas, uterine septae, suspicion of uterine wall weakness, or uterine cavity length <4 cm or >10 cm) or histological pathology, however Romer pre-treated both groups with two injections of gonadotrophin-releasing hormone analogues (GnRHa). Follow-up at 15 months found almost identical results in the two treatment arms of the study, with all 20 women expressing satisfaction with their treatment.

This study has severe methodological weaknesses – there is no power study to calculate the number of women needed to demonstrate if a statistically significant difference exists between the two treatments, and it shares the limitations of Myer's work, in using strict entry criteria and comparison with rollerball ablation.

The advantages of the balloon systems are that they seem to need little, if any, cervical dilatation but cause pain by uterine distension when performed under local anaesthetic. This is compounded by treatment times being relatively long. They seem to be restricted to a normal uterine cavity, which will exclude at least 30% of women in whom endometrial ablation is currently practised on as found in the Scottish Audit of Hysteroscopic Surgery.[21]

Microwave endometrial ablation

Microwave endometrial ablation (MEA) was introduced by Sharp in 1994. This method uses microwave energy delivered by an 8 mm diameter probe. It gives an instantaneous read out of surface temperature and aims to treat the endometrium to 80–90°C. This gives reliable tissue destruction to a depth of 4–5 mm. It must not be confused with the RAFEA which though often known as the 'microwave' method uses radiofrequency. No patient return electrode or modification of anaesthetic monitoring equipment is needed. The pilot study was of 23 patients with a normal sized uterus. Treatment time was 2 min and the success rate 83%.[30] Though it requires some manual manipulation in its performance, this is considerably less than with TCRE or ELA.

In Aberdeen, we have completed the first RCT comparing TCRE to MEA in 236 patients.[31] One major difference between this RCT and the others mentioned is that the patient inclusion criteria are the same as in all our previous studies with a uterine size of up to the size of a 10-week pregnancy and fibroids are included. The data on menstrual outcome and patient satisfaction shows no significant difference between the two methods. This method can be performed under local anaesthetic (LA), as, though the cervix needs dilating there is no uterine distension and the treatment time is short (Sharp, N: personal communication). We are now performing a RCT comparing MEA under local anaesthetic to MEA under general anaesthetic to assess the true acceptability of LA treatment.

Guidelines on endometrial ablation

The Cochrane Collaboration[8] has concluded that there is a significant advantage in favour of hysterectomy in the satisfaction rates (up to 4 years postoperatively) compared to endometrial destruction. The duration of surgery, hospital stay, and recovery time were all shorter for endometrial ablation patients. Most adverse effects, both minor and major were significantly more likely after hysterectomy. Repeat surgery, either endometrial ablation or hysterectomy was more likely after endometrial destruction than hysterectomy. Finally, the total cost of endometrial destruction was significantly lower than the cost of hysterectomy but the difference between the two procedures narrowed over time because of the high cost of re-treatment in the endometrial destruction group.

Structured, evidence-based guidelines on hysteroscopic surgery are now published by the Scottish Intercollegiate Guidelines Network (SIGN)[32] These use strict criteria and ensure that recommendations are strictly linked to the evidence and graded accordingly.[7] These will have an impact as there is still a severe under-provision of ablation services in the U.K. The days of anecdotal guidelines should be a thing of the past. With these guidelines in place, clinicians who have been awaiting authoritative, evidence-based statements on the role of endometrial ablation prior to offering such a service now have the information they need.

Conclusions

Endometrial ablation is now firmly established as a true alternative to hysterectomy. It should now be offered to all women wishing a surgical treatment for menorrhagia, though for many reasons this is still far from the case. The challenge is for purchasers of health care such as the health boards to now respond to the published evidence and guidelines such as produced by the Cochrane Collaboration and the SIGN to reduce the hysterectomy rate by insisting that endometrial ablation is widely available and by encouraging appropriate referral. A further challenge for the future is to see if one of the second generation methods will be as efficacious as the hysteroscopic methods especially in the uterus containing fibroids. It is vital that the progress made in evidence-based endometrial ablation over the past 10 years is not lost due to increased pressure from the medical equipment industry to get their new products into the market place.

REFERENCES

1. Garry R. Endometrial ablation and resection: validation of a new surgical concept. *Br J Obstet Gynaecol* 1997; **104**: 1329–1321.
2. Davis JA. Hysteroscopic endometrial ablation with the neodymium-YAG laser. *Br J Obstet Gynaecol* 1989; **96**: 928–932.
3. Magos AL, Baumann R, Lockwood GM, Turnbull AC. Experience with the first 250 endometrial resections for menorrhagia. *Lancet* 1991; **337**: 1074–1078.
4. Erian J. Endometrial ablation in the treatment of menorrhagia. *Br J Obstet-Gynaecol* 1994; **101** (Suppl 11): 19–22.
5. Nicholson SC, Slade RJ, Ahmed AIH, Gillmer MDG. Endometrial resection in Oxford: The first 500 cases – a 5-year follow up. *J Obstet Gynecol.* 1995; **15**: 38–43.
6. Parkin DE. Prognostic factors for success in endometrial ablation and resection. Lancet 1998; 351: 1147–1148.
7. Scottish Intercollegiate Guidelines Network (SIGN) Clinical Guidelines: criteria for appraisal for national use. Edinburgh. SIGN 1995.
8. Lethaby A, Shepperd S, Cooke I, Farquhar C. Endometrial resection and ablation versus hysterectomy for heavy menstrual bleeding. *Cochrane Database Syst Rev.* 2000 **2**: CD000329.
9. Dwyer N, Hutton J, Stirrat GM. Randomised controlled trial comparing endometrial resection with abdominal hysterectomy for the surgical treatment of menorrhagia. *Br J Obstet Gynaecol* 1993; **100**: 237–243.
10. Pinion SB, Parkin DE, Abramovich DR *et al.* Randomised trial of hysterectomy, endometrial laser ablation and transcervical resection for dysfunctional uterine bleeding *Br Med J* 1994; **309**: 979–983.
11. Gannon MJ, Holt EM, Fairbank J *et al.* A randomised trial comparing endometrial resection and abdominal hysterectomy for the treatment of menorrhagia *Br Med J* 1991; **303**: 1362–1364.

12. O'Connor H, Broadbent JA, Magos AL, McPherson K. Medical Research Council randomised trial of endometrial resection versus hysterectomy in management of menorrhagia. *Lancet* 1997; **349**: 897–901.

13. Crosignani PG, Vercellini P, Apolone G, De Giorgi O, Cortesi I, Meschia M. Endometrial resection versus vaginal hysterectomy for menorrhagia: long term clinical and quality of life outcomes. *Am J Obstet Gynecol* 1997; **177**: 95–101.

14. O'Connor H, Magos, A. Endometrial resection for the treatment of menorrhagia. *N Engl J Med* 1996; **335**: 151–156.

15. Phillips G, Chien PF, Garry R. Risk of hysterectomy after 1000 consecutive endometrial laser ablations. 1998; *Br J Obstet Gynaecol* **105**: 897–903.

16. Aberdeen Endometrial Ablation Trials Group. A randomised trial of endometrial ablation versus hysterectomy for the treatment of dysfunctional uterine bleeding: outcome at four years. *Br J Obstet Gynaecol* 1999: in press.

17. Cooper KG, Parkin DE, Garrett AM, Grant AM. A randomised controlled trial assessing the effectiveness of medical treatment versus transcervical resection of the endometrium (TCRE) for women with heavy menstrual loss. *Br J Obstet Gynaecol* 1997; **104**: 1360–1366.

18. Cooper KG, Parkin DE, Garret AM, Grant AM. Two-year follow-up of women randomised to medical management or transcervical resection of the endometrium for heavy menstrual loss; clinical and quality of life outcomes. *Br J Obstet Gynaecol* March 1999; **106**: 258–265.

19. Rogerson L, Duffy S. Management of menorrhagia-SMART study (Satisfaction with Mirena and Ablation: a Randomised Trial). *Br J Obstet Gynaecol* 2000; **107**: 1325–1326.

20. Gannon MJ, Day P, Hammadich N, Johnson N. A new method of measuring menstrual blood loss and its use in screening women before endometrial ablation *Br J Obstet Gynaecol.* 1996; **103**: 1029–1033.

21. Scottish Hysteroscopy Audit Group. A Scottish audit of hysteroscopic surgery for menorrhagia: complications and follow up. *Br J Obstet Gynaecol* 1995; **102**: 249–254.

22. Bhattacharya S, Cameron I M, Parkin DE *et al.* A pragmatic randomised comparison of transcervical resection of the endometrium with endometrial laser ablation for the treatment of menorrhagia. *Br J Obstet Gynaecol* 1997; **104**: 601–607.

23. Davis JR, Maynard KK, Brainard CP, Purdon TF, Sibley MA, King DD. Effects of thermal endometrial ablation: clinicopathologic correlations. *Am J Clin Path* 1998; **109**: 96–100.

24. Chullapram T, Song JY, Fraser IS. Medium-term follow up of women with menorrhagia treated by rollerball endometrial ablation. *Obstet Gynaecol* 1996; **88**: 71–76.

25. Overton C, Hargreaves H, Maresh M. A national survey of the complications of endometrial destruction for menstrual disorders: the MISTLETOE study. *Br J Obstet Gynaecol* 1997; **104**: 1351–1359.

26. Singer A, Almanza R, Gutierrez A, Haber G, Bolduc LR, Neuwirth, R. Preliminary clinical experience with thermal balloon endometrial ablation method to treat menorrhagia. *Obstet Gynaecol* 1994; **83**: 732–734.

27. Meyer WR, Walsh BM, Grainger DA, Peacock LM, Loffer FD, Steege JF. Thermal balloon and rollerball ablation to treat menorrhagia: a multicentre comparison. *Obstet Gynecol* **92**:(1) 98–103, July 1998.

28. Friburg B, Ahlgren M. Cavaterm™ endometrial ablation, results at 5-years follow up. Proceedings of the 7th Congress of the European Society of Gynaecological Endoscopy 1998; p5.

29. Romer T. Die therapie rezidivierender menorrhagien – Cavaterm-ballon koagulation versus roller-ball endometrium koagulation – eine prospektive randomiserte vergleichstudie. *Zentralblatt fur Gynakologie* 1998; **120**:(10) 511–514.

30. Sharp NC, Cronin N, Feldberg I, Evans N, Hodgson D, Ellis S. Microwaves for menorrhagia: a new fast technique for endometrial ablation. *Lancet* 1995; **346**: 1003–1004.

31. Cooper KG, Bain C, Parkin DE. Comparison of microwave endometrial ablation and trans-cervical resection of the endometrium for treatment of heavy menstrual loss: a randomised trial. The *Lancet* **354**: 27 Nov. 1999, p. 1859–1863.

32. Hysteroscopic surgery: a national clinical guideline. Scottish Intercollegiate Guidelines Network (SIGN) 1999.

15

Strategies to Avoid Complications in Laparoscopic and Hysteroscopic Surgery

T. C. Li
P. McGurgan
P. O'Donovan

Introduction

"Primum non nocere" – Above all, do no harm; attributed to Hippocrates, 460–375 B.C.

There is little doubt that minimal access surgery (MAS) presents many advantages over laparotomy; smaller scars, reduced post-operative pain, shorter hospital stay and speedier recovery. Any operation may be associated with complications; these may be divided into general risks, for example anaesthesia problems, and risks specific to the way the operation is performed. Minimal access surgery is no exception. Laparoscopic procedures, abdominal entry techniques, and the development of a pneumoperitoneum create specific risks that would not occur if an open abdominal or vaginal route had been used. Hysteroscopic procedures involve introduction of instruments into the uterus, and distension with media in a fashion not used conventionally. As a result, MAS has a potentially increased risk of iatrogenic complications, particularly during the learning phase of the surgeon. It is vital that every effort is made to reduce the complication rate of MAS procedures. This review focuses on practical and technological advances whereby complications may be decreased during MAS.

The scale of the problem

Obstetrics and gynaecology is the most intensely self-analytical of the specialities in modern medicine, minimal access surgery was born into this tradition; the result is a large volume of data, which can allow us to benefit from a vast range of experience.[1,2] The formation of national supervisory bodies, e.g., the Royal College of Obstetricians and Gynaecologists (RCOG) Working Party[3] and the American Association of Gynecologic Laparoscopists has provided the impetus for structured training and accreditation.

What then are the established rates of complications associated with MAS.? Different procedures have different complication rates. However as an overview the following data are presented. **Table 15.1** demonstrates the major complication rates for operative laparoscopy,[4] and **Table 15.2** gives the complication and emergency hysterectomy rate for the minimally invasive surgical techniques – laser, endothermal, or endoresection (MISTLETOE) study.[5] **Table 15.3** demonstrates the increase in laparoscopic and hysteroscopic complications noted by the American Association of Gynecological Laparoscopists.[2]

We can see that minimal access procedure-related complications are relatively infrequent. However, there is no room for complacency; rare complications for an individual surgeon can still represent a major problem on an international scale. We should not be lulled into a false sense of security by having no personal experience of complications, whilst using a technique which on large scale may be suboptimal.

The data in **Table 15.3** causes concern; minimal access surgical complications appear to be on the increase, and data from Chapron[6] and Querleu[7] in France reflect a similar trend. In this study, whilst the overall complication rate is low, there was a steep increase in complications as more advanced operative procedures were performed. We can only speculate as to the reasons; was it due to cases where the morbidity was intrinsically higher due to pre-existent pathology? Did this change over time reflect the attempt by less skilled surgeons to perform increasingly complex procedures, or less reticence by surgeons to report on their complications as MAS became more widely accepted in the surgical community? The lack of a definitive answer underlines the need for continuous audit of these techniques, and the appropriate emphasis on training and accreditation.

One of our main concerns is the fact that whilst tremendous advances in the ability to perform minimal access procedures have been made, there is a surprising lack of quality research on the optimum approaches to perform basic and safe laparoscopic and hysteroscopic surgery. In the absence of

Table 15.1 Major complications per 1000 operative laparoscopies.[4]

COMPLICATIONS		RATE
By instruments:	Veress needle	2.7
	Large trocar	2.4–2.7
	Accessory trocar	2.5–6
	Electrocautery	0.5–2.8
	Laser	1.2
	Pneumoperitoneum	7.4
By site of injury:	Vessels/bleeding	2.6–11
	Bowel	0.6–2
	Genitourinary	6.1
	Uterus	3.7
Other problems:	Death	0.05–0.3
	Hospitalisation >72 hours	4.2–27
	Hospital re-admission	3.1–5
	Infection	1.4–6.5

Table 15.2 Complications associated with endometrial ablation or resection.[5]

Technique	Complication rates (%)	Emergency hysterectomy
Resection alone	10.9	13/1000
Rollerball alone	4.5	3/1000
Combined resection/roller	7.7	5/1000
Laser	5.5	2/1000

established optimum techniques, we present an overview of different attempts to decrease the risk of complications in a MAS setting.

General principles of safe minimal access surgery

- Appropriate case selection
- Patient preparation
- Proper equipment
- Optimal exposure
- Knowledgeable use of electrical sources in MAS
- Awareness of the learning phase

Case selection

Proper case selection is one of the most important factors in reducing complication rates for both laparoscopic and hysteroscopic surgery.

Firstly, one must accept that not all cases are suitable for laparoscopic or hysteroscopic surgery. Surgeons must understand the limitation of laparoscopic surgery and not hesitate to resort to laparotomy whenever appropriate. Extensive, dense bowel adhesions, multiple intramural fibroids, grade IV endometriosis with complete obliteration of the Pouch of Douglas, or a haemodynamically unstable patient are examples of cases best dealt with by laparotomy rather than minimal access surgery. Furthermore, what may be technically possible may not be the safest option.

There are uncertainties as to whether some patients are suitable for minimal access surgery e.g. hysteroscopic surgery for large (>5 cm) type II submucous fibroids (**Table 15.4**), and laparoscopic surgery for rectovaginal endometriosis. Whilst there are claims by experienced surgeons that it is feasible to carry out these procedures by hysteroscopic or laparoscopic means, it is important to appreciate that what may be achieved by a few gifted surgeons may not be readily accomplished by the average practising, general gynaecologist.

Table 15.3 Comparison between complication rates between two A.A.G.L. surveys.[2]

Complication	Rate***/1000 cases		
Laparoscopic	**1988 survey**	**1991 survey**	**Change since 1988**
Major	15.4	N/A	–
Laparotomy for surgical trauma	4.2	8.9	↑ ×1.5
Laparotomy for haemorrhage	2.1	6.8	↑ ×2.6
Laparotomy for bowel/urinary tract damage	1.6	2.8	↑ ×1.7
Nerve injury	0.5	0.5	No change
Death	0.054	0.018	↓ ×3
Hysteroscopic**			
Uterine perforation (not requiring transfusion)	13	11.1	↓ ×0.9
Haemorrhage requiring transfusion	1.0	0.3	↓ ×3
Laparotomy to manage haemorrhage	0.5	1.4	↑ ×2.9
Laparotomy to manage visceral injury	0	0.3	
H_2O intoxication/			↑
Pulmonary oedema	3.4	1.4	↑ ×1.4
Death	0	0.1	↑

* ** Results are from a confidential survey with a 17% (*), and 15% (**) response rate. This may not represent true incidences

Table 15.4 Classification of submucous leiomyomas

Type	Location
0	Pedunculated
I	<50% intra-mural
II	>50% intra-mural

Thirdly, proper case selection is of particular importance in the 'learning phase'. As a rule start with simple cases. For example, in the case of laparoscopic adhesiolysis, start with patients who are not grossly obese and with only flimsy adhesive bands not affecting the bowel. When performing hysteroscopic resection of fibroids, start with small type 0 or type I submucous fibroids (**Table 15.4**). Once experience and confidence have been gained, more difficult cases may be undertaken.

Patient preparation

Appropriate patient preparation will make the operation easier and reduce complication rates.

1. Pre-operative counselling and accurate documentation: the most important factor in decreasing litigation is a fully-informed patient, particularly if there are known risk factors, (e.g. adhesions), to performing surgery. Patients may have unrealistic expectations about these new procedures; a leaflet explaining the procedure is a useful adjunct to a full discussion. A plan of "worst case scenario" should be made; for instance, the need for a laparotomy or hysterectomy in the event of a uterine perforation. When complications do occur, this should be fully documented, and remedial surgery instituted as soon as possible.[8]
2. Endometrial preparation in hysteroscopic surgery: the need for endometrial preparation prior to endometrial ablation is well recognised. However, there is no consensus on endometrial preparation for other hysteroscopic surgery such as removal of septae or submucous fibroids, but this is generally advisable except for those who are very experienced. The method of preparation varies, being either mechanical (curettage),[9] or pharmacological.[10] Gonadotrophin-releas-

ing hormone, (GnRH) analogues and danazol. GnRH analogues are very potent drugs, however they do add to the overall cost of the procedure, and may cause difficulties in cervical dilation.

3. Pre-operative bowel preparation: There is no need for routine bowel preparation in all cases of laparoscopic surgery. However, bowel preparation is advisable in patients undergoing advanced procedures, for example laparoscopic surgery for rectovaginal endometriosis.
4. Bladder catheterisation: in laparoscopic procedures lasting more than 45 min, it is important to insert a Foley catheter for continuous drainage to avoid bladder injury.

Proper equipment

It is essential to be properly equipped before embarking on laparoscopic surgery. The minimum requirements should include a good quality camera system, light source, and image recording facilities.

Both the surgeon and theatre nurse should be familiar with the equipment. If equipment is not working well, do not persevere with surgery – the procedure may have to be converted to an open procedure.

Optimal exposure

As for all surgical techniques, good exposure is vital. The surgeon must be able to clearly visualise the pelvic organs to perform safe surgery. Whenever there is difficulty in obtaining a clear view, stop the procedure and if possible improve the view to optimise exposure of the operative field.

Avoiding complications arising from the use of electrical sources in MAS

Complications of electrosurgery at laparoscopy may result from four situations, an accidental burn, direct coupling, capacitative coupling and insulation failure. There are general precautions to follow.[11]

1. Ensure good exposure, e.g. by dividing adhesions prior to definitive surgery so that important organs such as the bowel may be pushed away from the site of the surgery. Activate the electrical energy only when the tip of the instrument is in contact with the target tissue and in the view of the laparoscope using the lowest possible power setting.
2. The tip of the diathermy instrument may remain hot for several seconds after use. After its use, keep the instrument in view until it has cooled or whilst it is removed from the body. Dipping the tip in a pool of fluid in the Pouch of Douglas, or irrigating it may facilitate cooling.
3. Use bipolar instruments whenever possible, that do not involve use of a return plate and where only a small amount of tissue is included in the circuit. This means that bipolar can usually only desiccate and capacitance cannot occur. Monopolar systems do require a return plate, and the current flows through the whole body before exiting. Although monopolar is more versatile, capacitance and direct coupling may occur if precautions are not taken.
4. To avoid capacitative coupling, most importantly, do not use plastic abdominal wall grips (anchors) in conjunction with metal cannulae. Non-insulated instruments, e.g. laparoscope and irrigators, should be passed only through all metal cannulae/metal anchor combinations. Insulated instruments may be used in conjunction with all plastic, or all metal cannulae/metal anchor combinations. Also, when coagulating tissue to achieve haemostasis, deliver short sharp pulses of electrical power and avoid prolonged activation of the electrode.
5. Be aware of the warning signs of electricity leak, such as involuntary contraction of abdominal muscles, hissing sounds within the trocar or 'lightning' artefacts on monitors and electronic equipment. A reduction in the expected electrosurgical effect at a given power setting and energy mode may indicate that some of the electrical energy has dissipated

away from the tip of the active electrode. Do not keep increasing the power output. Instead, check the application of the neutral plate, and the insulation of the active electrode.

The easiest way to avoid direct coupling is to activate energy only when all of the active part of the instrument is visualised, and ensure that part of it is not in contact with any other instrument. Direct coupling can also occur due to insulation failure, which may be a defect in the instrument's insulation invisible to the naked eye. This can only be effectively confirmed by electrical tests on the instrument, and emphasises the need for regular inspection by testers to ensure the instruments integrity.

The use of contact quality monitoring of the return electrode (Valleylab, Boulder, Colorado) effectively eliminated alternate site burns. The introduction of "active shielding" of the electrosurgical devices in the 1990s (Electroscope, Boulder, Colorado) means that devices are now extremely safe; this instrument can detect direct coupling and insulation defects, and captures capacititavely coupled energy. By elimination, this leaves the surgeon solely responsible for any adverse effects.

The hysteroscopic use of electrosurgery has conventionally required a non-ionic distension medium for obvious reasons. Glycine 1.5% and sorbitol 3% are commonly used for operative hysteroscopy. As we know, considerable amounts of these non iso-osmotic substances can be absorbed systemically, with resultant morbidity and mortality (**Table 15.3**).

The use of a bipolar electrosurgical device (Versapoint™, Ethicon, USA) which operates in an ionic saline medium represents a considerable feat of engineering, and a valuable instrument for hysteroscopic surgery, the instruments small diameter means that operative procedures may be performed on conscious patients in an outpatient setting. Our experience agrees with the very positive initial reports;[12] care must still be taken to avoid fluid overload, although the osmotically-induced fluid shifts characteristic of other media are minimised.

Learning phase

It is well recognised that complication rates are higher for cases performed by surgeons during their learning phase. The following recommendations may help to reduce complication rates.

1. One should be competent and experienced in doing the procedure via laparotomy prior to embarking on an endoscopic approach.
2. There are different levels of complexity of laparoscopic and hysteroscopic surgery.[3] One should begin with simple procedures (level I and II) and not undertake complex procedures (level III and IV) until enough experience has been acquired (**Table 15.5**). The complication rate of advanced laparoscopic surgery is 4–8 times that of simple laparoscopic procedures.[13]
3. In some cases, hysteroscopic surgery may be safer with concurrent laparoscopic control, for example, resection of a type II submucous fibroid, (especially if situated over the cornual region), removal of uterine septum or dense intra-uterine adhesions (Asherman's syndrome). An experienced assistant, with a second camera and light source, continuously monitors the amount of light transmitted across the uterine wall and keeps the bowel away from the uterus. The amount of light transmitted should be compared with that via the cornual region – and should be no more than the latter. Combined synchronous laparoscopic control should be considered in all difficult hysteroscopic cases, and during the learning curve of beginners.
4. The RCOG has published a list of more than 100 preceptors in minimal access surgery in various parts of the United Kingdom. Gynaecologists should contact preceptors in their region to discuss individual training and preceptorship. The initial cases should be proctored by an experienced colleague or supervised by a recognised trainer until competence has been achieved.

Table 15.5 Examples of laparoscopic and hysteroscopic procedures by levels of training.[3]

Level	Laparoscopic procedures	Hysteroscopic procedures
I – Diagnostic procedures	Diagnostic laparoscopy	Hysteroscopy & target biopsy Removal of polyps/ IUCD*
II – Minor operative procedures	Sterilisation Needle aspiration/biopsy	Minor Asherman's Syndrome Proximal tubal cannulation
III – More complex (additional training)	Ovarian "drilling" Endometriotic ablation (AFS** Stage II/III) L.A.V.H./L.A.S.H.***	Endometrial resection/ablation Resection of submucous leiomyomas Resection of uterine septum
IV – Extensive (advanced level skills)	Myomectomy Endometriotic ablation (AFS** Stage III/IV)	

* Intra-uterine contraceptive device
** American Fertility Society
*** Laparoscopic assisted vaginal/sub-total hysterectomy

Complications specific to laparoscopy

There are two types of laparoscopic complications - those related to the mode of access, and those related to the performance of specific techniques. In this section we confine ourselves to the general principles of laparoscopic surgery with emphasis on the accepted and newer methods of avoiding complications.

The introduction of the Veress needle, formation of a pneumoperitoneum, and use of the primary and secondary trocars are the basic steps in the "classical" approach. **Table 15.6** demonstrates the Veress needle is responsible for a considerable proportion of the complications. In fact, every intra-abdominal structure can be, and has been injured by these methods. Unfortunately, this is an area which provokes the greatest controversy, yet there is a surprising lack of quality research on the optimum approaches to achieving a pneumoperitoneum. In the absence of established optimum techniques, we present an overview of different attempts to decrease the risk of complications in a MAS setting, which concurs with the Consensus Meeting of the British Society of Gynaecological Endoscopy.

Techniques for establishing a pneumoperitoneum

- The conventional approach
- Direct insertion
- Open techniques
- Gasless laparoscopy
- Alternative entry sites
- Radially expanding sleeves
- Insertion under direct vision – modified Veress needles – modified trocars

The conventional approach

This method is described in detail to compare other methods of entry, and explain the need for safer methods of entry. Compared to other techniques the conventional approach appears no better or, worse in the small trials performed. Its advantages lie in the fact that although it is a 'blind' procedure, it makes optimum use of the anatomical and physical environments we operate in, at least in theory, to prevent injury, and is advocated in various forms by respected surgeons.[19–21]

1. Prior to insertion of the Veress needle, check the needle is patent and the CO_2 insufflator

Table 15.6 Large studies of injuries due to Veress needle/trocar.[14]

Study	No. of laparoscopies	Haemorrhagic complications	Visceral perforation	Rate per 1000 cases
Querleu[7]	17,521	4	7	0.63
Mintz[15]	99,204	30 Veress, 18 Trocar	5 Veress, 26 Trocar	0.35
Bergqvist[16]	75,035	4 Veress, 1 Trocar	Not reported	0.07
Loffer and Pent[17]	32,719	Not reported	22	0.67
Tsaltas[18]	6,500	0	2	0.31

manometer correct by allowing CO_2 to perfuse through the device. Palpate the abdominal wall carefully for any pelvic mass. One should be aware that thin patients may be at greater risk of major vessel injury, as the aorta may lie only 3 cm below the umbilicus due to the lumbar lordosis.[22]

2. A skin incision is made at the base of the umbilicus – the abdominal wall is thinnest in this area (<1 cm usually), and the parietal peritoneum is most firmly attached here.[22]
3. The Veress needle is grasped like a dart, with the tap open – this allows air to enter the negatively-pressured abdominal cavity when the Veress is inserted.
4. The abdomen is lifted anteriorly and in a caudal direction, to avoid the retroperitoneal vessels at the lumbar lordosis.
5. The Veress is inserted a short distance (usually 3 cm) at an angle somewhere between the perpendicular and 45° towards the pelvis (aim for the sacral hollow in the midline), usually the experienced hand can feel the Veress incising the rectus sheath and peritoneum as two distinct resistances.
6. The intraperitoneal location may be confirmed by using a syringe. When the needle is intraperitoneal, drawing back on the syringe, then infiltrating 5–10 ml of saline will easily aid confirmation, the logic being that if aspiration of blood or bowel contents occur a major splanchnic organ has been entered. The ease of initial infiltration suggests that the needle is free in the cavity rather than against adhesions or elsewhere in the abdominal wall. Another technique is the hanging drop, whereby a small amount of saline is placed on the top of the Veress needle tap, the abdominal wall is again elevated, and if the Veress tip is intraperitoneal, the negative pressure thus created will cause the saline to be 'sucked' into the cavity. None of these techniques are foolproof.
7. When insufflating CO_2, we use a low flow initially. Once the manometer confirms low pressure, the flow is increased. We do not infuse a constant volume of CO_2, rather we depend on the intraperitoneal pressure to produce a firm 'bubble' of distended peritoneum, our insufflator has a pre-set cut off at 15–18 mmHg. This method utilises the logical approach formulated by Reich,[23] whereby the peritoneal cavity is assumed to be a variable size in each patient; therefore depending on the size of the cavity a variable amount of gas will be needed to reach a certain pressure. Reich advocates a pressure of 25 mmHg, as studies have demonstrated that the distance between the anterior abdominal wall and bowel is 10 cm at this pressure (compared to 6 cm distance at 10 mmHg), so increasing the 'bubble' size and hence safety margin prior to the insertion of the primary trocar.
8. It is well accepted that the most dangerous moment in laparoscopic surgery is the insertion of the primary trocar, which is almost always inserted in a blind fashion.[24] Like the Veress, the trocar is inserted into the base of the umbilicus, where the abdominal wall is thinnest. The trocar is held in a 'palmed' fashion, that is, the top of the trocar is enclosed by

the palm, whilst the index finger follows the vertical axis, until only 1–2 cm of the sharp tip is exposed. The trocar is inserted initially vertically in the midline, then towards the pelvis (aim for the sacral hollow) in the midline, with the gas tap open thereby allowing immediate confirmation that the cavity has been entered. This allows a good degree of control over this potentially fatal instrument.

9. Once the laparoscope is inserted, and initial confirmation of correct placement is achieved, the surgeon performs an anatomical tour of the pelvis. This covers all four quadrants, and is used to identify any pathology and to ensure that no iatrogenic injury has occurred during the procedure. Only after this procedure should the intended operation take place.

Direct insertion

As **Table 15.6** shows, approximately a third to a half of trocar-related injuries are due to the Veress needle. This is considered significant enough to warrant the banning of the Veress in New York State. The advocates of the direct technique include a number of highly experienced laparoscopists.[25–27] They make use of the negative pressure in the abdomen elicited by elevating the abdominal wall. A primary trocar, with the gas tap open is then inserted usually subumbilically, and the laparoscope immediately inserted to view the cavity when entered. The open gas tap allows the bowel to move posteriorly as the atmospheric air enters the peritoneal cavity. Once safe entry is confirmed, and a panoramic view of the pelvis obtained, rapid insufflation can begin. Not surprisingly with two such dichotomous procedures, trials have been performed comparing direct with conventional methods.[26–29] The results are inconclusive, but in Jansen's study,[29] which was one of the largest (70,607 laparoscopies) direct insertion caused more serious morbidity. This technique lacks any ability to avoid abdominal wall adhesions, and has the potential to cause large, unrecognised "through and through" injuries to the bowel. That is, perforating both anterior and posterior walls of the bowel with the trocar sleeve, which will not be noted unless the instrument is slowly withdrawn under direct vision. In conclusion, this remains an accepted method for the moment in experienced hands. However, the balance of evidence supporting it is weak.

Open techniques

It was a natural progression for surgeons to attempt to circumvent the potential complications posed by blind entry. This was first described by Hasson,[30] using only blunt instruments, by performing an intra-umbilical minilaparotomy incision. When the rectus sheath is divided, two stay sutures are inserted, which are later used to anchor the Hasson (blunt) cannula. One would expect the use of this blunt open technique to significantly reduce iatrogenic injury. Whilst studies have demonstrated that the risk of major blood vessel injury is reduced, the incidence of bowel injury does not appear to be decreased,[31] and in some studies may be higher. This is probably due to observer bias, as the Hasson technique is usually selected for high risk cases, and demonstrates that, like open laparotomy, adherent bowel may be injured upon abdominal entry. Most general surgeons have adopted this technique over the conventional one, and with experience they find that time taken to perform the minilaparotomy is compensated by the rapid insufflation allowed, and it is officially recommended as the technique of choice for all laparoscopy in New York State.

A variation of this approach is performed by Semm,[32] whereby an open "cut down" is performed subumbilically, to the level of the peritoneum. A 5 mm telescope is then placed at this level; if the area below the light is clear of bowel, no light will be reflected and the area will appear dark. On the other hand, adhesions against the peritoneum will reflect light if present, and this will then appear as a bright area. No large studies exist to confirm the safety of this method, however it does possess a reasonable logic; this idea is further developed in the latest instruments.

Gasless laparoscopy

The open technique is taken a step further by the use of gasless laparoscopy whereby the need for a pneumoperitoneum is avoided by using mechanical means to distend the abdominal cavity. As always, the abdomen must first be entered, usually by a Hasson open approach and the inner peritoneal surface of the peritoneal cavity digitally palpated to ensure there is no adherent bowel, a variety of devices are then inserted and used to elevate the cavity by external traction.[33] Again, common sense would suggest that this method is unlikely to reduce bowel injury over other methods, and of note, intra-abdominal adhesions are classed as a relative contra-indication to the procedure. Studies have been small, and poorly designed in general, hence it is difficult to compare this to other techniques. The potential benefits are due to the fact that the cardiovascular effects of pneumoperitoneum are avoided and there is no loss of vision secondary to loss of pneumoperitoneum when tissue is removed for example by posterior colporrhaphy. General surgeons have been interested by this method in cancer surgery, due to the possibility of tumour metastasis being increased by pneumoperitoneum.[34]

Alternative entry sites

The Veress needle started life as an instrument for creating pneumothoraces in cases of pulmonary tuberculosis, by its inventor the respiratory physician, Janos Veress in the 1930's.[35,36] So, it is hardly surprising that surgeons have expanded this versatile instrument's anatomical sites further. Alternative sites include:

- Subumbilical
- Midway between the umbilicus and symphysis pubis
- Suprapubic[37]
- Palmer's point[38]
- Ninth left intercostal space in the midclavicular line[39]
- Pouch of Douglas[40]
- Trans-uterine[41]

All of the sites which are abdominal but subumbilical, must perforate the parietal peritoneum which is only loosely adherent to the abdominal wall, this tends to 'tent', that is, follow the axis of the Veress rather than be perforated by the needle. The result is either an extraperitoneal CO_2 insufflation and unsuccessful entry, or a Veress needle entering the pelvis deeply with all its attendant risks.

The Pouch of Douglas or trans-uterine[40,41] approaches are favoured by a few laparoscopists in the presence of previous abdominal surgery, however if adhesions are present they may also be pelvic, and the patients who need laparoscopy commonly have pathology distorting the pelvic anatomy in the first instance. Anatomically, there is a danger of damaging the pelvic vessels laterally or over the sacral promontory. The fact that these techniques are contra-indicated if there is a history of adhesive disease or endometriosis limits their practical use.

In the upper abdomen, the left hypochondrium is usually devoid of adhesions, also the parietal peritoneum is sufficiently adherent. Palmer's point,[38] 3 cm inferior to the left costal margin in the mid clavicular line, or the ninth left intercostal space in the anterior axillary line[39] which is below the pleural cavity, are therefore reasonable alternatives to the intra-umbilical site if adhesions are suspected. Care must be taken to ensure that there is no splenomegaly, and if using the intercostal space, that the Veress is inserted on the superior border of the tenth rib to avoid the neurovascular bundle on the ribs inferior undersurface. These two locations are widely advocated. They also allow the primary trocar to be inserted in Palmer's point – which can then be used to detect where it is safe to enter the lower abdomen under direct vision.

Radially expanding sleeves

The use of radially expandable sleeves (Step, Innerdyne, Sunnyvale, Ca. USA) is an attempt to allow a more controlled and safer entry whilst minimising anterior abdominal wall trauma **(Figures**

15.1 and 15.2). This is achieved by using a blunt trocar (1.5 mm diameter) containing the expandable sleeves, which is inserted in the conventional technique, through a 3 mm skin incision to enter the abdominal cavity. A tapered dilator is then inserted, that expands the sleeve up to 12 mm if necessary, and creates a tissue tract by splitting tissue layers along paths of resistance, which promotes a cosmetic result.[42] Otherwise, operative laparoscopy is performed as usual. This approach is 'blind' initially, however, it allows a controlled, and potentially safer entry; we await larger studies to confirm these theoretical advantages.

Insertion under direct vision

The next logical step in attempts to make the process of laparoscopic entry safer was to take advantage of the developments in fibreoptics, and develop instruments that could fit in either the "sleeves" of an adapted Veress needle, or a threaded trocar (Endotip™, Karl Storz, Tuttlingen, Germany), similar in principle to Semms method.[32]

The "optical" Veress cannulae attempt to make the process of laparoscopic entry safer by taking advantage of the developments in fibreoptics. The first modified Veress was produced by Karl Storz (Tuttlingen, Germany), but there are now a variety of instruments on the market. Our experience has been with the optical Veress (Karl Storz, Tuttlingen, Germany),[43–6] a reusable robust device, and the Microlap™ (Nikomed, Hampshire, UK),[47–50] which is very similar to the usual disposable Veress (**Figure 15.3**). All the instruments use mini-laparoscopes which fit in the "sleeves" of an adapted Veress type needle.

The Optical Veress has a diameter of 2.1 mm and is 10.5 cm long. This is usually inserted as in the conventional technique and uses a 1.2 mm diameter semi-rigid fibreoptic minilaparoscope. The Microlap has a 2 mm diameter and is 14 cm long; it uses a 1.98 mm fibreoptic laparoscope and has an anchor engagement device at the distal end to prevent accidental displacement once peritoneal entry is confirmed. This technique removes much of the uncertainty (and time) associated with the various

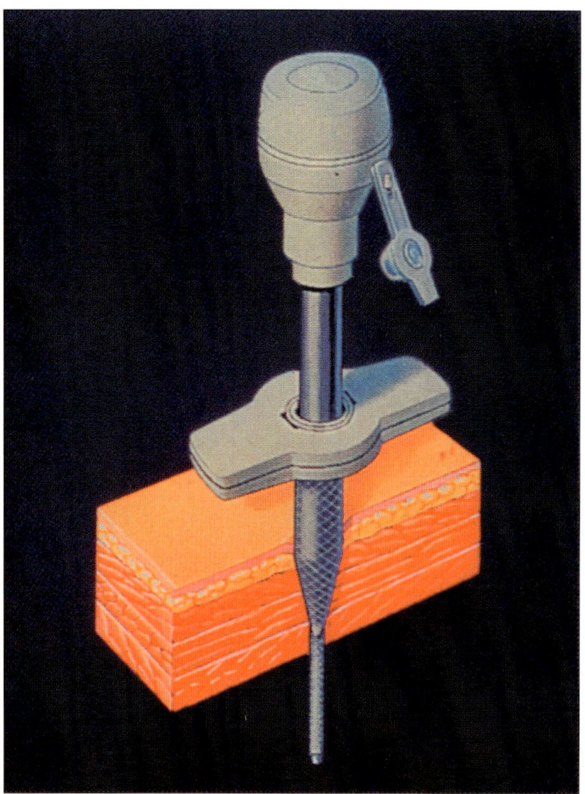

Figure 15.2 Schematic diagram of radially expandable sleeves through the abdominal wall (Step, Innerdyne, Sunnyvale, Ca. USA).

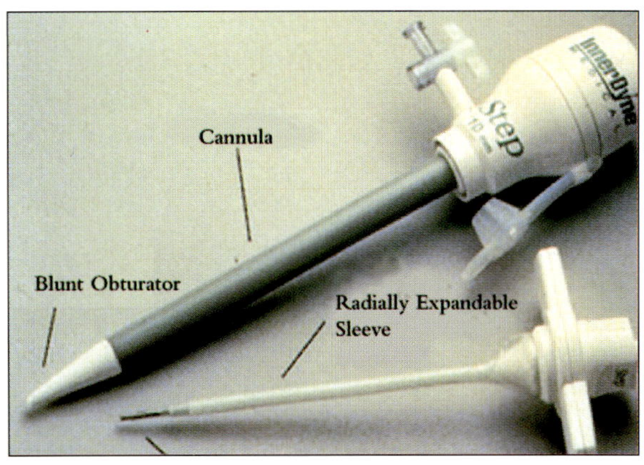

Figure 15.1 Radially expandable sleeves (Step, Innerdyne, Sunnyvale, Ca. USA).

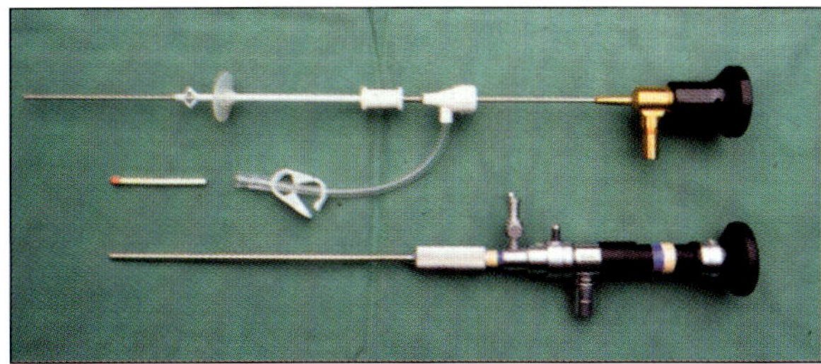

Figure 15.3 "Optical" Veress cannulae: the microlap (Nikomed, Hampshire,UK) above and the optical Veress (Karl Storz, Tuttlingen, Germany) below, alongside a matchstick to demonstrate their relative dimensions.

indirect tests described in the conventional technique to confirm peritoneal entry. However, the fact still remains that an initially blind technique is being used to gain entry into the cavity and the time required for insufflation can be long if only using the optical Veress. Like other units, we have modified this technique somewhat by using the optical Veress in Palmer's point in our high risk patients.[43,44,50]

These instruments' small calibre, combined with surprisingly good image quality, have led to the development of micro/minilaparoscopy on conscious patients, particularly in the American managed patient care system.[51–53] This is a controversial area in laparoscopic surgery at the moment and we await evidence on its superiority over conventional laparoscopy under general anaesthesia (with all its attendant risks), before attempting it.

The above techniques have been further refined to use a modified form of Semm's approach,[32] that is, entering the peritoneum with the optical Veress, using the minilaparoscope directly as the Veress is inserted. The difficulty encountered here is that the small diameter lens is easily obscured by artefacts such as blood as the abdominal wall layers are passed.

This idea is modified by the Endotip™ (Karl Storz, Tuttlingen, Germany): here the trocars in a range of diameters (6–1 mm) have a specially designed thread which allows a controlled "screw" entry once a "cut down" to the sheath has been performed (**Figures 15.4 and 15.5**). The laparoscope has a movable wedge located along its axis, which is positioned such that the camera is focused to the threaded tip of the Endotip, which allows direct vision to be maintained. At the level of the peritoneum, Semm's principle is followed; if the area below the light is clear of bowel, no light will be reflected and the area will appear dark. On the other hand, adhesions against the peritoneum will reflect light if present, and this will then appear as a bright area. Although the camera is protected to some extent by the threaded trocar, it can be obscured by artefacts such as blood as the abdominal wall layers are passed. This new instrument awaits large-scale studies, however we foresee it making a significant step towards laparoscopic safety. Studies so far have been enthusiastic, but of note the largest series used a conventional Veress to develop a pneumoperitoneum technique, before using the Endotip.[54]

Complications specific to hysteroscopy

Operative hysteroscopy is a new and valuable technique in the management of non-malignant pathology of the uterine cavity. As with any surgical procedure, there are potential complications due to the mode of access, and then to the actual surgical procedure performed. In this section we

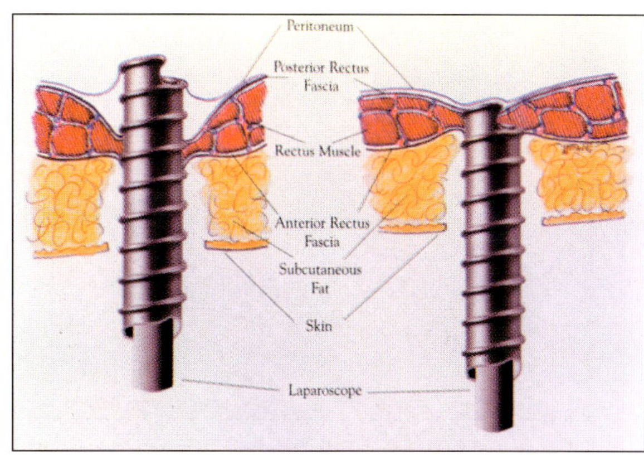

Figure 15.4 The Endotip™ (Karl Storz, Tuttlingen, Germany).

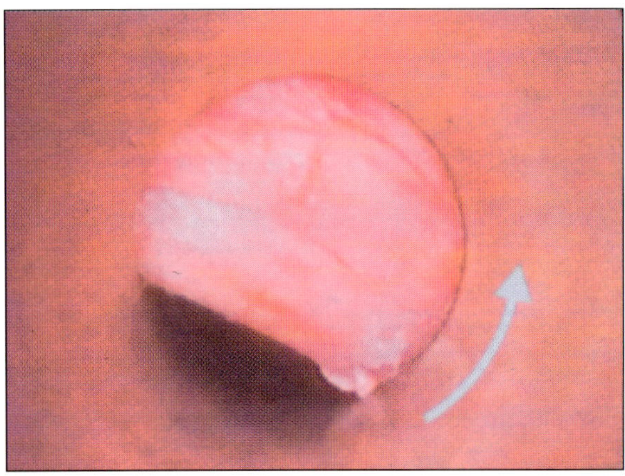

Figure 15.5 Abdominal wall fascia realigning in an anatomical fashion after the Endotip™ (Karl Storz, Tuttlingen, Germany) is removed.

confine ourselves to the general principles of hysteroscopic surgery with emphasis on the accepted and newer methods of avoiding complications. Appropriate training in this new field is vital, with staged levels of procedures, progressing only after adequate experience is developed at each stage in training (**Table 15.5**). The three intrinsic complications to any hysteroscopic procedure are dilating the cervix, the use of distension media, and the possibility of uterine perforation.

Dilation and perforation

As gynaecologists, we are trained to dilate the cervix, however the patients for operative hysteroscopy will often have received GnRH analogues. Whilst these drugs are an important part of pre-operative endometrial preparation, they can have a significant stenotic effect on the cervix. In these instances options include traditional methods such as laminaria stents (Lamicel, Cabot Medical, Penn., USA). Pharmacological methods are more commonly administered, for example prostaglandins such as PgE_2 or $PgF_2\alpha$. GnRH analogues also decrease the uterine size; this increases the risk of initial perforation during dilation and possible subsequent perforation by the instrument during operative hysteroscopy. The management of perforation depends largely on the instrument being used. If a perforation occurs during uterine sounding, a conservative approach can be followed, by stopping the procedure, treatment with antibiotics and overnight stay. After perforation with a large dilator, or operative hysteroscope it is usually advisable to perform a laparoscopy to evaluate the extent of trauma. Occasionally, it may be necessary to perform a laparotomy, particularly if perforation by a "hot" instrument has occurred, or even a hysterectomy if bleeding is heavy. The incidence of perforation during operative procedures is experience dependent, and is estimated at 1–2% of operations.[55]

Distension media

Gas or liquid distension media are needed as a prerequisite for hysteroscopic surgery, in order to keep the uterine walls separated and obtain a clear view. It is the use of these media which creates complications specific to hysteroscopy.

The use of CO_2 was first described by Rubin in 1925. Its advantages are that it is cheap, easily available in theatres, non-flammable, and relatively soluble in blood. It has a similar refractive index to air and allows good quality images to be obtained. The disadvantages of CO_2 are that it causes bubbling in the presence of excess fluid or any bleeding, this effectively limits its use to diagnostic hysteroscopy. If intravasation occurs, deaths have been reported due to CO_2 gas embolism – therefore flow rates of less than 100 $ml.min^{-1}$ are fixed (a flow rate of 30–40 $ml.min^{-1}$ is usually satisfactory).

Liquid distension media include high viscosity fluids such as dextran 70 (Hyskon), and low viscosity fluids, for example 5% dextrose, 1.5% glycine, 3% sorbitol, and 0.9% saline. Different experts have their preferences, Baggish prefers Hyskon, due to its immiscibility with blood, and the high viscosity decreases the risk of extravasation. The potential problems with the compound are due to its high viscosity. This makes it difficult to work with, and necessitates immediate washing if instruments are touched by it. Although extravasation is uncommon, a volume of only 300 ml is sufficient to cause pulmonary oedema. This is because dextran 70 is hydrophilic and in the circulation it osmotically shifts six times its own volume of water into the intravascular compartment. The compound also has an effect on blood coagulation, rarely causing a disseminated intravascular coagulation type consumptive coagulopathy, and has been linked to adult respiratory distress syndrome.[56] At present, there is a suspicion that these features are due to an allergic type reaction.

Low viscosity fluids are more commonly used in the UK, although they are miscible with blood, they are not associated with any coagulopathic, or allergic complications. Dextrose 5% is rarely used as it has no advantage over saline, but has the additional side-effect of being hypo-osmolar. The solutions mainly used for operative hysteroscopy are 1.5% glycine and 3% sorbitol. Both of these are non-ionic, and therefore suitable for electrosurgery. Glycine, used originally by the urologists, is hypo-osmolar, and excess absorption results in a dilutional hyponatraemia, which can be further complicated by a subsequent hyperammonaemia due to glycine's intrahepatic metabolism causing the "TURP Syndrome". As with all of these compounds vigilance is mandatory, and deaths have been reported.[2] Sorbitol is similar to glycine being hypo-osmolar (approx. 170 mOsmol), it also has metabolic complications, causing a hyper-glycaemia due to its breakdown. Mannitol[57] is a relatively new medium being used, its advantage is that it is iso-osmolar (approx. 285 mOsmol), and it is a natural osmotic diuretic. Little experience exists in the literature so far of any complications, but mannitol will cause a volume overload if large intravasation occurs.

Until recently operative hysteroscopic surgery was limited to requiring a non-ionic medium, as electrosurgery in an ionic environment could not be performed, and the current would simply disperse throughout the medium. However, Versapoint, (Ethicon, USA) can operate in an ionic saline medium (**Figures 15.6** and **15.7**).

This represents a considerable feat of engineering, and we feel this will ultimately become a valuable instrument for hysteroscopic surgery, the instruments small diameter (5 French) means that operative procedures may be performed on conscious patients in an out-patient setting. Our experience[12] agrees with the very positive initial reports, however, care must still be taken to avoid fluid overload, although the osmotically-induced fluid shifts characteristic of other media are minimised.

It is essential that all theatres performing hysteroscopic surgery should have a system for monitoring fluid deficits during the procedure, and a protocol for the management of excessive deficits (**Table 15.7**).[58]

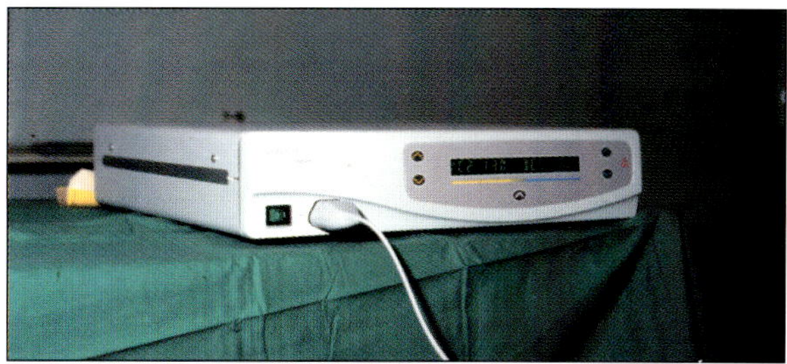

Figure 15.6 Versapoint (Ethicon, U.S.A.) 'smart' generator which automatically controls power output to the tissue impedance.

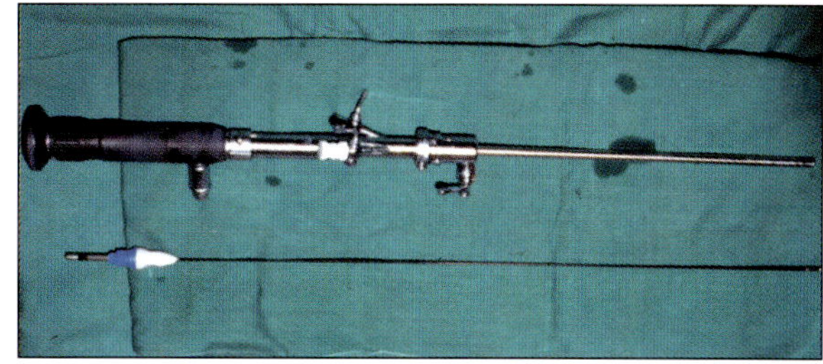

Figure 15.7 Versapoint (Ethicon, U.S.A.) bipolar electrode (5 French) beside a hysteroscope for relative size comparisons.

Table 15.7 Management for iatrogenic hysteroscopic fluid overload.

Deficit	Management
<1 L	Continue surgery
<1.5 L	Expedite procedure, check electrolytes, catheterise to monitor input: output
<2 L	Give frusemide 40 mg intravenously, terminate procedure if possible
>2 L	Terminate procedure, recheck haematocrit and electrolytes

Prevention is better than cure, and there are many devices attempting to calculate the amount of fluid absorbed during the procedure. These range in sophistication from syringes, calibrated fluid bags hung at a certain height over the level of the uterus (60–100 cm) with a collecting bucket or pouch in the sub-perineal drapes, to calibrated spring weight gauges. If any of these simpler devices are used the fluid balance must be checked every 5 min.

A method for the biochemical assessment of absorbed fluid is the addition of a small (2%) amount of ethanol to the distension media, this is measured to assess systemic fluid absorption by analysing the alcohol expired by the patient. There is very little literature on this area, being mostly small trials with poor design,[59] and the potential complications of systemic alcohol in a post-operative patient are cause for concern.

There are a wide variety of pump systems, ranging from simple pumps where a constant rate of flow of fluid is produced at a given pump rate, up to sophisticated pressure controlled pump systems. There are a variety of these devices available. Our experience is with the pressure limited rotary pump system (this avoids the catastrophic complications due to the gas driven variety); the Hamou Endomat (Karl Storz, Tuttlingen, Germany). Our experience agrees with Hamou's findings[60] of decreased fluid absorption, and decreased morbidity (**Figure 15.8**). At present, there is no consensus on hysteroscopic monitoring, however in France, government legislation forbids hysteroscopic surgery unless a pump system is being used.

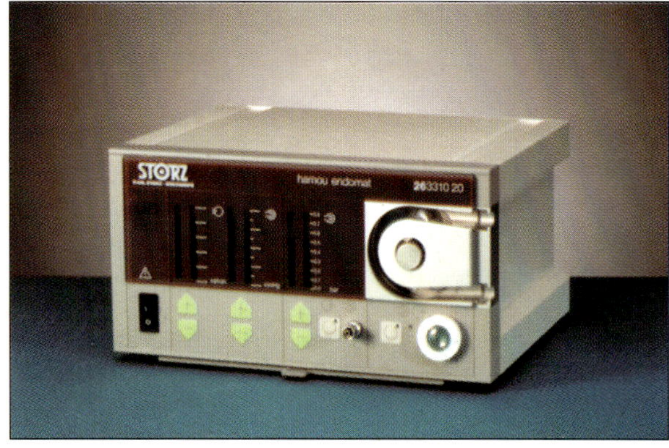

Figure 15.8 Hamou Endomat (Karl Storz, Tuttlingen, Germany) a pressure limited rotary pump system.

Conclusions

This review is an evaluation of the different methods used to decrease the risk of complications in minimal access surgery. We have focused on the prevention of those complications which are related to the basic principles of laparoscopic and hysteroscopic surgery, rather than a discourse on specific operative complications.

Despite the tremendous advances in this area of gynaecological surgery, and the appropriate emphasis on training, accreditation, and critical appraisal of new techniques, there is a surprising lack of consensus on even the most basic techniques, this has been addressed recently by the British Society of Gynaecological Endoscopists. Due to lack of quality research on what are the safest approaches, we have been unable to give any didactic opinions. Instead, we offer a critical account of current practices, and look forward to the time when we can give more definitive answers. Minimal access surgery has now proved its superiority over conventional open surgery in a range of operations; it is now time to firmly establish what the acceptable and safest methods are for performing these operations.

Extensive international surveys have shown that laparoscopic and hysteroscopic surgery are associated with very few complications, but these surveys have noted a slight rise in complications. The reasons for this are not clear; it may reflect the advances in our surgical ability, where the morbidity will be intrinsically higher as a result of operating on cases with extensive pathology. Less reassuringly, it may indicate the attempt by less skilled surgeons to perform increasingly complex procedures, or less reticence by surgeons to report on their complications as MAS becomes more accepted in the wider surgical community. Our inability to explain this trend underlines the need for continuous audit of these techniques, and the appropriate emphasis on training and accreditation.

We have attempted to give as comprehensive an overview of the equipment as possible. There have been remarkable and welcome developments in this area, notably in improving the safety aspects of these potentially lethal devices. Good quality trials to confirm clinically the theoretical advantages these instruments possess are awaited.

Key points for clinical practice

General

- Appropriate case selection is vital.
- Patient preparation both physically and psychologically are equally important.
- Confidence in surgery depends on appropriate training, and the use of quality equipment with which the surgeon and theatre staff are familiar.

Laparoscopic surgery

- In the absence of definite opinions on the safest mode of entry, it is the responsibility of every surgeon to adopt techniques with which they are competent and are accepted as safe and reasonable practice.
- The potential for injury should always be at the forefront of the surgeon's mind, and a panendoscopy of the abdominal cavity should be routine at the start and end of every laparoscopic procedure.
- Patients after laparoscopic surgery should recover rapidly, if this is not the case, potentially major complications should be suspected until proven otherwise.

Hysteroscopic surgery

- Beware the difficult cervical dilation, in our experience, the degree of force is proportional to the complication rate.
- Select the distension media to suit the procedure and the patient, always monitor flow rates and fluid balance.
- If the uterine cavity collapses, this is uterine perforation until proven otherwise. Have a low threshold for investigating iatrogenic trauma if this occurs in operative procedures.

REFERENCES

1. Chamberlain G, Carron Brown JA. RCOG. Report on the confidential enquiry into gynaecological laparoscopy, Royal College of Obstetricians and Gynaecologists Press, 1978.
2. Hulka JF, Peterson HB, *et al.* American Association of Gynecologic Laparoscopists' Survey 1972–1993 *J Am Assoc Gynecol Laparoscopists.*
3. Report of the R.C.O.G. working party on training in gynaecological endoscopic surgery, Royal College of Obstetricians and Gynaecologists Press, 1994.
4. Asch R, Studd J. 1999 Progress in reproductive medicine. Nezhat *et al.* (Edit.) New York: Pantheon Publishing.

5. Overton C, Hargreaves J, Maresh M. A national survey of the complications of endometrial destruction techniques for menstrual disorders: the MISTLETOE study. Minimally invasive surgical techniques – laser, endothermal or endoresection. *Br J Obstet Gynaecol* 1997; **104**(12): 1351–1352.

6. Chapron, Ch., de Poncherville, L.Pierre, F., French survey on gynaecologic laparoscopy. *Human Reproduction.* 1998; **13**(7): 1761.

7. Querleu D, Chevallier L, Chapron C, Bruhat, MA. Complications of gynaecological laparoscopic surgery. A French collaborative study. *Gynaecol Endosc* 1993; **2**: 3–6.

8. Report of the audit committee's working group on communication standards gynaecology: surgical procedures. Royal College of Obstetricians & Gynaecologists 1995.

9. Lefler H, Sullivan G, Hulka J. Modified endometrial ablation: electrocoagulation with vasopressin and suction curettage preparation. *Obstet Gynecol* 1991; **77**: 949–953.

10. Fraser I, Healy D, Torode H, Song J, Mamers P, Wilde F. Depot goserelin and danazol pre-treatment before rollerball endometrial for menorrhagia. *Obstet Gynecol* 1996; **87**: 544–550.

11. Vancaillie TG. Electrosurgery at laparoscopy: guidelines to avoid complications. *Gynaecol Endosc* 1994; **3**: 143–150.

12. O'Donovan P, McGurgan P, Jones SE. Versapoint™: a novel technique for operative hysteroscopy in a saline medium. American Association of Gynecologic Laparoscopists. Abstract: Atlanta 1998.

13. Goodwin, H. *Minimal Access Surgery Journal of the M.D.U.* Feb 1998; **14**:(1).

14. Rosen D, Lam AM, Chapman M, Carlton M, Cario GM. Methods of creating pneumopreitoneum, *Obstetric Gynecol Survey*. 1998; **53**(3): 167–174.

15. Mintz M. Risks and prophylaxis in laparoscopy: a survey of 100,000 cases. *J Reprod Med* 1977; **18**: 269–272.

16. Bergvist D, Bergvist A. Vascular injuries during gynecologic surgery. *Acta Obstetrica Gynecol Scand* 1987; **66**: 19–23.

17. Loffer FD, Pent D. Indications and contraindications and complications of laparoscopy. *Obstet Gynecol Survey* 1975; **30**: 407–423.

18. Tsaltas J, Healy DL, Lloyd D. Review of major complications of laparoscopy in a free standing gynecologic day case hospital. *Gyn Endosc* 1996; **5**: 265–270.

19. Hill DJ. Complications of the laparoscopic approach. Baillières *Clin Obstet Gynaecol.* 1995; **8**: pp. 865–879.

20. Garry, R. Complications of laparoscopic entry. *Gynaecol Endosc.* 1997; **5**: pp. 319–329.

21. Sutton CJ A practical approach to laparoscopy. Endoscopic surgery for gynaecologists. 2nd Ed. Sutton and Diamond. WB Saunders, London 1998.

22. Hurd WH, Bude RO, DeLancey JO, Gauvin JM, Aisen AM. Abdominal wall characterisation with magnetic resonance imaging and computed tomography. The effects of obesity on the laparoscopic approach. *J Reprod Med* 1991; **36**: 473–476.

23. Reich H, Garry R. Advanced laparoscopic surgery. *Laparoscopic Hysterectomy*. Ch.4, p.51 Oxford: Blackwell Science. 1993.

24. Phipps JH. Complications of laparoscopic surgery. Avoidance and management. *Yearbook of the Royal College of Obstetrics and Gynaecology*. London: RCOG. 1995: pp. 67–78.

25. Dingerfelder JR. Direct laparoscopic insertion without prior pneumoperitoneum. *J of Reprod Med* 1978; **21**: 45–47.

26. Byron JW, Fujiyoshi CA, Miyazawa K. Evaluation of the direct trocar insertion technique at laparoscopy. *Obstet Gynaecol* 1989; **74**: 42–48.

27. Hill DJ, Maher PJ. Direct cannula entry for laparoscopy *J of the AAGL* 1996; **4**: 77–79.

28. Mehzat FR, *et al.* Comparison of direct insertion of disposable and standard reusable laparoscopic trocars and previous pneumo-peritoneum with Veress needle. *Obstet Gynaecol* 1991; **78**: 148–150.

29. Jansen FW, Kapiteyn K, Trimbos-Kemper T, Hermans J, Trimbos JB. Complications of laparoscopy: a prospective multicentre observational study. *Br J Obstet Gynaecol.* 1997; **104**: 595–600.

30. Hassan HM. Window for open laparoscopy. *Am J Obstet Gynecol.* 1980; **137**: 869–870.

31. Hulka J, Peterson H, Phillips J, Surrey M. 1995 Operative laparoscopy. A.A.G.L. 1993 membership survey **2**: 133–136.

32. Semm K. Operative pelviscopy. *Br Med Bull* 1986; **42**: 284–295.

33. Hill DJ, Maher PJ, Wood EC, Barnetson B. Gasless laparoscopy. *Austral New Zeal J Obstet Gynaecol* 1993: **34**: 79–80.

34. Watson DI, Mathew G, Ellis T, Baigne CF, Rofe AM, Jamieson GG. Gasless laparoscopy may reduce the risk of port site metastases following laparscopic tumour surgery. *Arch Surg*. Feb 1997; **132**(2): 166–168.

35. Veress J. Neues instrument sur Ausfuhrung von Brust-oder. *Dt Med Wshr* 1938; (**64**): 1480–1481.

36. Baskett TF. On the shoulders of giants. RCOG Press 1996. London.

37. Kleppenger RK. Closed techniques for equipment insertion. Manual of endoscopy American Association of Gynecologic Laparoscopists Edits. Martin D.C. *et al*: 1990; pp. 15–22.

38. Palmer R. Safety in laparoscopy. *J Reprod Med* 1974; **3**: 1–5.

39. Reich H, Levie M, McGlynn F *et al*. Establishment of pneumoperitoneum through the left ninth intercostal space. *Gynaecol Endosc* 1995; **4**: 141–143.

40. Neely MR, McWilliams R, Makhlouf H.A. Laparoscopy: routine pneumoperitoneum via the posterior fornix. *Obstet Gynecol* 1975; **45**: 459–460.

41. Morgan HR. Laparoscopy: Induction of pneumoperitoneum via transfundal procedure. *Obstet Gynecol* 1979; **54**: 260–261.

42. Bhoyrul S, Mori T, Way LW. Radially expanding dilatation. A superior method of laparoscopic trocar access. *Surg Endosc* 1996; **10**(7): 775–778.

43. Okeahialam MG, O'Donovan PJ, Gupta JK. Microlaparoscopy using an optical Veress needle inserted at Palmer's point. *Gynecol Endosc* 1999; **8**(2): 115–116.

44. Audebert AJM, Gomel V. Role of microlaparoscopy in the diagnosis of peritoneal and visceral adhesions and in the prevention of bowel injury associated with blind trocar insertion. *Fertil Steril* 2000; **73**(3): 631–635.

45. Fuller PN. Microendoscopic surgery. *Am J Obstet Gynecol* June 1996 **174**(6): pp. 1757–1761.

46. Miannay E, Lanvin D, Querleu D. Security using a micro-optic introduced by the Veress needle *J Gynecol Obstet Biol Reprod* March 1998; **27**(2): 185–190.

47. Downing BG, Wood C. Initial experience with a new 2 mm microloaparoscope. *Aust NZ J Obstet Gynaecol* 1995; **35**(2): 202.

48. Faber, BM, Coddington, CC. Microlaparoscopy: a comparative study of diagnostic accuracy. *Fertil Steril*. May 1997; **67**(5).

49. Hauesler, G. *et al*. Diagnostic accuracy of 2 mm microlaparoscopy. *Acta Obstet Gynecol Scand* 1996; **75**: 672–675.

50. Bauer O, Kaipker W, Felberbaum R, Gerling W, Diedrich K. Small diameter laparoscopy using a laparoscope *J Assis Repro Gene* 1996; **13**(4).

51. Love BR, McCorvey R, McCorvey M. Low cost office laparoscopic sterilisation. *J Am Assoc Gynecol Laparos* 1994; **1**: 379–381.

52. Risquez F, Pennehoaut G, McCorvey R, Love B, Vazquez A, Partamian, Lucena E, Audebert A, Confino E. Diagnostic and operative laparoscopy: a preliminery multicentre report. *Human Repro*. 1997; **12**(8): 1645–1648.

53. Palter SF, Olive DL. Office microlaparoscopy. *J Am Assoc Gynecol Laparos* 1996; **3**(3): 359–364.

54. Ternamian AM. A trocarless, reusable, visual-access cannula for safer laparoscopy; an update. *J Am Assoc Gynecol Laparos*. 1998; **5**(2): 197–202.

55. Hulka J, Peterson H, Phillips J, Surrey M. 1995 *Operative hysteroscopy. A.A.G.L.* 1993 Membership survey **2**: 133–136.

56. Manager D, Gerson JI, *et al*. Pulmonary oedema and coagulopathy due to Hyskon. *Anesth Analg* 1989; **68**: 686–687.

57. Kim AH, Keltz MD, Arici A, Rosenburg M, Olive DL. Dilutional hyponatraemia during hysteroscopic myomectomy with sorbitol-mannitol distension media. *J Am Assoc Gynec Laporos*. 1995; **2**(2): 237–242.

58. O'Connor H. 1998 How to avoid complications at hysteroscopic surgery. *In: Recent advances in obstetrics and gynaecology*. Edit. J. Bonnar 20th edition: Churchill Livingstone, Edinburgh.

59. Allweiner D, *et al*. Addition of ethanol to the distension medium in surgical hysteroscopy as a screening test to prevent "fluid overload". *Geburtshilfe und Frauenheilkunde*. 1996; **56**(9): 462–469.

60. Hamou J, Fryman R, McLucas, B, Garry R. A uterine distension system to prevent fluid intravasation during hysteroscopic surgery. *Gynecol Endosc* 1996; **5**: 131–136.

16

Microwave Endometrial Ablation in the Out-patient Setting

N. Sharp

Introduction

Endometrial ablation evolved as a surgical technique to enable women with menorrhagia to have an effective, safe, surgical alternative to hysterectomy. The "first generation" techniques (laser, resection and rollerball) have been described as "the most carefully evaluated of surgical procedures".[1] Whilst national audits and randomised controlled trials (RCTs) have confirmed their efficacy and safety,[2–10] these procedures still have a number of inherent disadvantages:

1. they require a distension medium which has caused iatrogenic complications (and fatalities) in a small number of patients;
2. the techniques used require a high level of surgical skill and training;
3. laser equipment is highly specialised and expensive;
4. although there are reports of using the "first generation" techniques in an out-patient setting, the time taken to perform the procedure (usually 30 min), and the size of the operative hysteroscope (usually 8 Fr) mean that most units prefer patients to have a general anaesthetic.

Over recent years a number of technologies have emerged to try and overcome the problems associated with the 'first generation' techniques for the treatment of menorrhagia whilst retaining their safety and efficacy.

Microwave endometrial ablation (MEA) is one of the fastest treatments, with a mean treatment time under 3 min, whilst still being very effective. The treatment has been extensively evaluated both by large cohort series with long-term follow-up,[11,13] and compared to rollerball/resection in a pragmatically designed RCT.[14] The inherent simplicity, safety and speed of treatment has enabled the author to evolve from a day case theatre treatment under general anaesthetic to day case local anaesthesia with sedation and now to out-patient treatment under local anaesthesia alone. The evolution of MEA to an out-patient/office procedure has found to be satisfactory for many women and will be described in this chapter.

Indications for MEA

MEA is indicated for women with dysfunctional uterine bleeding (DUB) with or without associated dysmenorrhoea, who do not wish to have a hysterectomy and whose family is complete.

Physics

Microwave endometrial ablation uses waveguide technology to deliver microwave energy at a frequency of 9.2 GHz through the uterine cervix into the uterine cavity where it is absorbed by the endometrium – causing rapid heating. A coaxial cable takes the energy from a magnetron source to the microwave applicator. (**Figure 16.1**) The energy released at the active tip is only 22 W, but despite this low power, therapeutic temperatures (70–80°) are registered within 45 sec.

The microwave frequency is chosen to limit the penetration of energy into the tissues to no more than 6 mm. Within this narrow zone, tissue temperatures of 100°C are reached, with superheated steam being formed at microscopic level at the instrument tissue interface. A lower temperature is registered by the thermocouple as it is heat-sunk on the applicator shaft and covered by the fluoropolymer sheath. This 'discrepancy' is accommodated by the equipment design and temperature

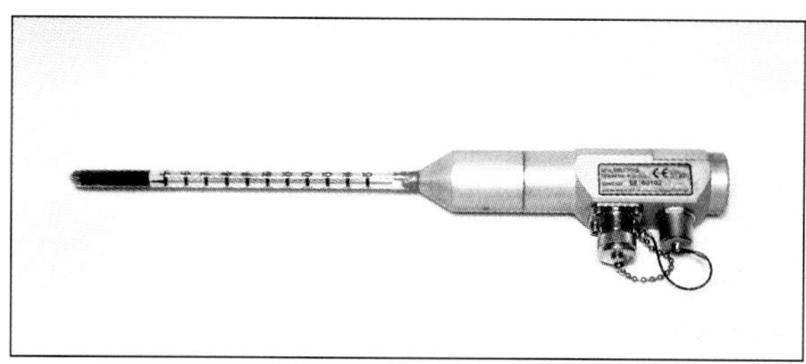

Figure 16.1 Microwave applicator.

display. It is this very precise high-energy field which makes MEA such a quick and effective technique. Further descriptions of the physical principles and basic research stages may be found elsewhere.[11,12]

Patient selection

To make a diagnosis of DUB, intra-uterine pathology needs to be excluded. All patients in our clinic have a transvaginal ultrasound scan (TVS) to assess the uterus and particularly the endometrial cavity, and an out-patient endometrial biopsy is taken with a Pipelle (Pipelle de Cornier). Their menstrual symptoms are scored using a simple 10 question validated menstrual questionnaire (**Table 16.1**) to enable objective analysis and improvement in symptomatology to be determined.[13]

Table 16.1 Menstrual score chart

	SCORE
Dysmenorrhoea	2
Days of bleeding	
7–10	1
> 10	2
Average length of cycle	
If > 28	0
If 24–27	1
If < 24	2
Heavy days	
For each	1
Sanitary protection	
If doubled	2
Frequency of changing	
If > 2 hourly	1
If > hourly	2
Clots	1
Flooding	1
Housebound or time off work	2
Pre-operation	
Duration of problems > 5 years	1
Post-operation	
Any menstrual loss	1

Endometrial or fibroid polyps

If the TVS indicates an endometrial or fibroid polyp suitable for removal then we either remove it prior to MEA to see if menstruation improves, or immediately prior to the MEA procedure to ensure the ablation is not compromised by the polyp's presence and to get a histological diagnosis.

Uterine fibroids

Although many of the 'second generation' endometrial ablative techniques require a normal-sized regular uterine cavity, a significant proportion of women presenting with menorrhagia have uterine fibroids. The finding of fibroids on TVS is not a contra-indication to MEA, and most patients with fibroids are suitable for MEA, but they need to be aware that fibroids will not be affected significantly by the procedure. It is only in cases where the cavity is distorted to such a degree that the applicator tip is prevented from being applied to the entire cavity surface that MEA is unsuitable. Occasionally, it will be necessary to undertake hysteroscopy to assess the cavity adequately. Hysterectomy is usually only recommended for symptoms such as pressure effects: frequency of micturition or altered bowel habit; pelvic congestion symptoms, or a uterine size greater than 12 weeks gestation. Our data suggest that the presence of fibroids does not compromise the success of the treatment. We use 5 cm as the upper limit for fibroids impinging onto the uterine cavity to be suitable for MEA.

Caesarean section

A Caesarean section scar represents an inherent weakness in the uterus. In the majority of cases the uterine scar heals well, but in a small proportion of cases the scar will be defective.

The uterine scar is easily visualised on a sagittal section using TVS and its thickness can be readily measured. In those few cases with defective healing the endometrial outline will be seen 'tenting' up into the scar area. These inward 'steps' can also be visualised at hysteroscopy.

Laboratory studies with tissue substitutes have shown that tissue defects opening into the microwave field can have a focusing effect, with tissue changes occurring 1–2 mm beyond the 5–6 mm ablation zone in relation to these defects. For this reason we err on the side of caution and exclude women whose caesarean section scar thickness measures less than 8 mm because of the theoretical risk of microwave energy transgressing the scar, with risk of bladder damage, although this has never been a problem in clinical practice. For these reasons we believe that a routine TVS in all women with a history of caesarean section is an important pre-operative precaution.

Psychology

Careful personality selection is required for patients undergoing MEA in the outpatient setting. Whilst most patients are understandably a little nervous, a woman who is highly anxious or fearful may not cope with the procedure and will probably prefer a general anaesthetic.

Similarly, it has also been our experience that women with deep-seated emotional conflicts can react in an unexpected fashion e.g. hyperventilation causing carpopedal spasm or intractable pain after MEA.

If such a problem is suspected (e.g. history of mental illness, abuse, or adverse pregnancy outcome) then general anaesthesia should be considered.

Contra-indications to MEA

- Abnormal endometrial histology
- Other uterine or pelvic pathology which would make hysterectomy a better choice
- Previous uterine surgery e.g. myomectomy or previous endometrial resection (Caesarean section – see above).
- Continued fertility needs.

Special precautions for MEA

- Uterine retroversion – care is required to ensure correct instrumentation placement in the cavity
- Chronic steroid use – increased risk of uterine perforation.
- Connective tissue disorder e.g. osteogenesis imperfecta, Ehlers-Danlos Syndrome – increased risk of uterine perforation.
- Uterine abnormality e.g. a bicornuate uterus – the author recommends abdominal ultrasound control during the MEA treatment to ensure treatment of both uterine cavities.

Equipment

- Suitable facility e.g. colposcopy suite or out-patient hysteroscopy facility
- Recovery area
- Microwave Generator (Microsulis, Waterlooville, Hants, UK.)
- Microwave applicators (**Figure 16.1**)
- D&C set (cervical dilators, vulsellum forceps etc.)
- Sterile steel rule
- Dental syringe
- Speculum (Marina Medical Instruments, Hollywood, USA) (**Figure 16.2**)
- Transvaginal ultrasound scanner
- Pulse oximeter
- Oxygen supply and masks
- Nitrous oxide/oxygen – "Entonox" supply with demand valve
- Patient distractions and a supportive environment e.g. music source, ability to have a companion present
- Needles, syringes, cannulae, IV giving sets, IV fluids etc.
- Arrest trolley with defibrillator and intubation equipment.

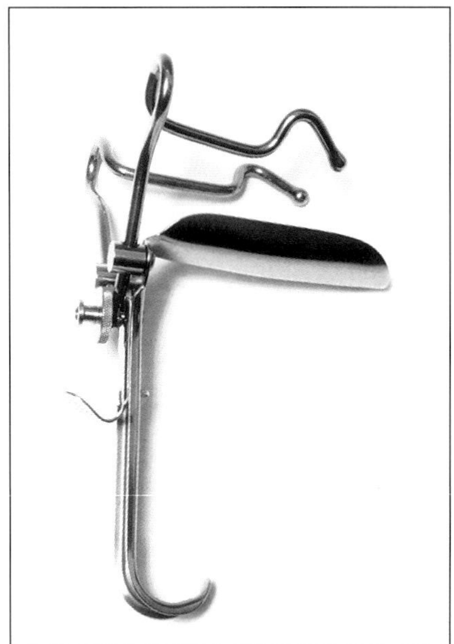

Figure 16.2 Speculum for use where access is difficult.

Drugs

- Diclofenac (Voltarol) 100 mg suppository (Geigy) Ibuprofen tabs
- Prilocaine 3% with Felypressin (Citanest with Octapressin) 2.2 ml glass cartridges (Astra)
- Bupivacaine 0.5% (Marcain) (Astra)
- Midazolam (Hypnoval) 10 mg amps (Roche)
- Alfentanil (Rapifen) 1 mg amps (Janssen)
- Anexate (Flumazenil) 500 µg (Roche) (Reversant for Midazolam)
- Naloxone (Narcan) 400 µg (Du Pont) (Reversant for Alfentanil)
- Atropine 600 µg (To correct bradycardia)

Analgesia

Effective analgesia for MEA is provided by a combination of non-steroidal anti-inflammatory agent and a local anaesthetic cervical block. A diclofenac suppository is self-administered by the patient 1 h beforehand. Whilst we have not undertaken a formal study of diclofenac use, experience has shown an increased awareness of discomfort in patients where it has been omitted (either through oversight or contraindication). Discussion with other workers in the field of endometrial ablation supports this finding and the same conclusion has been arrived at independently by others.[15] Peak plasma concentrations occur within an hour of administration.

Cervical block

Local anaesthetic uterine block is achieved with a four quadrant block technique.[16] Having exposed the cervix, a small amount of Prilocaine with Felypressin is injected into point A, (**Figure 16.3**) using a dental syringe. After waiting a short time, the cervix is then grasped at this point with the volsellum forceps, and the block is completed with one cartridge being used for each quadrant. The needle is inserted into the centre of each quadrant (point X, **Figure 16.3**) parallel to the cervical canal and up to the needle hilt, before injecting the cartridge contents. Quadrants 2 and 3 are probably the most important, blocking the insertion of the uterosacral ligaments. This block technique aims to establish a ring block at the internal cervical os. It is necessary to wait for 1–2 min to achieve the full anaesthetic effect.

Using this technique it is possible to dilate the cervix with no discomfort in almost all cases.

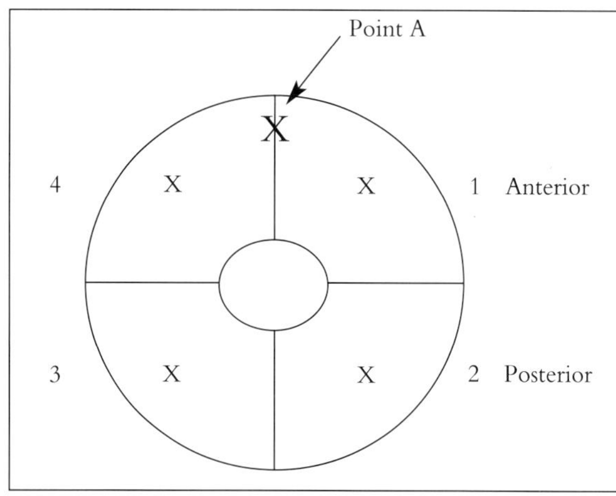

Figure 16.3 Schematic diagram of the cervix.

Despite an effective cervical block, there will be a small proportion of women who still retain some sensation at the uterine fundus. This seems to be an inherent feature and may have to be accepted. The woman should be warned that there may therefore be some initial discomfort during the treatment phase but that this should pass quickly. The use of "Entonox" may be useful for these women. The fact that the discomfort is transient and that uterine pain is a familiar symptom to most women, usually enables the patient to cope with inhalational analgesia alone.

Once the fundal area is treated any discomfort usually passes. With experience and confidence, the additional use of sedation becomes infrequent. However, intravenous cannulation should always be performed prior to undertaking MEA, and for those few women who need additional intravenous medication, the fully recumbent position is required and oxygen is administered with pulse oximetry prior to sedation. Sedation is achieved with a bolus of 3–5 mg of Midazolam and 0.3–0.5 mg of Alfentanil given concomitantly. Both of these agents may cause respiratory depression and experience with these agents should be gained in the company of a trained anaesthetist.

At completion of the MEA procedure, a repeat four quadrant block with 5 ml of 0.25% bupivicaine per quadrant using a standard 20 ml syringe and needle gives a prolonged post-operative analgesia.

It is advisable for patients to have an analgesic available at home as a proportion will still have some uterine discomfort later on. Our advice is for them to use whichever proprietary brand they prefer of their own – those containing Ibuprofen or other non-steroidal anti-inflammatory being particularly effective.

Procedure

Having established the cervical block, the uterine cavity is sounded in the usual way and the sounding checked against a sterile steel rule. The cervix is then dilated to 9 mm and the sounding checked again with the 9 mm dilator.

The microwave applicator (**Figure 16.1**) is then connected to the microwave source with a coaxial cable, and to the temperature display screen with a second cable connected to the data acquisition port. The temperature display screen should show the ambient temperature. The microwave applicator is then introduced to the uterine cavity until the tip reaches the fundus. The previous cavity measurements should conform to the measurement on the applicator shaft. This strict triple check ensures that there is no risk of inadvertent perforation. Using a foot switch the surgeon energises the magnetron and microwave energy at 22 W is delivered from the applicator tip.

Rapid heating is readily seen on the temperature display. After a few moments, 60°C is registered and the applicator is then moved slowly and steadily from side to side to evenly heat the fundus and cornual areas. Once the whole fundal area has achieved therapeutic temperatures, the applicator is slowly withdrawn in 3 mm decrements maintaining the steady side-to-side motion to distribute the energy evenly into the endometrium. As the applicator is moved from a warm to a cool area the temperature is seen to fall, indicating that the applicator should be held still momentarily to ensure treatment of that area when the temperature will be seen to rise. Once the therapeutic temperature is achieved again the applicator is moved once more.

The treatment proceeds in this fashion with slow steady applicator withdrawal. The temperature profile typically shows a 'saw-tooth' wave form (**Figure 16.4**). Once the applicator tip reaches the lower uterine cavity a yellow band on the applicator shaft appears at the external os as a warning to the surgeon. When the active tip reaches the internal os, a black band on the applicator appears externally and indicates that the power should be switched off and the applicator withdrawn, com-

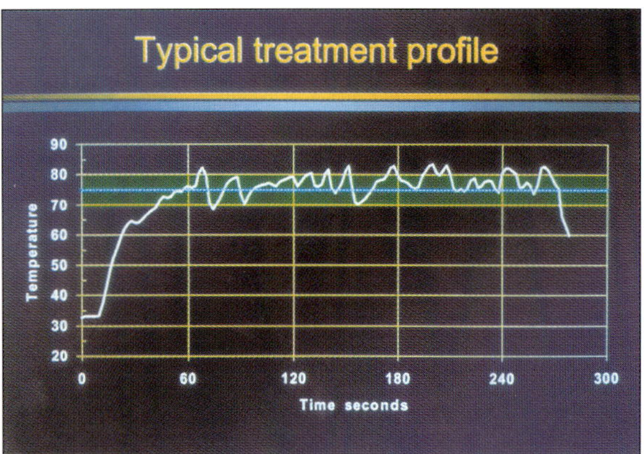

Figure 16.4 Typical patient treatment profile.

pleting the treatment and preventing endocervical heating.

The procedure is 'clean' – there is no bleeding and hysteroscopic fluids are avoided. The procedure is quick; treatment is completed in less than 3 min for an average-sized uterus. Larger cavities require slightly longer treatment times.

Staffing

To conduct an outpatient/office treatment session, four people are required.

1. *Surgeon* – to perform the treatment.
2. *Assistant* – to operate the equipment, connect the cables and generally aid the surgeon. This is a doctor in training or member of nursing staff.
3. *Treatment nurse* – to look after patient and distract their attention with conversation during the process. They also administer inhalational analgesia or intravenous sedation under the surgeon's instruction.
4. *Recovery nurse* – to attend to the patient during the post-treatment period.

Discussion

Safety

Microwave endometrial ablation is inherently safe for a number of reasons.

- Physics – tissue penetration is limited strictly by the microwave frequency chosen.
- Low power – only 22 W is required.
- Low energy – a combination of low power and short treatment time means a very low energy dose.
- Continuous thermometry – the surgeon knows the tissue temperature at all times.
- Non-earthing – no risk of earthing injury.
- Continuous applicator withdrawal – no risk of inadvertent uterine perforation during treatment.
- No fluid overload – hysteroscopic fluids are not required, in addition the microwave system incorporates a number of safety inter locks.
- No risk of operative haemorrhage.

In addition to its inherent safety, microwave endometrial ablation has a number of other features that make it attractive to the gynaecological surgeon and to the patient:

- safe
- effective
- quick
- clean
- interactive
- easy to learn
- reusable.

Outcome

Over 400 women have been treated in our unit over a 5-year period, with no major complications. Results have been consistent with good medium- and long-term outcomes.

Amenorrhoea is achieved in 37% and satisfaction in 84% of cases at 3-year follow-up.[11] Most treatment failures present 6 months after treatment, and very few beyond 18 months. Of those women requesting repeat treatment, 4 out of 5 had a satisfactory result after retreatment, resulting in an overall satisfaction rate in excess of 90%.

Dysmenorrhoea is also usually improved.[11,13,14] Moderate (55.8%) or severe (27.9%) dysmenorrhoea pre-operatively (total 83.7%) had improved to 11.6% and 6.8% (total 18.4%) respectively at 3 years. This represents an 80% reduction in the incidence of dysmenorrhoea in addition to the 84–90% improvement in menstrual loss.

The speed and simplicity of the MEA treatment enable it to be readily adapted to the outpatient or office setting, with its reduced costs. With increasing emphasis on the cost of healthcare provision, the ability to offer good, effective care in a lower cost environment is becoming a major factor when selecting a preferred treatment option.

For these reasons MEA compares very favourably with other existing ablative techniques.

Acknowledgements

The author would like to thank Mr B. Butters at Microsulis PLC (Commercial sponsor). Also Mr David Hodgson MRCOG & Mr Michael Ellard MRCOG during their research fellowships, and their helpful comments during the preparation of this chapter.

Pharmacopoea

Astra Pharmaceuticals Ltd, Kings Langley, Herts, UK

Du Pont Pharmaceuticals, Stevenage, Herts, UK

Geigy Pharmaceuticals, Horsham, W. Sussex, UK

Janssen Pharmaceuticals, Wantage, Oxon, UK

Roche Products Ltd, Welwyn Garden City, Herts, UK

REFERENCES

1. Garry, R. Endometrial ablation and resection: validation of a new surgical concept. *Br J Obstet Gynaecol* 1997; **104**: 1329–1321.
2. Overton C, Hargreaves H, Maresh M. A national survey of the complications of endometrial destruction for menstrual disorders: the MISTLETOE study. *Br J Obstet Gynaecol* 1997; **104**: 1351–1359.
3. Scottish Hysteroscopy Audit Group: A Scottish audit of hysteroscopic surgery for menorrhagia: complications and follow up. *Br J Obstet Gynaecol* 1995; **102**: 249–254.
4. Dwyer N, Hutton J, Stirrat GM. Randomised controlled trial comparing endometrial resection with abdominal hysterectomy for the surgical treatment of menorrhagia. *Br J Obstet Gynaecol* 1993; **100**: 237–243.
5. Pinion SB, Parkin DE, Abramovich DR *et al.* Randomised trial of hysterectomy, endometrial laser ablation and transcervical resection for dysfunctional uterine bleeding *Br Med J* 1994; **309**: 979–983.
6. Gannon MJ, Holt EM, Fairbank J *et al.* A randomised trial comparing endometrial resection and abdominal hysterectomy for the treatment of menorrhagia *Br Med J* 1991; **303**: 1362–1364.
7. O'Connor H, Broadbent JA, Magos AL, McPherson K. Medical Research Council randomised trial of endometrial resection versus hysterectomy in management of menorrhagia. *Lancet* 1997; **349**: 897–901.
8. Crosignani PG, Vercellini P, Apolone G, De Giorgi O, Cortesi I, Meschia M. Endometrial resection versus vaginal hysterectomy for menorrhagia: long term clinical and quality of life outcomes. *Am J Obstet Gynecol.* 1997; **177**: 95–101.
9. O'Connor H, Magos, A. Endometrial resection for the treatment of menorrhagia. *N Engl J Med* 1996; **335**: 151–156.
10. Aberdeen Endometrial Ablation Trials Group. A randomised trial of endometrial ablation versus hysterectomy for the treatment of dysfunctional uterine bleeding: outcome at four years. *Br J Obstet Gynaecol* 1999; **106**(4): 360–366.
11. Hodgson DA, Feldberg IB, Sharp NC, Cronin N, Evans M. Microwave Endometrial Ablation – Development, Clinical trials and outcomes at three years. *Br J Obstet Gynaecol* 1999; **106**: 684–694.
12. Sharp NC, Feldberg IB, Hodgson DA, Butters B, Cronin N. Microwave endometrial ablation. *Endoscopic surgery for Gynaecologists*, Second Edition, Sutton and Diamond EDS, WB Saunders 1998, Ch 63: 630–637.
13. Sharp NC, Cronin N, Feldberg IB, Evans M, Hodgson D, Ellis S. Microwaves for menorrhagia:

A new fast technique for endometrial ablation. *Lancet* 1995; **346**:1003–1004.

14. Cooper KG, Bain C, Parkin DE. Comparison of microwave endometrial ablation and transcervical resection of the endometrium for treatment of heavy menstrual loss: a randomised trial. *Lancet* 1999; **354**(9193): 1859–1863.

15. Nagele F, Lockwood G, Magos AL. Randomised placebo controlled trial of mefenamic acid for pre-medication at outpatient hysteroscopy: a pilot study. *Br J Obstet Gynaecol.* 1997 July; **104**(7): 842–844.

16. Ferry J, Ranklin L. Transcervical resection of the endometrium using intracervical blocks only: a review of 278 procedures. *Aust NZ J Obstet Gynecol* 1994: **34**: 457–461.

17

The Filshie Clip:

current uses and development

Sharif M. F. Ismail
G. M. Filshie

Introduction

Since its development by Marcus Filshie in Nottingham in 1981,[1] the Filshie clip has proved to be a popular device for female sterilisation and yet has the best potential for reversal as it results in minimal tubal damage.[2] Currently, new and innovative uses of this clip are being developed. This chapter provides an overview on the use of Filshie clip for sterilisation and explores possible future applications.

Historical background

The clip was developed by Mr Marcus Filshie in Nottingham in 1981, helped by Don Casey following research studies, to provide a simple and effective method of sterilisation.[1] Several prototypes were evaluated, ending in mark VI, which is the device currently used.

Since its introduction, the clip has become the market leader in the United Kingdom and is used in 85% of female sterilisations in Canada. Since its approval by the Food and Drug Administration in 1996, 35,000 female sterilisation procedures have been carried out in the United States of America.[3] Scottish gynaecologists have agreed to recommend it as the method of choice for laparoscopic sterilisation.[4] It has become the preferred method for female sterilisation in the guidelines endorsed by the All State Family Planning Associations as well as the Australian Federation of Family Planning Associations.[5]

Where the clip is not popular, this is often the result of other factors, for example, the low rate of sterilisation generally in Italy and Spain,[2] is mainly a result of the position of the Roman Catholic church, which does not approve of the procedure.[6] The same applies to Moslem countries, where sterilisation is not a popular method of contraception.[7] Although contraception is allowed under Islam, the consensus view is that permanent methods are not preferred, unless pregnancy is to be avoided for medical reasons. With the availability of in-vitro fertilisation and the good results of reversal, sterilisation is becoming less 'absolute' as a method of contraception. This depends, of course, on the availability, as well as the affordability, of assisted conception and reversal procedures. As a result, sterilisation is a method for individual, rather than mass, contraception.

The clip in current use is mark VI (**Figure 17.1**), and is a titanium clip lined with silicone rubber. It consists of two jaws joined by a hinge pin. The upper jaw is curved and the lower one has a hooked tip. It is 14 mm long, 3.7 mm wide and weighs just 0.36 g. It exerts pressure, occluding the tube without lacerating it. It is applied using a 7.4 mm applicator, which is usually accompanied by its own portal.

Advantages

The clip is simple to apply, compared with other methods of sterilisation, and the equipment is also easy to maintain.[8] There is no risk of thermal damage.[9] It is also effective, and no correctly applied clip has yet been shown to have failed.[10] Reported failure rates were 0.27% for interval sterilisation[11] and 0.9 to 8.5% for postpartum sterilisation.[12] Since it causes minimal destruction of the tube, 4 mm,[1] it has excellent potential for reversal, with a reported success rate of 80%.[2]

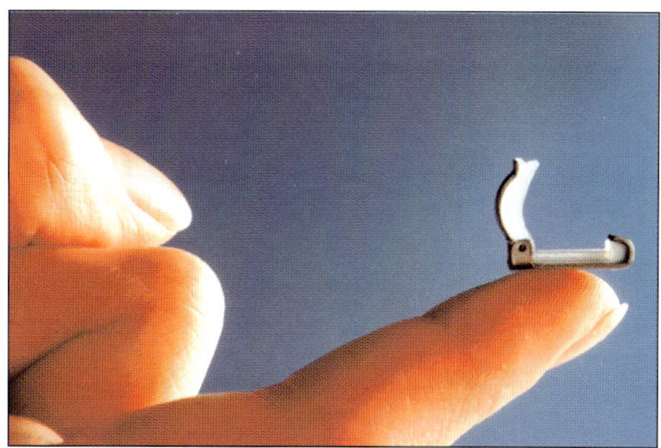

Figure 17.1 The Filshie clip. (Reproduced with the kind permission of Femcare Ltd.)

This potential for reversibility represents an important factor in patient choice, as more women would be happy to be sterilised if the procedure is seen as being reversible.[13] The clip is long enough to be placed on Fallopian tubes of different shapes and sizes, including postpartum ones,[14] and because of this versatility, its use is associated with reduced need for additional clips per tube.[15]

Recommendations for proper use

Figure 17.2 (below) shows the clip being applied to the Fallopian tube.

Problems encountered in applying the clip can be avoided by following the guidelines listed below:

- Avoid gripping handle of the applicator too firmly during insertion of the loaded clip through the second portal, so as to avoid closing the clip prematurely.
- Keep the curved jaw up, and open the applicator slowly, so as to avoid dropping the open clip into the abdomen.
- If a dropped clip is seen, it is better grasped by the applicator (or grasping forceps) and kept in a secure place, such as the anterior fornix, for later retrieval. No attempt should be made to pull a clip that is not properly located in the applicator out through either the laparoscope or the secondary puncture, as it may fall into the abdominal cavity and become difficult to find. As the clip is non-allergic, there is little harm in leaving it in the peritoneal cavity.
- Apply the clip on the isthmus, the narrowest portion of the tube and therefore the region most likely to be occluded effectively. This is also important, since anastomosis is most successful at this area, if sterilisation is to be reversed.[16]
- Check the anatomy of the pelvis carefully before applying the clip, so as to identify the tube and avoid clipping the round ligament. This also helps to identify the rarely encountered cases of double tubes, or uterus.
- The clip needs to be perpendicular to the tube and sterilisation should therefore only be carried out by those well trained in laparoscopy.
- The clip should be applied slowly, with a firm grip, to ensure its closure.
- After applying the clip, the applicator should not be opened and/or withdrawn rapidly, as it can come out with the clip, leading to transection of the tube. If this happens, a clip will need to be applied to each end of the transected tube.
- If there is any doubt as to the application of the clip, a second clip should be applied adjacent to the first.
- If any difficulty is encountered when applying the clip, such as in the presence of peritubal adhesions, then an alternative approach, such as salpingectomy, should be considered.
- A visual checking that the clip has been applied to the isthmic portion of the tube is essential at the end of the procedure.

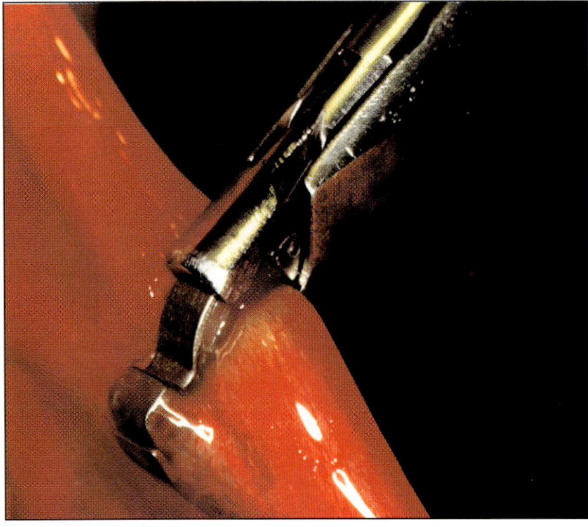

Figure 17.2 The Filshie clip being applied to the Fallopian tube. (Reproduced with the kind permission of Femcare Ltd.)

When to apply the clip

In practice, sterilisation is commonly carried out as an interval procedure, 6 weeks to 3 months after delivery. It can, however, be used safely in the postpartum period, under local anaesthesia through a minilaparotomy incision at the level of the umbilicus,[17] or under general anaesthesia through a suprapubic minilapratomy incision.[18] Postpartum use is generally perceived to carry a higher failure rate, though the CREST study showed that the risk of failure may actually be lower.[19] The use of postpartum sterilisation may have some appeal in the developing countries, where access to health-care facilities is often fraught with difficulties, and it would be better to perform sterilisation while patients remain in the hospitals or health centres after birth. Filshie reported a failure rate of 3 in 593 cases, or 0.5%.[20] The technique can also be used after abortion.

Analgesia
In developed countries, the procedure is often performed under general anaesthesia.[7] It can be carried out as a day case, with the use of short-acting anaesthetic agents (with their associated anti-emetic properties), to enable patients to be discharged on the same day, even if the procedure is carried out in the afternoon[21] In addition, the clip can be applied effectively under local anaesthesia in an out-patient setting. This requires careful selection, as well as counselling, of patients, to exclude those who would need general anaesthesia due to underlying medical conditions or because they would not tolerate the procedure when performed under local anaesthesia.[22] This enhances the cost-effectiveness of sterilisation, making it more suitable for developing countries, and eliminates morbidity and mortality risks associated with the use of general anaesthesia.[23] Post-operative pain relief can be helped by using local anaesthetic, either as an infiltration,[24] or intraperitoneal instillation over the clip after application.[25] Although local anaesthetic gel application to the clip has been associated with reduced pain, it does not affect analgesic requirements.[26]

Approach
Various approaches can be used. For the double puncture technique, a small suprapubic incision is necessary to accommodate the 7 mm applicator, in addition to a subumbilical incision for the laparoscope. For the single puncture technique, a single subumbilical incision is necessary to introduce the 7.3 mm laparoscope.[11] The clip is also the easiest to use if sterilisation is be carried out vaginally (through the posterior fornix) for rapid and efficient sterilisation,[27] though this is not a commonly used approach.

Minilaparotomy may be more suitable for developing countries, where it is often difficult to maintain sophisticated laparoscopic equipment.

Complications
In addition to failure, which is usually due to misapplication of the clip,[10] there have been a few reports of rather unusual complications associated with the use of the clip for sterilisation. These complications include persistent post-operative pain,[28] recurrent pelvic abscess associated with a detached clip,[29] delayed transurethral expulsion of the clip,[30] torsion of the clip presenting as acute abdomen,[31] torsion of the fallopian tube[32] and prolapse of the clip following vaginal hysterectomy.[33] Failure can be followed by resterilisation, when it is advisable to obtain a specimen for histopathological examination and alert the histopathologist to check the patency of the tube, for medicolegal reasons.[10] There was also one case of appendicitis with a clip found in the appendix.[34] Interestingly, the clip was not one of the methods of female sterilisation followed by pelvic inflammatory disease in a recent review.[35]

New developments

New models are being developed to reduce the glare effect of the applicator. A twinclip loading applicator (**Figure 17.3**) will be available as well, allowing the application of two clips without having to reload the applicator. A larger clip is being assessed for postpartum applications.

The clip is also being assessed as a surgical clip for endoscopic surgery. Potential uses include:

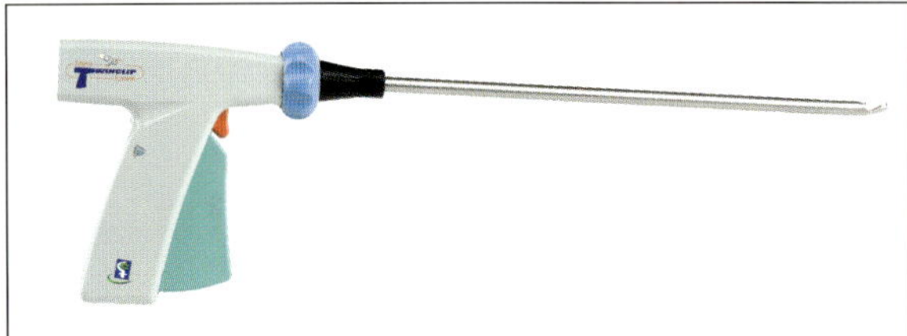

Figure 17.3: The twinclip loading applicator. (Reproduced with the kind permission of Femcare Ltd).

- Laparoscopic salpingectomy, as in ectopic pregnancy, where a clip can be applied on either side of the tube, or across the tube and mesovarium.
- Laparoscopic oophorectomy, when the uterus is to be retained, where the ovarian as well as the infundibulopelvic ligaments can be dissected, skeletonised, clipped and divided.
- Laparosocpic hysterectomy, where the uterine arteries can be dissected, skeletonised, clipped and divided.
- Laparoscopic oophorectomy can be carried out after hysterectomy, where the infundibulopelvic ligament is dissected, skeletonised, clipped and divided.
- Colposuspension procedures can be assisted by anchoring the sutures above the rectus sheath, using the clip.
- The clip can also be applied to the cystic artery and the cystic duct during laparoscopic cholecystectomy, as well as the appendix, during laparoscopic appendectomy.

These potential uses promise lower cost (compared with stapling devices), quick and easy operations (compared with tying as well as the application of loops), no risk of burns or need for small secondary incisions, for application portals, with better cosmetic results and less need to take muscle sutures to avoid incisional hernia. If the use of the Filshie clip in these applications proves to be even remotely as popular as in sterilisation, then the future will see a new and effective surgical tool in endoscopic surgery. This will depend on designing the proper model, carefully researching its use and identifying the best techniques for its application.

Conclusion

The Filshie clip has proved to be a popular device for female sterilisation. Its appeal lies in its simplicity, effectiveness and high potential for reversal, as well as its ability to be applied in a variety of circumstances and settings. Its use in a wide range of endoscopic procedures is currently the subject of intensive research, and it is hoped that it will prove to be a valuable tool in the treatment of several conditions.

REFERENCES

1. Filshie GM, Casey D, Pogmore JR, Dutton AGB, Symonds EM, Peake ABL. The titanium/silicone rubber clip for female sterilisation. *Br J Obst Gynaecol* 1981; 88(**6**): 655–662.
2. Filshie GM. Reversal of female sterilisation using the Filshie clip. *Arch Gynaecol* 1985; (suppl) (**237**): 173.
3. Penfield AJ. The Filshie clip for female sterilisation; A review of world experience. *Am J Obstet Gynaecol* 2000; 182(**3**): 485–489.
4. Penny GC, Souter V, Glasier A, Templeton AA. Laparoscopic sterilisation. *Br J Obst Gynaecol* 1997; 104(**1**): 71–77.
5. Kovacs GT. Female sterilisation. *Med J Aust* 1994; 161(**11**): 612–614.
6. Filshie GM. Sterilisation. *Obstet Gynaecol* 1999; 1(**1**): 26–32.
7. Hendrix NW, Chauhan SP, Morrison JC. Sterilisation and its consequences. *Obstet Gynaecol Survey* 1999; 54(**12**): 766–777.
8. Davies GC, Letchworth AT, Diamond I. A comparison of Filshie and Hulka-Clemens clips in sterilisation operations. *Obstet Gynaecol* 1990; 10(**3**): 251–252.
9. Kandwala SD. Laparoscopic sterilisation; A comparison of current techniques. *J Reprod Med* 1988; 33(**5**): 463–466.
10. Filshie GM. Update in female sterilisation. *Curr Obstet Gynaecol* 1995; 5(**3**): 169–173.
11. Rioux J-E. Female sterilisation and its reversal, In: Filshie M, Guillebaud J: *Contraception; Science and*

Practice 1989; Butterworths, London, United Kingdom, 275–291.

12. Chi I-C, Gates D and Thapa S. Performing tubal sterilisation during women's postpartum hospitalisation; A review of the United States and international experiences. *Obstet Gynaecol Survey* 1992; 47(**2**): 71–79.

13. Hoffman JJ. Sterilisation reversal; Assessment of demand and results, In: Brosens I and Winston R (eds.): Reversibility of female sterilisation. *Academic* 1978; London, United Kingdom.

14. Rioux J-E, Yuzpe AA. Modern approaches to female sterilisation. *Contemp Ob/Gyn* 1997; 42(**9**): 2–8.

15. Toplis PJ, Newman RB. Laparoscopic sterilisation; A comparison of Hulka-Clemens and Filshie clips. *Br J Fam Plann* 1988; 14: 43–45

16. Winston RML. Reversal of female sterilisation. *IPPF Med Bull* 1978; 12(**6**): 1–2.

17. Chi I-C, Gates D, Bunce S, Rivera R, Apelo R, Ramos R, de la Vega JL. Timing of postpartum tubal sterilisation using the Filshie clips; an analysis of data from two developing-country centres. *Contraception* 1991; 43(**1**): 33–44.

18. Graf A-H, Staudach A, Steiner H, Spitzer D, Martin A. An evaluation of the Filshie clip for postpartum sterilisation in Austria. *Contraception* 1996; 54(**5**): 309–311.

19. Petterson HB, Xia Z, Hughes JM, Wilcox LS, Tylor LR, Trussell J. The risk of pregnancy after tubal sterilisation; Findings from the US Collaborative Review of Sterilisation. *Amer J Obstet Gynaecol* 1996; 174: 1161–1168.

20. Filshie GM. Postpartum use of the Filshie clip for female sterilisation. *Adv Contracept* 1987; (**3**): 175.

21. Ratcliffe F, Lawson R, Millar J. Day-case laparoscopy revisted; Have post-operative morbidity and patient acceptance improved? *Health Trends* 1994; 26(**2**): 47–49.

22. Mackenzie IZ, Turner E, O'Sullivan, Guillebaud J. Two hundred out-patient laparoscopic sterilisations using local anaesthesia. *Br J Obst Gynaecol* 1987; 94(**5**): 449–453.

23. Roberts H. Good practice in sterilisation; New British guidelines will help. *BMJ* 2000; 320: 662–663.

24. Fiddes TM, Williams HW, Herbison GP. Evaluation of post-operative analgesia following laparoscopic application of Filshie clips. *Br J Obst Gynae* 1996; 103(**11**): 1143–1147.

25. Kelly MC. An assessment of the value of intraperitoneal bupivacaine for analgesia after laparoscopic sterilisation. *Br J Obst Gynaecol* 1996; 103(**8**): 837–839.

26. Barclay K, Calvert JP, Catling SJ, Edwards ND, Rees A. Analgesia after laparoscopic sterilisation; Effect of 2% lignocaine gel applied to Filshie clips. *Anaesthesia* 1994; 49(**1**): 68–70.

27. Hartfield VJ. Female sterilisation by the vaginal route; A positive reassessment and comparison of 4 tubal occlusion methods. *Aust NZ J Obstet Gynaecol* 1943; 33(**4**): 408–412.

28. Robson S, Henshaw R. Intractable pelvic pain following Filshie clip application. *Aust NZ J Obstet Gynaecol* 1997; 37(**2**): 242–243.

29. Robson S, Kerin J. Recurrence of pelvic abscess associated with a detached Filshie clip. *Aust NZ J Obstet Gynaecol* 1993; 33(**4**): 446–448.

30. Kesby GJ, Korda AR. Migration of a Filshie clip into the urinary bladder seven years after laparoscopic sterilisation. *Br J Obst Gynae* 1997; 104(**3**): 379–382.

31. Ong NC, Higgins JR, Tan HJ. Torsion of a Filshie clip presenting as an acute abdomen. *Gynaecol Endosc* 1998; 7(**6**): 333–334.

32. Meniru G, Barik S, Jones M. Isolated torsion of the fallopian tube following sterilisation. *J Obstet Gynaecol* 1993; 3(**3**): 208.

33. Buckett W. Prolapse of Filshie clips following vaginal hysterectomy. *Acta Obstet Gynaecol Scan* 1998; 77(**4**): 471–472.

34. Denton GWL, Schofield JB, Gallagher P. Uncommon complications of laparoscopic sterilisation. *Ann R Coll Surg* 1990; 72: 210.

35. Levgur M, Duvivier R. Pelvic inflammatory disease after tubal sterilisation: a review. *Obstet Gynaecol Survey* 2000; 55(**1**): 41–50.

18

Recent Advances in Electrosurgery

Versapoint^{TM} technology

M. Farrugia
P. McGurgan
D. L. McMillan
P. J. O'Donovan

Introduction

Electrosurgery is the generation and delivery of an alternating current between an active and a return electrode in order to raise the tissue temperature for the purposes of desiccation and cutting. The tissue effect achieved is dependent on a number of factors, which include peak voltage, the frequency of the alternating current, modulation, type of tissue, shape of the electrode and the time energy is applied for. In operative hysteroscopy, the energy source and the distension medium used are closely linked. The use of a cheaper and more versatile electrosurgery generator instead of laser energy has been offset by the risk of serious complications resulting from the use of non-ionic distension media. Versapoint™ bipolar technology has combined electrosurgery with a safer distension medium, saline.

Principles of electrosurgery

Electrosurgery is the most commonly used energy source for both open and endoscopic surgery, yet the underlying basic principles are often poorly understood. Without knowledge of the biophysics of electrical energy, the surgeon is unable to utilise the appropriate waveform and settings to achieve the best effect.

The effect of an electrical current passing through tissue is to generate heat and raise the temperature of the tissue. This tissue effect is directly related to the rise in temperature irrespective of the energy form used. At a temperature between 80–100°C, tissue desiccation is achieved (coagulation). At above 100°C, steam is generated, and >200°C, the tissue cells are completely vaporized (cutting).

Electricity is the flow of electrons through a conducting body. The amount of electrons flowing–current, (I, amperes) depends on the voltage (V, volts) and the resistance of the conducting body (R, ohms), as dictated by Ohm's Law:

$$V = I \times R$$

Using water flowing from a pipe as an analogy, the flow (current) is dependent on the pressure (Voltage) and the diameter of the pipe (resistance). When an alternating current is used, the resistance to flow of current is termed impedance. Wattage, or power delivered, is dependent on voltage and current

$$W = V \times I$$

Wattage is usually expressed on electrosurgical generator panel meters. Any combination of voltage and current may result in one power setting, i.e. 40 W could be 40 V × 1 A or 4000 V × 0.01 A. The clinical significance of wattage is that it gives no indication of the voltage used, and in laparoscopy, this may be up to thousands of volts.

Power density is of particular importance as the size and shape of the active electrode compared to the return electrode determines the tissue effect. The larger the active electrode surface area, the lower the power density, and vice versa. When the power density is constant, time becomes the major factor determining the degree of tissue destruction and thermal spread.

As mentioned previously, the temperature reached by the target tissue will determine the resulting tissue effect. The commonly used modes of cutting, coagulation and blend currents are achieved by modulating the waveform and voltage of the current used. Cutting or non-modulated current results in very high tissue temperature with tissue vaporization. The peak voltage is usually low. In desiccation mode, bursts of current are separated by intervals where no current flows, allowing the heat to dissipate into the tissue to achieve haemostasis. A blended current is a mixture of modulated and non-modulated current, allowing a greater degree of heat dissipation during cutting **(Figure 18.1)**.

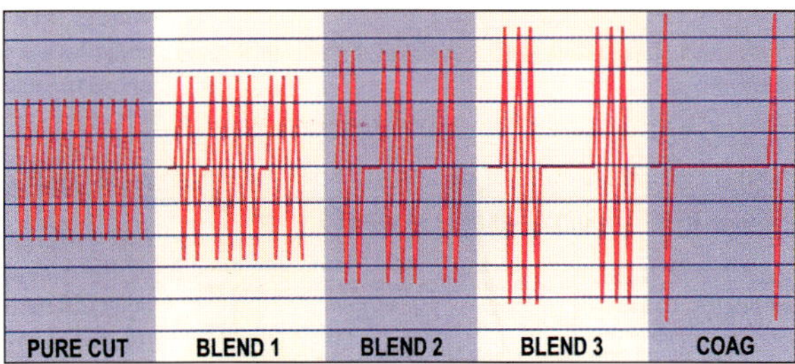

Figure 18.1 Non-modulated (cutting), blended and modulated (coagulation) current waveforms for conventional electrosurgery.

Monopolar surgery

Current flow in monopolar surgery is from an active electrode, through tissue and returned to the generator via a large surface area plate. The high power density at the active electrode creates the desired tissue effect while the very low power density at the return electrode ensures the safe return of current. The plate does not 'earth' the patient but simply provides a low resistance return to complete the electrical circuit.

Bipolar surgery

With the use of two electrodes placed close to each other, current is passed though the tissue placed in between the two electrodes. Bipolar electrosurgery is commonly used in endoscopy in the form of bipolar coagulating forceps, with a modulated current used to achieve tissue desiccation. The passage of a non-modulated (cutting) current is ineffective. This is a safer form of electrosurgery as the patient's body is not part of the electrical circuit. Thermal spread is less likely to occur, as the area of tissue contact is limited when compared to the desiccation mode in monopolar electrosurgery.

Distension media

The use of distension media in hysteroscopic surgery is a continuing source of iatrogenic complications[1] and fatalities have resulted from excessive absorption of hypotonic distension media.[2]

Laser energy is versatile and can travel in any medium that does not absorb or impair the passage of the light energy, therefore physiological media e.g. 0.9% saline or Ringer's lactate are ideal. Unfortunately, laser energy is expensive to generate and deliver into the uterine cavity, and requires extensive training for its safe use.

The cheaper alternative of electrosurgery made operative hysteroscopy more accessible to many gynaecologists. However, as conventional electrosurgery requires a non-ionic distension media, this was at the potential expense of more iatrogenic complications. Hyponatraemia, hyperammonaemia, pulmonary and cerebral oedema, and cardiac arrhythmias have all been reported from the use of glycine, sorbitol and mannitol.

The use of physiological media, such as 0.9% saline, aim to reduce the potential complications of fluid overload, and prevent any osmotic complications, as excretion by the kidneys is all that is necessary for their elimination. However, the unpredictable rate of fluid loss still dictates that fluid balance should be carefully monitored. Very rapid absorption into the body can potentially embarrass the cardiovascular system causing pulmonary oedema. Diuretics may be necessary if over 2 L of fluid are lost and it is prudent to terminate surgery if 2.5–3 L are lost. Although these guidelines are not evidence based, there is no doubt that excessive absorption of normal saline can be fatal.[3]

Versapoint™ technology

Versapoint™ electrodes utilise a revolutionary design where the active and the return electrodes are 'staggered' or placed in-line, with a ceramic insulator or spacer in between (**Figure 18.2**). Both a non-modulated and a modulated current can be employed, giving the bipolar electrodes the versatility to cut and desiccate, as in monopolar surgery. Therefore, one can say that Versapoint™ behaves like a high-power density monopolar electrode with the safety of a bipolar coagulating forceps.

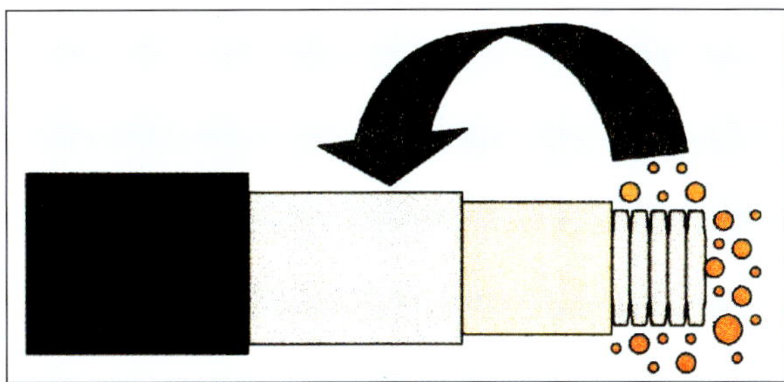

Figure 18.2 Bipolar electrode design.

On activation of Versapoint™, small steam bubbles form at the active electrode as the tip approaches boiling point. The vapour pocket around the tip creates a high resistance to the flow of current. The generator increases the voltage to compensate and arcing occurs within the pocket. As tissue comes into contact with the vapour pocket, the tissue forms part of the return circuit. Tissue adjacent to the vapour pocket has increased resistance due the thermal effect of the hot saline. The current flows out of the saline and back to the return electrode, choosing the path of least resistance (**Figure 18.3**). Hence, there is minimal lateral thermal spread and charring.

During desiccation mode, a vapour pocket does not form and tissue forms part of the return circuit. In contrast to conventional electrosurgery generators, the voltage used during coagulation is less than that used during cutting.

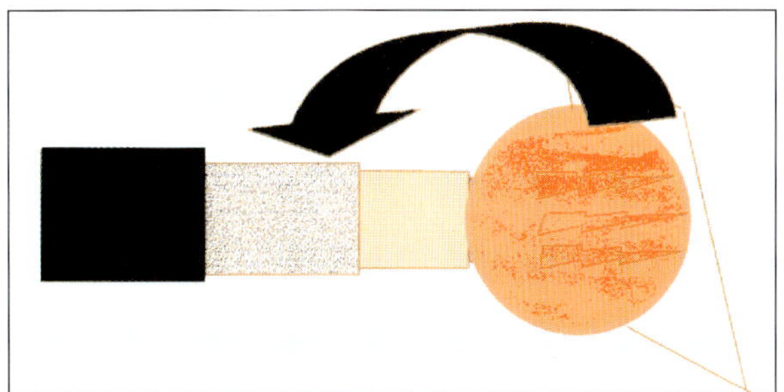

Figure 18.3 Current return path during tissue vaporization.

Versapoint™ generator

The Versapoint™ generator (**Figure 18.4**) is a dedicated electrosurgical system specifically designed for use with Versapoint™ electrodes. The electrodes will not connect to or function correctly with other generators.

The generator operates in a similar way to traditional ones commonly used in operating theatres. A footswitch operates 'cutting' and 'coagulation' modes. A reusable connector cable attaches the electrodes to the generator. Once a specific electrode is recognized, the Versapoint™ system automatically provides the surgeon with appropriate power levels for a particular electrode. The operator may alter the values, but generally it is not necessary to do so.

The voltage settings with Versapoint™ electrodes are generally less then those used in laparoscopic surgery. The generator has three pre-set non-modulated current settings, VC1, VC2 and VC3, two blend current settings BL1 and BL2 and one modulated current setting DES. On connecting an electrode to the generator, the default setting is VC1, which gives maximal tissue effect. With VC2 and VC3, the vapour pocket is smaller, resulting in a lesser tissue effect.

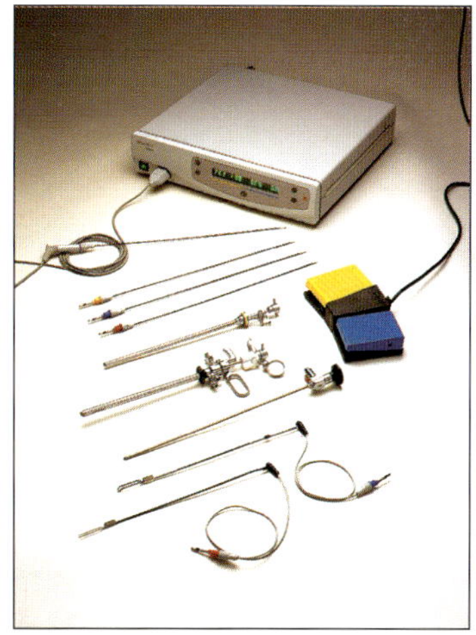

Figure 18.4 The Versapoint™ electrosurgical generator.

The voltages used are:[4]

VaporCut1, VC1	340V rms
VaporCut2, VC2	307V rms
VaporCut3, VC3	254V rms
Blend1, BL1	340V rms
Blend2, BL2	307V rms
Desiccate, DES	120V rms

The generator has several inbuilt safety features. During start-up, an internal check system notifies the correct functioning of the generator and the cable. The unit recognizes individual electrodes, and the power levels are limited to within a given range. The operator cannot raise power levels beyond the safety limits, and should an electrical leak to earth occur, the generator will automatically reset to zero power output.

Versapoint™ electrodes

There are currently five available bipolar electrodes. A set of three 1.6 mm diameter electrodes with different tip configurations can be used with any hysteroscope that has a 5–7 F (1.6–2.0 mm) operating channel. The 0° electrode and the bipolar loop can only be used with a Gynecare resectoscope.

Spring, twizzle and ball electrodes

These three electrodes (**Figure 18.5**) are 1.6 mm in diameter and 35 cm long. They are colour coded for easy recognition. The tips are made of a Rhodium/Palladium alloy and each configuration is most suited for a particular task.

The spring electrode is 1.2 mm in diameter and 1.6 mm long. Its active electrode has a large surface area, which makes it suitable for tissue vaporization and debulking. Leiomyoma vaporization is best carried out with this electrode. The default power output settings are VC1 130 and DES 24.

The twizzle electrode is 0.6 mm in diameter and 3.0 mm long and is ideally suited for delivering 'laser-like' energy to cut tissue. Endometrial polyps or Type 0 leiomyomas are easily resected using this electrode with minimal adjacent tissue destruction. The default power output settings are VC1 100 and DES 50.

The ball electrode has a spherical tip of 1 mm diameter. This allows precise tissue vaporization and desiccation. The ball is most suited for resecting uterine septae or intra-uterine synechiae. The default power output settings are VC1 50 and DES 24.

The Versapoint™ bipolar resectoscopic system

To complete the bipolar operative hysteroscopy system (**Figure 18.6a and b**) two more electrodes have been developed to effectively treat larger intra-cavity pathology and resect or ablate the endometrium. The 0° electrode and the bipolar

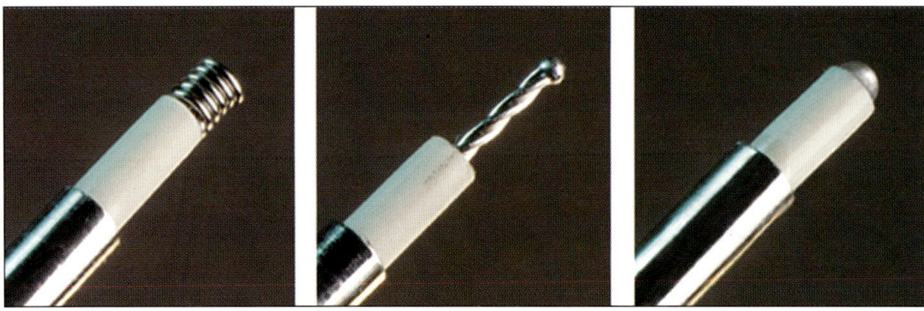

Figures 18.5 The spring, twizzle and ball Electrodes (left, middle and right espectively).

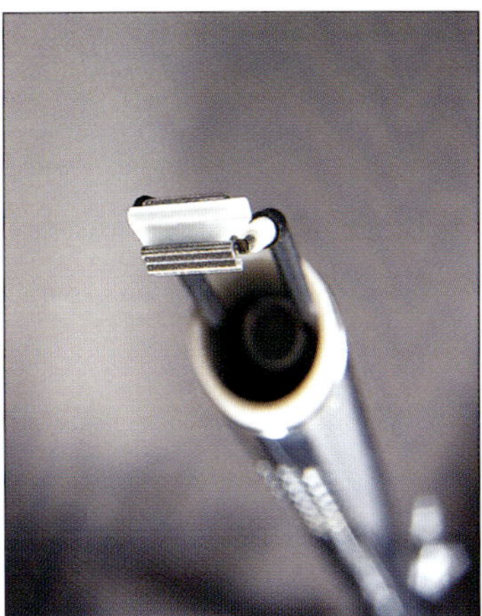

Figure 18.6a The 0° Electrode.

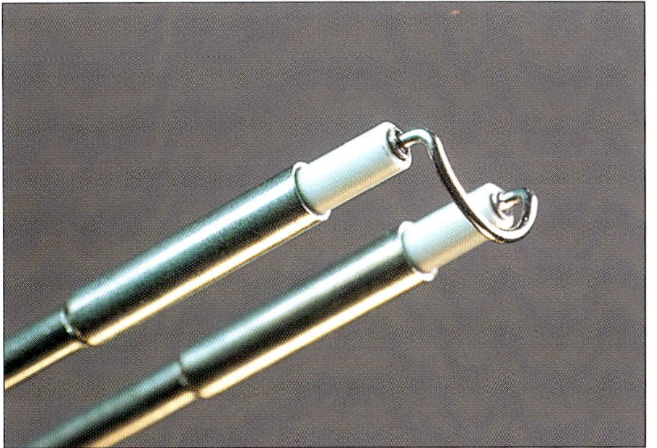

Figure 18.6b The bipolar loop.

loop use a dedicated continuous flow resectoscope with a wide angle 30° hysteroscope. The outer sheath diameter of the Resectoscope is 27 F (9.0 mm).

The 0° degree electrode is 8 mm wide and ablates tissue without any residual chips. The bipolar loop operates in a similar way to a monopolar electrode and has the same characteristics. As tissue contact is not necessary for activation, the electrodes do not 'stick' in tissue whilst cutting. There is minimal thermal damage to the resected strips, providing excellent material for histological examination. The default power settings for both electrodes are VC1 170 and DES 80.

Clinical experience

The Versapoint™ bipolar electrosurgical system is a new technology and there are few reported cases in the medical literature. To date, 49 cases treated with Versapoint™ have been reported in the United States[3,5,6] and 125 patients treated in Europe.[7] The majority of patients have had endometrial polyps or leiomyomas resected or ablated, whilst a smaller number of patients have had intra-uterine septae or synechiae removed. Endometrial ablation using the Versapoint™ 5F electrode has also been reported.[8]

The Outpatient Hysteroscopy Clinic at Whipps Cross Hospital was established in 1989 and its role expanded to a twice-weekly evening session for the investigation and treatment of abnormal uterine bleeding. Since the introduction of the Versapoint™ system, 125 patients with benign focal intra-uterine pathology have been treated.

The inclusion criteria for treatment were benign intra-uterine pathology not larger than 4 cm diameter. The exclusion criteria were bleeding at the time of hysteroscopy, a painful diagnostic hysteroscopy or suspected malignancy. A successful treatment was defined as one where the pathology was removed completely within a 20 min operating time. Treatment failed if the pathology was not completely removed for any reason or the treatment time was over 20 min.

Local anaesthesia was used in 27 patients (21.6%). This consisted of a local cervical block using about 10 ml of 1% lignocaine. The indications for the administration of local anaesthetic were patients' request or the need for cervical dilatation. The latter was necessary in 12 patients (9.6%).

At hysteroscopy, 86 patients were found to have endometrial polyps. Ten of these women had multiple polyps, two patients had four polyps, and four patients had three polyps. In total, 104 polyps were diagnosed, 84 of these were completely resected in one sitting. The procedure failed in five patients

Table 18.1 Pathology treated

Type of pathology	Number of patients	Number of lesions	Failures	Success%
Endometrial polyps	86	104	5	94.2
Type 0 fibroids	21	21	3	86
Type 1 fibroids	10	10	3	70
Type 11 fibroids	8	8	4	50

(6%). Subsequent admission as a day-case under general anaesthesia was necessary in all five failures.

Leiomyomata were treated in 39 patients. 21 patients had type 0 myomas, 10 had type I fibroids while eight had type II fibroids. The procedure was successful in 18 (85%) of the patients with type 0 fibroids, seven (70%) in type I fibroids and 4 (50%) in type II fibroids. Seven patients needed a second hysteroscopy after the administration of 1–2 doses of a GnRH analogue (goserelin 3.6 mg subcutaneously), while three were rescheduled for resection of the fibroid under general anaesthesia.

The overall success rate of the procedures was 88%. The failure rate was 12% (15 patients). Of these, seven had their surgery successfully completed in a second session. Eight patients (6.4%) needed admission for a day-case procedure under general anaesthesia.

There were no major complications. Most patients complained of lower abdominal cramping during the procedure, but this improved immediately as the surgery ended. Post-operative discomfort responded to simple analgesia and 124 patients were comfortable going home within 1 hour after the procedure. One patient required admission for pain control after partial resection of a type 0 fibroid: she was discharged home after an overnight stay. Two patients complained of heavy bleeding in the first 2 days following the procedure, which responded to oral tranexamic acid.

The Versapoint™ system is very easy to set-up and use in an outpatient setting[9] and it is immediately available for use if saline is used as distension medium for diagnostic hysteroscopy. The conversion from a diagnostic to an operative procedure does not require removal of the hysteroscope from the uterine cavity. The generation of bubbles is the norm during electrode activation, and periodic flushing out of the accumulated bubbles is necessary to prevent obstruction of vision and keep the electrode completely immersed in saline. The duration of activation should be kept to a minimum to prevent overheating.

Conclusion

The Versapoint™ bipolar electrosurgical system is a new and exciting development for hysteroscopic surgery. It offers a complete range of instruments, which will be suitable for most intra-cavitary operations. The 5F electrodes are best suited for outpatient treatment without anaesthesia and in uteri where cervical dilatation is best avoided. Where the pathology is sufficiently large, the 0° electrode and the bipolar loop provide a fast and effective treatment using a safer distension medium, saline.

REFERENCES

1. Istre O, Skajaa K, Schoensby AP, Forman A. Changes in serum electrolytes after transcervical resection of the endometrium and submucous

fibroids with the use of glycine 1.5% for uterine irrigation. *Obstet Gynecol 1992;* **80**(2):189–191.

2. Arieff AI, Ayus JC. Endometrial ablation complicated by fatal hyponatraemic encephalopathy. *JAMA* 1993; **270**: 1230–1232.

3. Vilos GA. Intrauterine surgery using a new coaxial bipolar electrode in normal saline solution (Versapoint™): A pilot study. *Fertil Steril* 1999; **72**(4): 740–743.

4. VersaPoint™ hysteroscopic bipolar electrosurgical system user manual, gynecare, a division of Ethicon, a Johnson & Johnson Company. pp. 21–22.

5. Kung RC, Vilios GA, Thomas B, Penkin P, Zaltz AP, Stabinsky SA. A new bipolar system for performing operative hysteroscopy in normal saline. *J Am Assoc Gynecol Laparosc* 1999; **6**(3): 331–336.

6. Lindheim SR, Kavic S, Shulman SV, Sauer MV. Operative hysteroscopy in the office setting. *J Am Assoc Gynecol Laparosco* 2000; **7**(1): 65–69.

7. Farrugia M, McMillan DL. Versapoint™ in the treatment of focal intra-uterine pathology in an outpatient setting. *Références en Gynécologie Obstétrique*. 2000; **2**, 7.

8. P. O'Donovan, P. McGurgan. Evaluation of operative micro-hysteroscopy with bipolar electrosurgery in a saline medium. *J Am Assoc Gynaecol Laparosc* 1998; **5**, 3 (Suppl), S35: 125.

9. Syed R. Retrospective analysis of 500 consecutive cases of microhystero scopy with the Microspan hysteroscope. *J Am Assoc Gynecol Laparosc* 1999; **6**(3): S54.

Index

Note: references to figures are indicated by 'f' and references to tables are indicated by 't' when they fall on a page not covered by the text reference.